A Pattern Approach to Lymph Node Diagnosis

A Pattern Approach to Lymph Node Diagnosis

Anthony S.-Y. Leong, MB, BS, MD, FRCPA, FRCPath, FCAP, FASCP, FHKAM (Pathol), Honorary FHKCPath, Honorary FRCPT

Director, Pathology Laboratories, Sunway Medical Center, Petaling Jaya, Malaysia

Professor of Pathology, Jeffrey Cheah School of Medicine, Monash University, Sunway Campus, Malaysia

Formerly
Medical Director, Hunter Area Pathology Service, Newcastle
Professor and Chair, Discipline of Anatomical Pathology
University of Newcastle, New South Wales, Australia

Springer

Anthony S.-Y. Leong, MD
Director
Pathology Laboratories
Sunway Medical Center
Petaling Jaya
Malaysia

Professor of Pathology
Jeffrey Cheah School of Medicine
Monash University
Sunway Campus
Malaysia
aleong45@gmail.com

ISBN 978-1-4419-7175-3 ISBN 978-1-4419-7176-0 (eBook)

DOI 10.1007/978-1-4419-7176-0
Springer New York Dordrecht Heidelberg London

Library of Congress Control Number: 2010935338

Printed on acid-free paper

Springer is part of Springer Science+Business Media (www.springer.com)

Preface

The development of sophisticated ancillary techniques for lymph node diagnosis has made hematopathology a specialized discipline in many developed countries. Immunohistology, electron microscopy, and molecular diagnostic techniques are expensive procedures and require specialized resources and technical skills, commodities that are not readily available in many laboratories other than those in large medical facilities. The general or community hospital pathologist is thus still required to make a histological diagnosis based on microscopic observations of the biopsied lymph node, or at least, to decide if the pathological changes represent a reactive or neoplastic process before referring the material for an expert opinion. Importantly, as the pathologist to first encounter the excised lymph node, he or she is responsible for triage of the specimen. This requires familiarity not only with the different technologies employed in the proper examination of the sampled material but also with the appropriate preparation of the specimen and what each adjunctive technique has to offer.

There are many large and excellent textbooks on lymph node pathology that define and describe diseases of lymph nodes in great detail. These take the conventional approach of separately describing each of the reactive and neoplastic entities that involve the lymph node and lymphoid tissues, and their accompanying immunophenotypic profiles, and cytogenetic and molecular characteristics. This approach is contrary to the conventional method applied in histologic diagnosis which is one of pattern recognition performed through a systematic assessment of the various anatomical compartments of the tissue for changes in architecture, expansion of a population of normal cells, or accumulation or presence of abnormal populations of cells. In the lymph node, such anatomical compartments are not clearly visible. Such a method of assessment is even more important for the lymph node as anatomical compartmentalization reflects immune and cellular function. To the trainee and general/community pathologist, the lymph node may represent a morass of small and large lymphocytes without clearly visible compartmentalization. This problem is further compounded by the fact that neoplastic lymphoid cells invariably have cytologic features similar and even identical to their normal counterparts, so that cellular density, composition, and compartmentalization become important aspects of the histologic assessment. Reactive processes can produce exuberant expansions of different lymph node compartments, and the changes are dynamic, adding further to difficulties of diagnosis.

The pattern approach to lymph node diagnosis has been previously proposed but such an approach has not been adopted before in a textbook. The advent of immunohistology and the availability of a comprehensive range of sensitive antibodies that are immunoreactive in routinely fixed, paraffin-embedded sections make it much easier to adopt such a diagnostic approach which more truly reflects the manner in which pathologists routinely examine lymph nodes. Invariably, as some neoplasms and most reactive conditions involve more than one compartment and produce more than one pattern of change, there will be some degree of overlap with this method of diagnostic approach. However, in this book, this is kept to a minimum and each entity is discussed under its primary pattern of presentation and will be briefly mentioned, especially in differential diagnoses, when it produces alternative and less-frequent patterns of histologic change.

Immunohistology is now an established ancillary diagnostic technique that is employed by most routine laboratories, although the range of antibodies available will vary. We will not only discuss the minimal repertoire of antibodies required for lymphoma diagnosis but also provide detailed immunoprofiles for complete characterization of each neoplastic process. Clinical, molecular, and cytogenetic characteristics will also be discussed as they often aid diagnosis and provide further understanding of the neoplastic process. Electron microscopy, which is less contributory in the area of lymphoma diagnosis, will be touched on where appropriate.

It is the primary aim of this book to demonstrate that a systematic approach to lymph node examination can be achieved through recognition of morphological patterns produced by different disease processes. A level of confidence and familiarity with lymph node pathology can be attained through the adoption of such an approach that is employed largely in every other organ system in the body. This book is thus directed at trainee and general/community pathologists who have first contact with the excised lymph node and are required to make an initial judgment on the morphologic changes, especially if deciding to refer the specimen on for expert opinion. The classification system employed throughout this book is that of the 2008 World Health Classification. This book is not intended to supplant the many excellent texts available on lymph node pathology and is not intended to provide new information or knowledge. Its purpose is to instruct the reader in a method of examination that employs the recognition of patterns and colors. The discussion of each diagnostic entity is accompanied by ample color illustrations that highlight the diagnostic features. In addition, text boxes summarizing the salient features are provided. This is essentially a "how-to" manual that also integrates current information about specific neoplastic entities. References have been deliberately excluded as they distract from the primary purpose and the reader is referred to the 2008 WHO book for a comprehensive and appropriate reference listing and to other selected references.

Anthony S.-Y. Leong, MD

Contents

Acknowledgments

The contributions of Michael R Lewis, MD, MBA, Department of Pathology, University of Vermont and Fletcher Allen Health Care, Burlington, Vermont, USA, to **Chapters 6**, 7, and **9**, and specifically to the immunohistology and flow cytometry components of **Chapter 3** are gratefully acknowledged. He also made valuable suggestions to other parts of this book.

Dr Leonard Tan, Department of Pathology, The Singapore General Hospital, Singapore, generously contributed figures 7.147–7.152.

Section I

Chapter 1

Introduction

Key words: Knowledge-based, systematic approach, classification, capsule, perinodal tissue, follicles, sinuses, paracortex, hilum, pattern, tinctorial characteristics.

The formulation of histologic diagnosis in lymph nodes, as in other tissue/organ sites, is knowledge-based and is applied in combination with visual recognition. These processes are not mutually exclusive. The pathologist firstly must be acquainted with the entities that can occur at the specific tissue site with an appreciation of their relative frequencies, as "common things occur commonly." In addition, the pathologist should be fully cognizant of the spectrum of histologic features that are manifested by each pathological entity and be able to recognize them, the latter skill commonly known as "pattern recognition." While a specific entity may display a number of diagnostic features, they all may not be present in every case, and very few are specific or pathognomonic. The relative importance of each morphologic feature, like the minimum number or most important set of morphologic features that permits a definite diagnosis, is determined by published data, the skills and experience of the pathologist, and the clinical setting. The availability of ancillary diagnostic techniques lends greater objectivity to the outcome. The diagnostic process is therefore extremely complicated. Because there is currently limited understanding of how the human brain computes all this information to formulate a diagnosis, it is impossible to teach or learn the diagnostic process in the same manner that the human brain functions. Furthermore, there is also invaluable intuitive or "gut" feeling possessed by experienced pathologists that defies definition. Undoubtedly, the unraveling of the brain processes in the formulation of histologic diagnosis through the examination of tissue sections will greatly contribute to the design and building of a computer for this function. Thankfully, for those

A.S.-Y. Leong, *A Pattern Approach to Lymph Node Diagnosis*,
DOI 10.1007/978-1-4419-7176-0_1, © Springer Science+Business Media, LLC 2011

in the profession of making histologic diagnoses, this development is yet a few years away.

While the pattern approach to diagnosis is taught and practiced with almost every other tissue or organ in the body, the lymph node remains a mystery to most residents or registrars starting out in pathology and even to those pathologists with limited experience in the area. To many, the lymph node can appear to be a morass of small and large lymphoid cells without obvious compartmentalization. One aim of this book is to demonstrate that lymph node compartments can be recognized histologically, especially with the aid of immunohistochemical markers, and that this knowledge can be employed effectively to localize and identify pathological changes in different compartments in order to facilitate histological diagnosis. In addition to the patterns and tinctorial characteristics that may reflect various pathological entities, there are also defining histological features that, because of their pathological occurrence in lymph nodes, can be useful pointers to specific diagnoses or disease processes. A pattern approach to lymph node diagnosis has been mooted in the past, but because it was based largely on routinely stained sections, this method of diagnosis did not gain much popularity. However, the advent of sensitive and specific antibodies that allow accurate localization of lymphocyte subtypes and other relevant cells has been a pivotal development that renders the lymph node compartments and their diagnostic alterations more readily recognizable.

It is the primary purpose of this book to teach one method of approach to the diagnosis of lymph node pathology through the systematic examination of the anatomical compartments of the lymph node, and to provide and integrate the information available about each neoplastic entity that occurs primarily in lymph nodes, according to the 2008 World Health Organization (WHO) classification. Reactive conditions are also considered in detail, and the application of various ancillary diagnostic techniques, especially immunohistochemistry, will be described for the specific identification of the neoplastic entities and their differentiation from reactive conditions.

Knowledge-Based Diagnosis

As young pathologists lack extensive experience or intuition to call upon, their ability to formulate specific diagnoses has largely to be knowledge-based, complemented by the acquired ability to recognize morphological patterns and cytological features (image recognition). Familiarity with contemporary classifications and with the definition of specific entities is therefore essential in lymphoma diagnosis.

The classification of non-Hodgkin lymphoma has seen many changes since its inception and especially so over the past two decades. The worthiness of any classification system remains in its applicability, reproducibility, ease of usage, clinical relevance, and biological appropriateness. The REAL classification of 1994, now superseded by the World Health Organization (WHO) classification, addresses these issues. Both classifications provide clear definitions of the diagnostic entities that can be recognized with the aid of available ancillary techniques. Besides Hodgkin lymphoma, and histiocytic and dendritic cell neoplasms, the WHO classification contains the subtypes of non-Hodgkin lymphoma and includes leukemias. The classification employed in this book will be the 2008 WHO classification, but only those entities that occur primarily in lymph nodes or those that commonly involve them secondarily will be described in detail. Others that present primarily in extranodal sites and rarely in the lymph node will be described briefly and only when appropriate (**Table 1.1**).

Table 1.1
Tumors of lymphoid tissues in the 2008 WHO classification

B cell neoplasms
B-lymphoblastic leukemia/lymphoma
Chronic lymphocytic leukemia/small lymphocytic lymphoma
B cell prolymphocytic lymphoma[a]
Splenic B cell marginal zone lymphoma[a]
Hairy cell leukemia[a]
Splenic B cell lymphoma/leukemia, unclassifiable[a]
Lymphoplasmacytic lymphoma
Heavy chain diseases[a]
Plasma cell myeloma, solitary plasmacytoma of bone, extraosseous plasmacytoma[a]
Extranodal marginal zone lymphoma of mucosa-associated lymphoid tissue (MALT lymphoma)[a]
Nodal marginal zone lymphoma
Follicular lymphoma
Primary cutaneous follicle center lymphoma[a]
Mantle cell lymphoma
Diffuse large B cell lymphoma, including T cell/histiocyte-rich large B cell lymphoma, primary cutaneous DLBCL, leg type[a] and EBV-positive DLBCL of the elderly
DLBCL associated with chronic inflammation
Lymphomatoid granulomatosis[a]
Primary mediastinal (thymic) large B cell lymphoma[a]
Intravascular large B cell lymphoma[a]
ALK-positive large B cell lymphoma
Plasmablastic lymphoma
Large B cell lymphoma arising in HHV8-associated multicentric Castleman disease
Primary effusion lymphoma[a]
Burkitt lymphoma
B cell lymphoma, unclassifiable
T cell neoplasms
T-lymphoblastic lymphoma/leukemia
T cell prolymphocytic leukemia[a]

Table 1.1 (continued)

Aggressive NK cell leukemia[a]
Systemic EBV-positive T cell lymphoproliferative disease of childhood
Hydroa vacciniforme-like lymphoma[a]
Adult T cell lymphoma/leukemia
Extranodal NK/T cell lymphoma, nasal type[a]
Enteropathy-associated T cell lymphoma[a]
Hepatosplenic T cell lymphoma[a]
Subcutaneous panniculitis-like T cell lymphoma[a]
Mycosis fungoides/Sezary syndrome[a]
Primary cutaneous CD30-positive T cell lymphoproliferative disorders including lymphomatoid papulosis[a], primary cutaneous anaplastic large cell lymphoma[a]
Primary cutaneous gamma–delta T cell lymphoma[a]
Primary cutaneous CD8 positive aggressive epidermotropic cytotoxic T cell lymphoma[a]
Primary cutaneous CD4 positive small/medium T cell lymphoma[a]
Peripheral T cell lymphoma, unspecified
Angioimmunoblastic T cell lymphoma
Anaplastic large cell lymphoma, ALK positive
Hodgkin lymphoma
Nodular lymphocyte predominant
Classic Hodgkin's Lymphoma
– Nodular sclerosis
– Lymphocyte rich
– Mixed cellularity
– Lymphocyte-depleted
Histiocytic and dendritic cell neoplasms
Histiocytic sarcoma
Langerhans cell histiocytosis/sarcoma
Interdigitating dendritic cell sarcoma
Follicular dendritic cell sarcoma
Fibroblastic reticular cell tumor
Indeterminate dendritic cell tumor
Disseminated juvenile xanthogranuloma

[a] Entities that are primarily extranodal and involve lymph nodes only uncommonly

In addition to the neoplasms listed above, post-transplant lymphoproliferative disorders (PTLD) now have a place in the 2008 WHO classification and include (1) early lesions – plasmacytic hyperplasia and infectious mononucleosis-like PTLD, (2) polymorphic PTLD, (3) monomorphic PTLD (B- and T/NK cell types), and (4) classical Hodgkin lymphoma-type PTLD.

In the formulation of diagnoses, it is thus essential to be familiar with the list of diagnostic entities and their definitions in order to match a specific diagnostic label with the observed morphological features. This "best-fit" process is a combination of knowledge-based assessment and pattern recognition.

Systematic Examination of the Lymph Node

As with other tissues, to be able to recognize morphological abnormalities, the pathologist must have a firm knowledge of the normal anatomy and functional compartmentalization of the lymph node. The pattern approach to lymph node diagnosis is based primarily on the recognition of involvement of these specific compartments. This recognition process is relatively easy to perform in many other organ systems. For example, the uterus has clearly recognizable compartments such as the endometrium, composed of stroma and glands, and the myometrium, composed of smooth muscle and connective tissue. In a similar manner, the intestine can be divided into epithelium, lamina propria, muscularis mucosae, submucosa, muscularis propria, and subserosa/serosa. In contrast, the lymph node is made up of compartments that are often indistinct and blurred in the routine H&E-stained section. Furthermore, lymph nodes are dynamic, and these compartments rapidly change in size, shape, and appearance in benign reactions. Compounding this is the fact that every neoplastic cell has a benign counterpart with similar cytological features, so that the ability to recognize individual neoplastic cells is often lost. For these reasons, the need to clearly delineate each compartment in order to localize and identify the pathological changes is an essential but difficult task in lymph node sections.

It cannot be overemphasized that the lymph node must be examined in a methodical fashion in order to identify the pathologic process. It is important to appreciate that the recognition of changes in the various compartments is best accomplished with the low-power objective. While trainee pathologists feel more comfortable looking through the high-power objective lens (×40), cytological features are of secondary importance in lymph node diagnosis, and much more information, particularly regarding alterations in pattern, is gained using scanning or low-power lens (×2 and ×4 objectives). Furthermore, changes, particularly benign alterations, which are by far more frequent than neoplastic diseases, are characterized by focal changes in different compartments and may be missed in high-power examination.

Sequentially, at scanning magnification, the capsule, subcapsular and medullary sinuses, follicles, mantle zones, marginal zones, interfollicular areas, and medulla or hilum of the lymph node should be scrutinized. Importantly, it is necessary to compare the compartments with each other for disproportional size and abnormalities. A suggested order of examination and questions to be answered is listed in **Table 1.2**.

Table 1.2
Systematic examination of anatomical compartments

Structure/feature	Question
Size of node	Is it enlarged? Is the shape normal?
Capsule	Is it thickened? Is it breached?
Perinodal tissue	Is it infiltrated? Is there a reaction? Are there vascular abnormalities?
Hilum	Is it involved by an abnormal infiltrate?
Follicles	Are they hyperplastic, atrophic, or showing lysis? What is their distribution? Is there polarization? Is the mantle zone normal? Are marginal zone cells hyperplastic? Are vessels normal? Are there abnormal deposits present? Are there similar cells within neoplastic follicles and without, especially centroblasts?
Paracortex	Is it hyperplastic/expanded? Are there nodules present? What are the cells contributing to the expansion? Are there abnormal cells? Is there necrosis? Are vessels prominent? Are they abnormal?
Sinuses	Is the sinus architecture preserved? Are they infiltrated? What cells are infiltrating? Polymorphous or monomorphous? Are there histiocytes present? Are they phagocytic or epithelioid? Is there pigment or foreign material present? Are the plasma cells abnormal? Are there multinucleated giant cells present?
Defining feature	Are any of the following features present? • Granulomas • Foreign material – pigmented, refractile, birefringent • Necrosis • Hemorrhage • Mast cells, clear cells • Vascular proliferation • Spindled cells • Fibrosis and hyaline deposition • Glandular inclusions, epithelial cells, nevus cells • Hematopoietic cells • Protozoa

Throughout the process of examining the tissue section, the pathologist needs to answer the following questions:

Is the tissue normal or abnormal?

Is this a reactive or neoplastic process?

If neoplastic, is this a primary lymphoid neoplasm or metastatic tumor?

If it is lymphoid, what type of lymphoma does it represent?

The first two questions are answered by low-power examination of the entire lymph node section, looking for changes in architectural features, patterns, color, and the location of normal and abnormal cells in the various compartments. The last question is also important in the diagnostic algorithm. If the process is assessed to be a lymphoid neoplasm, then it should be possible to subtype the lymphoma; otherwise the diagnosis of lymphoma should be questioned.

Cell Type Identification

At scanning magnification, the pathologic focus in the section can be recognized because it is often localized, sometimes corresponding to a specific compartment, and show a tinctorial property that is different from the neighboring areas. Similarly, when cells of different types occur in compact groups, they can be identified at low magnification on the basis of their color or tinctorial properties. For example, small lymphocytes are black to dark blue because of their compact chromatin and scanty cytoplasm; plasma cells are purple because of moderate quantities of basophilic cytoplasm, and their nuclei with coarse chromatin are dark blue; blast cells have a bluish tinge imparted by their slate grey nuclei and scanty pale cytoplasm; transformed lymphoid cells have a similar appearance with larger quantities of cytoplasm producing a basophilic tinge which, in a background of small lymphocytes, produces a mottled pattern; eosinophils have a brick red color; mast cells, interdigitating reticulum cells, Langerhans cells, and monocytoid B cells have moderate quantities of pale cytoplasm, producing areas of pallor; and epithelioid histiocytes produce pink areas because of the color of their ample cytoplasm, as may carcinoma cells. Thus subtle differences in color can be recognized and employed to aid the localization of focal pathologic changes (**Table 1.3** and **Figs. 1.1**, **1.2**, **1.3**, **1.4**, **1.5**, **1.6**, **1.7**, **1.8**, **1.9**, **1.10**, **1.11**, **1.12**, **1.13**, and **1.14**).

Cell Size and Cellularity

Differences in fixing and processing impart variable shrinkage to the tissue so that it is always necessary to compare cell sizes in the same tissue section. Red blood cells, macrophages, and endothelial cells serve as useful internal controls for cell size. For example, to qualify as a "large cell," it is necessary that the nucleus of the lymphoid cell exceeds the diameter of endothelial cells or macrophages or is twice that of red cells.

Density of cellularity is an important parameter. Hypercellularity is a feature of most malignant proliferations, regardless of their cell of origin. Hypercellularity is reflected by one or more of the following features: obliterated nodal sinuses, increase in the number of follicles or follicular structures, expansion of the cortex and/or paracortex, engorgement of the nodal sinuses, pericapsular infiltration, increase in cellular density, and proliferation of one cell type to produce a monotonous infiltrate. Compact

Table 1.3
Tinctorial characteristics of different cell types

Cell type	Tinctorial characteristic
Small lymphocytes	Black or dark blue
Blast cells	Shades of dark blue
Transformed lymphoid cells	Pale blue
Plasma cells	Purple
Eosinophils	Brick red
Epithelioid histiocytes	Pink
Interdigitating reticulum cells	Pale pink
Monocytoid B cells	Pale pink
Mast cells	Pale pink

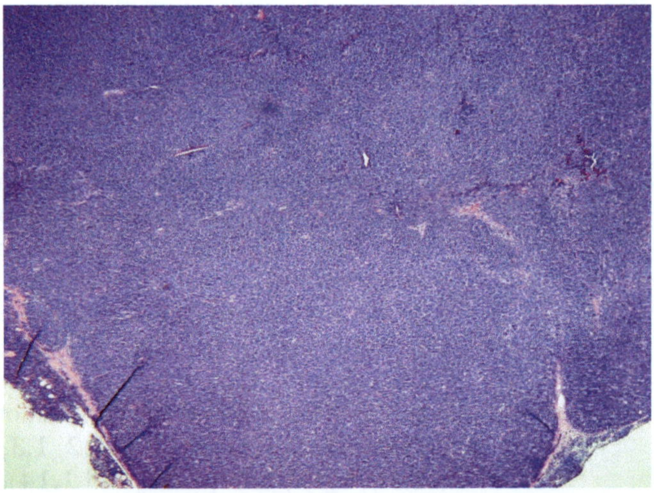

Fig. 1.1. Chronic lymphocytic leukemia/small cell lymphoma diffusely replacing the lymph node. The infiltrate is frequently "wall-to-wall" and the *dark blue* color is characteristic of small lymphoid cells.

hypercellular areas suggest a neoplastic process, but this is by no means foolproof, as some benign conditions, including viral lymphadenitis, systemic lupus erythematosus, and abnormal immune responses, may also be hypercellular.

Immunohistology

The availability of highly sensitive antibodies reactive in fixed tissue makes it possible to employ immunostaining to aid in the identification of abnormal cell populations seen in lymph node sections. This additional tool greatly aids the assessment of the various lymph node compartments which may otherwise be blurred in H&E-stained sections. Such markers will be discussed

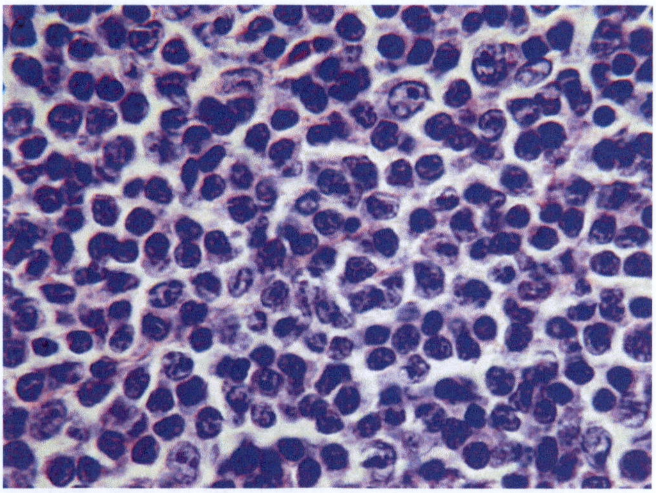

Fig. 1.2. The small lymphocytes have scanty cytoplasm and *dark blue* nuclei due to the coarse chromatin.

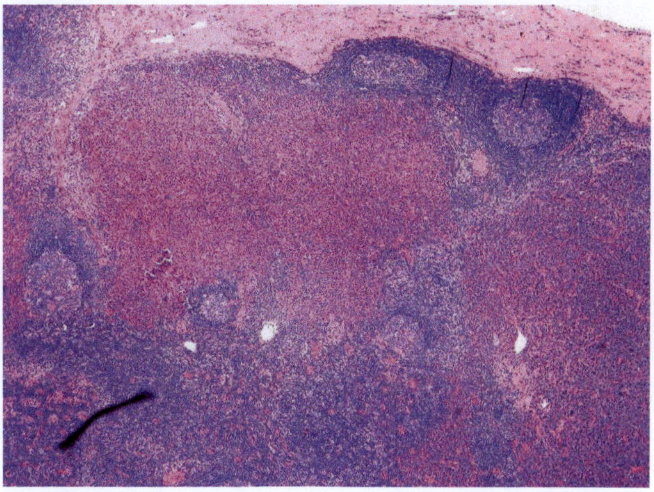

Fig. 1.3. Plasma cells display a *purple color* different to the background of *dark blue* small lymphocytes.

in greater detail in a separate chapter, and diagnostic markers will be discussed in conjunction with the specific histological entities.

Cytological Preparations

Unlike other tissues, the lymph node is most likely to be received fresh in the laboratory, and the handling of such specimens is described separately. It cannot be overemphasized that properly prepared imprints from freshly cut lymph node surfaces are the best source of material for cytologic examination. Such imprints arc best air-dried and stained with Giemsa or fixed in a mixture of 10% formalin and 100% ethanol (50:50 by volume) and stained with the H&E protocol employed for frozen sections. The

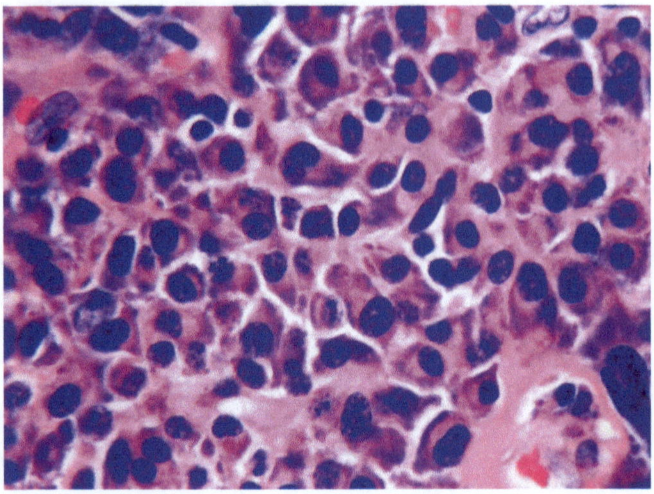

Fig. 1.4. Plasmacytoma. The *purple color* is due to the moderate quantities of cytoplasm and *dark blue* nuclei.

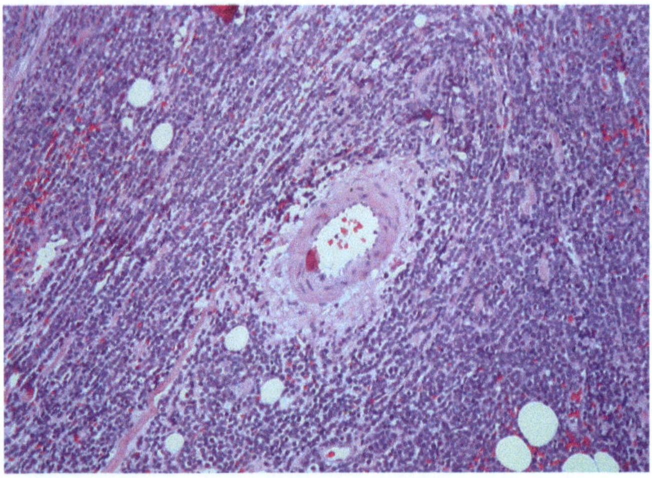

Fig. 1.5. Lymphoblastic lymphoma. The cells have a slate *blue color* due to the staining of the nuclei and scanty cytoplasm.

cytomorphology in the latter preparations will closely resemble that of fixed, paraffin-embedded tissues, unlike air-dried preparations that generally show larger cells and are stained with Giemsa, which produces different tinctorial properties to H&E. If immunostaining is anticipated, it is best to air-dry the imprints before fixing in 1% formal saline (van der Griendt fluid) for 2–14 h before antigen retrieval and immunostaining. This protocol removes most of the background staining that otherwise occurs with other fixatives and protocols. It used to be common practice to obtain cytospin preparations from homogenized nodal tissue in tissue culture fluid. Such preparations allow a study of cell cytology and histochemical and immunohistochemical

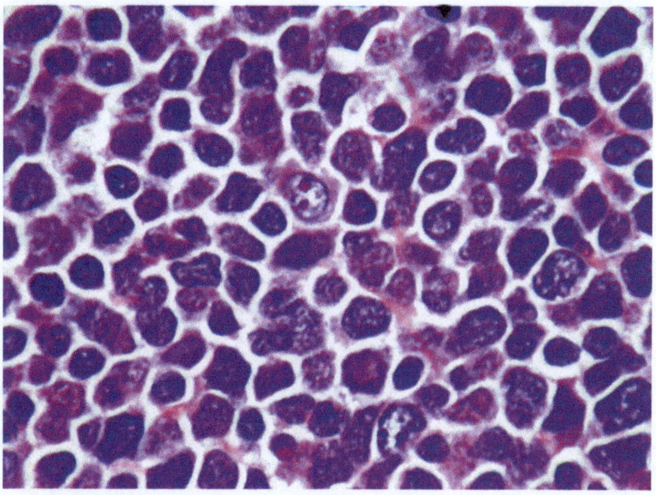

Fig. 1.6. The slate *blue color* of lymphoblasts is due to the nuclei characteristics and scanty dense basophilic cytoplasm.

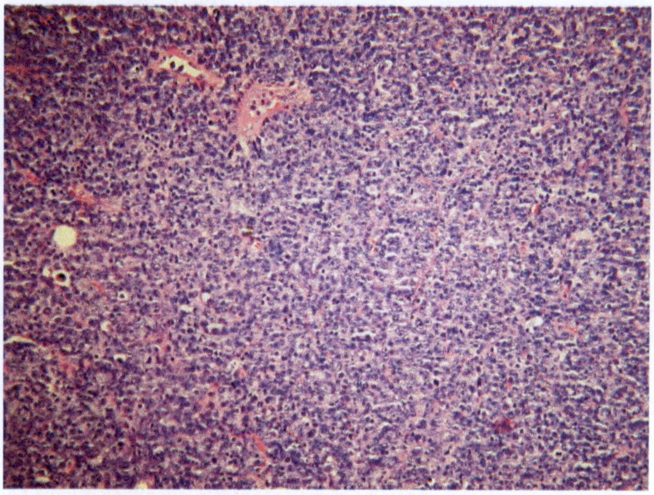

Fig. 1.7. Immunoblastic sarcoma has a *grey blue color*. The cells are larger and have more cytoplasm that is basophilic.

staining following air drying or fixation in acetone at 4°C. With the availability of a range of sensitive antibodies immunoreactive in fixed paraffin-embedded sections, this practice is no longer followed.

Compared with other cell types, lymphoid cells are fragile and very prone to significant cytologic distortions in paraffin-embedded sections as a result of fixation and retraction artifacts. While B5 was a favored fixative because it produced sharper nuclear and cytoplasmic details, it also resulted in significant shrinkage so that cell volumes could be as much as 20% less than those in formalin-fixed sections. B5 fixative should no longer be employed as it contains mercury, a toxic environmental pollutant.

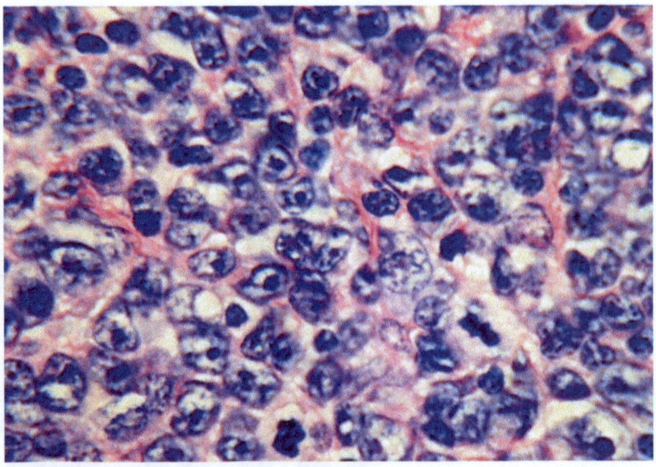

Fig. 1.8. Immunoblasts have large vesicular nuclei, central basophilic nucleoli, and moderate quantities of *pale blue* cytoplasm.

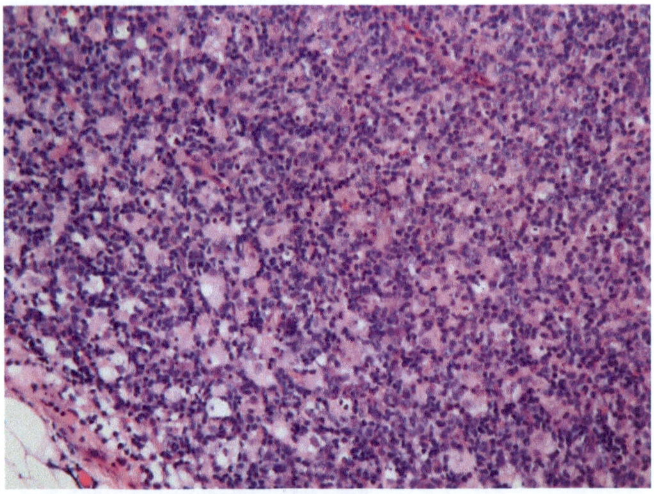

Fig. 1.9. Hyperplastic immunoblasts in the cortex and paracortex produce a mottling because of their moderate quantities of *pale blue* cytoplasm

Furthermore, this fixative produces high background staining in immunohistochemical preparations. Because of all the foregoing reasons, the pathologist is very much dependent on optimally fixed and thin, paraffin-embedded sections supplemented by cytological preparations for the diagnosis of lymph node pathology.

The Pattern Approach to Diagnosis

Clearly there can be more than one way of teaching image recognition in lymph node diagnosis, and the pattern approach has been chosen for this book. When combined with the recognition of key identifying features, it forms the basis of image recognition

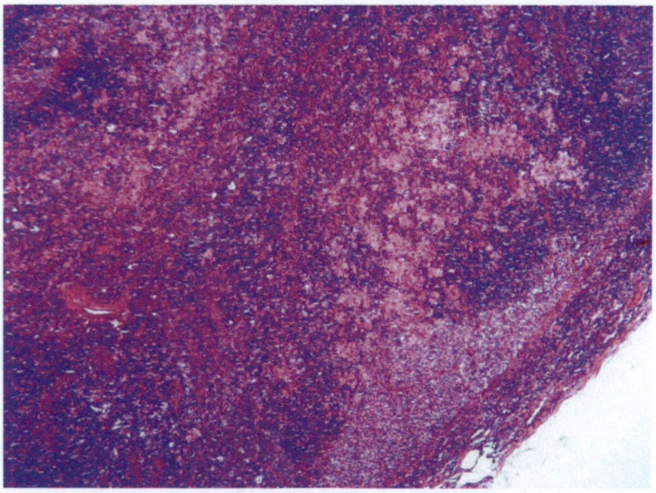

Fig. 1.10. Monocytoid B cells distend sinuses as areas of pallor (MB), whereas epithelioid histiocytes occur as clusters of *pink* from their cytoplasmic staining.

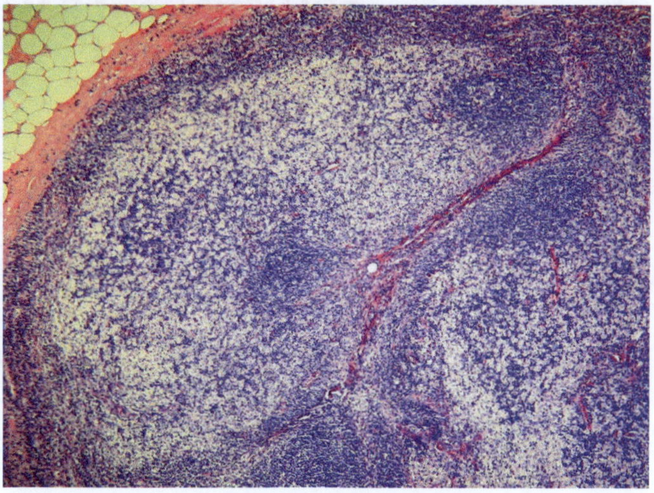

Fig. 1.11. Hyperplastic interdigitating reticulum cells in the paracortex produce nodular areas of pallor due their abundant pale cytoplasm and vesicular nuclei.

in pathology. If these skills are applied with the knowledge and experience accrued over time and exposure, it should be possible for most pathologists to gain sufficient confidence and skills in the area of lymph node diagnosis.

The two major patterns in lymph node pathology are a follicular or nodular pattern and a diffuse pattern of infiltration. These patterns conform to recognizable anatomical compartments of the node, and identification of these patterns, combined with knowledge of the diagnostic entities that produce such patterns, will form the basis of instruction in this book. Other patterns such as sinusoidal, interfollicular/paracortical, and focal patterns can be recognized and have been described to be useful, but these

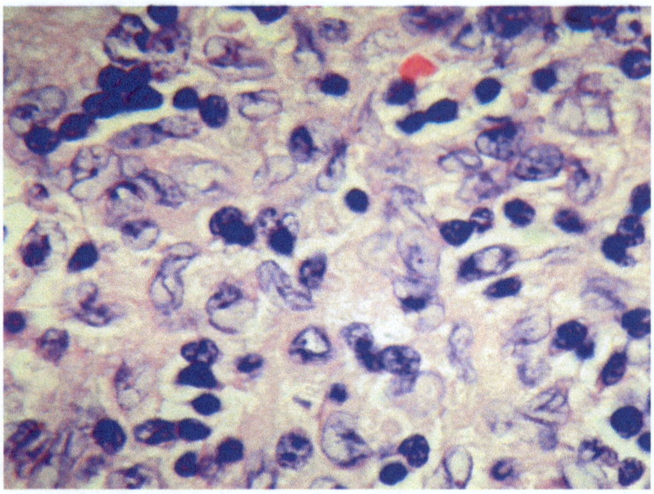

Fig. 1.12. The pallor is imparted by the abundant pale cytoplasm and large pale nuclei of the dendritic cells which display prominent folds of their thin nuclear membranes.

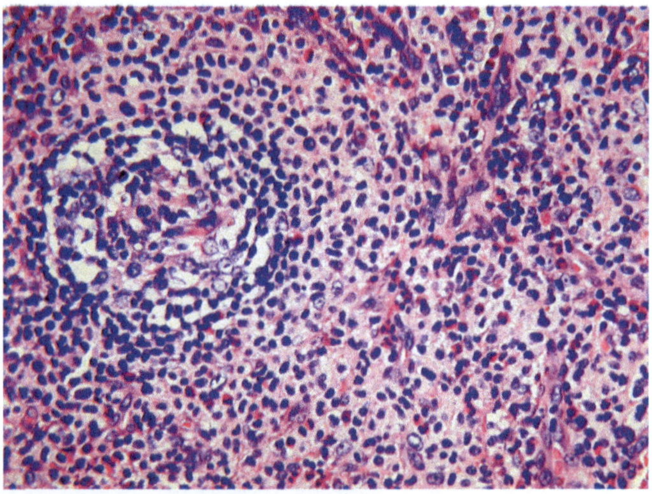

Fig. 1.13. Mast cells have moderate quantities of pale cytoplasm.

are variations of a partially diffuse pattern and will be discussed as such.

An important aspect of pattern recognition in the lymph node is the identification of microscopic defining features that often provide important clues to the pathological process and diagnosis. These defining features are often focal but can be diffuse throughout the lymph node. A large number of diseases, mostly non-lymphoid in nature, are identified by the presence of such defining features. Invariably, there will be overlap in the patterns produced by some conditions, and the main discussion of each entity will be conducted under its primary mode of presentation.

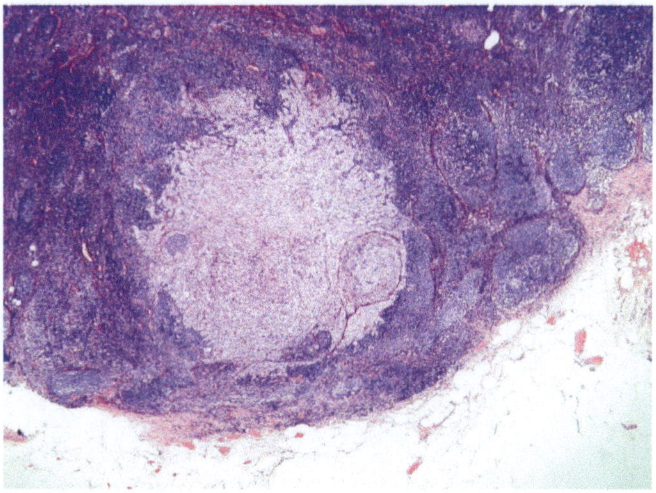

Fig. 1.14. Metastatic carcinoma cells stain *pink* because of their abundant cytoplasm allowing distinct localization.

Despite the extensive interest in biological neural networks and cognitive modeling, our understanding of how the brain processes and integrates the knowledge-based data and visually acquired information in order to formulate a tissue diagnosis is still very rudimentary. As we cannot replicate this learning process, an algorithmic approach to diagnosis is adopted at the end of each section by listing a set of questions that help to consider diagnostic entities that can present with the morphological features observed. This list also serves as a comprehensive reminder or checklist of entities to be considered in differential diagnoses. While the experienced pathologist seemingly arrives at a diagnosis almost instantaneously after examination of the tissue sections, on the occasion when this goal cannot be achieved, he or she carefully considers, in a similar manner, each entity in the differential diagnosis.

The layout of this book will be in accordance with the primary pattern of presentation of the diagnostic entity. Differential diagnosis will be discussed. Appropriate illustrations of each major diagnostic entity will be provided. There will be a level of overlap in the discussion, but this will be kept to a minimum, highlighting only important points. The intention is not to add new knowledge to the subject but to present this book as a "how-to" manual, providing instruction on how to examine lymph nodes and integrate available knowledge to arrive at a "best-fit" diagnosis. As such, the entities will be well illustrated, but references will not be provided, and the reader is referred to the 2008 WHO classification, which contains a comprehensive list of pertinent references.

Selected Reading

Swerdlow SH, Campo E, Harris NL, et al. (eds). WHO classification of tumors of hematopoietic and lymphoid tissues. 4th Edition. Lyon, France: International Agency for Research on Cancer, 2008.

Chapter 2

Handling of the Lymph Node Biopsy

Key words: Triage, imprint, cytology, molecular, cytogenetics, immunohistology, flow cytometry, electron microscopy, bacterial culture.

Introduction

As with other diagnostic situations, failure to obtain an optimal biopsy is the greatest obstacle to achieving a correct diagnosis. The sample should be representative of the lesion, and, more so in lymphoid disorders, it needs to be optimally preserved and processed for a number of ancillary investigations that have become essential for the proper assessment of lymphoproliferative disorders. A timely and accurate diagnosis of optimally preserved representative material that allows the examination of relevant prognostic and predictive parameters is essential for correct management.

The Biopsy

The biopsy sample must be removed with minimal damage to the tissue. The sample should be representative. Often, when a group of superficial lymph nodes are enlarged, it is the deepest or largest node that reflects the pathology, the others often being reactive. Lymph nodes should be excised intact if possible, with minimal trauma to the specimen as lymphoid cells are fragile and

A.S.-Y. Leong, *A Pattern Approach to Lymph Node Diagnosis*,
DOI 10.1007/978-1-4419-7176-0_2, © Springer Science+Business Media, LLC 2011

readily develop artifacts of traction and pressure, especially when the lymph node is fibrotic or removed from confined spaces such as the mediastinum.

Needle or core biopsies taken under imaging guidance are used increasingly, especially when lesions are intra-abdominal or retroperitoneal as it removes the need for laparotomy and the procedure is associated with low morbidity. The limited material restricts the use of some ancillary techniques of examination, but a properly fixed core of tissue can provide good morphological preservation and allow immunohistochemical examination for the precise identification of most common lymphomas. Fine-needle aspiration biopsy has a limited role. It is useful for identifying metastatic disease, confirming recurrence, and staging in some types of lymphoma but is inadequate for subtyping of lymphoma and differentiating most lymphomas from reactive processes. Aspirated samples are useful for flow cytometry as an adjunct to a needle core biopsy sample.

The site of lymphadenopathy does not correlate with a specific etiology. However, some general comments can be made about nodes involved by lymphoma. They tend to be non-tender and often remain mobile, present as generalized lymphadenopathy or involve localized nodes in the neck, axilla or inguinal region, produce asymmetrical enlargement of the mediastinum, or form large palpable or viscera-displacing masses in the abdomen or retroperitoneum. Lymph nodes involved by Hodgkin lymphoma, while non-tender are often fixed and matted. Solitary tender nodes in other sites are generally associated with systemic infections or localized infection in the draining area, e.g., scalp infections produce hyperplasia of occipital or cervical nodes, infections in the hands produce enlargement of epitrochlear nodes, and inguinal lymphadenomegaly may be due to lymphogranuloma venereum, syphilis, and gonococcal, herpetic and mycoplasmal infections. Infections and metastatic carcinoma generally produce tender nodes that may or may not be fixed to surrounding tissues.

Lymph Node Triage

Lymph node specimens need to be assessed individually with regard to the investigations that may be required. As the amount of tissue available may be limited, apportionment of the specimen for the various ancillary investigations will depend on the differential diagnoses considered. It is therefore necessary to formulate a list of possible diagnoses based on the age, gender, relevant clinical history and physical findings, and the biopsy site as soon as the fresh specimen arrives in the laboratory. For convenience, many laboratories develop fresh lymph node protocols which can be modified according to the quantity or volume of material received. While optimally preserved cytomorphology and immunohistochemistry are the minimal requirements today, consideration should be given to flow cytometry, cytogenetics, and molecular studies. Electron microscopy is less often performed. In the case of infectious diseases, bacterial or viral cultures will be needed, and electron microscopy and storage of fresh frozen tissue may be the requirements for additional studies or research.

An example of a fresh lymph node protocol is provided below in **Table 2.1**.

Table 2.1
Fresh lymph node protocol

1.	Slice, with a new scalpel, the node at 2-mm intervals perpendicular to its long axis.
2.	Prepare touch imprints by gently pressing a clean glass slide on the freshly cut surface of the node, taking care not to drag. Do not prepare more than two imprints per cut surface. The imprints may be air-dried and stained with Diff-Quick or Giemsa, fixed in ethanol for Papanicolaou stain, or fixed in a 10% formalin–100% ethanol mixture (50:50 by volume) for hematoxylin–eosin stain. Imprints fixed in 10% formal-saline and air-dried are particularly useful for immunostaining; alternatively, rehydrated air-dried specimens can be used.
3.	The slice from which imprints are prepared can be frozen for storage and used as required.
4.	Fresh tissue from one pole of the specimen is submitted for flow cytometry.
5.	The other pole is submitted fresh for molecular studies.
6.	If required, fresh material is submitted for cytogenetics and diced tissue fixed in 2.5% glutaraldehyde at 4°C for electron microscopy.
7.	The remaining tissue should be fixed overnight for histology and immunohistochemistry. Fixed tissue can also be employed for some molecular studies.

Note: Should there be anticipated delays in transporting the fresh specimens for flow cytometry or molecular studies, they should be placed in physiological saline, Hanks solution, or RPMI 1640 culture medium at 4°C.

Chapter 3

Immunohistology and Other Diagnostic Techniques

Key words: Immunoglobulins, B cell markers, T cell markers, NK/T cell markers, precursor B cell markers, precursor T cell markers, monocyte/macrophage markers, Langerhans cell markers, FDC markers, DRC markers, Reed–Sternberg/Hodgkin cell markers, myeloid markers, mast cell markers, histochemistry, flow cytometry, molecular analysis, gene expression profiling.

Introduction

While morphologic examination of H&E-stained sections remains the cornerstone of lymph node diagnosis, a wide variety of ancillary investigations have served to better define the malignant lymphomas and leukemias. Importantly, they have contributed to a conceptual understanding of the lymphomas, particularly those of B cell lineage. Among the more common techniques that are useful in diagnosis are immunohistology, flow cytometry, cytogenetics, and molecular analysis, with histochemistry, electron microscopy, and bacterial and viral cultures providing useful diagnostic information in more specific situations. Gene expression profiling and proteomics are still research tools but have enhanced our knowledge and facilitated the introduction of new immunohistochemical markers.

While ancillary techniques assist in the accurate diagnosis and typing of the lymphoproliferative disorders, it cannot be overemphasized that suboptimal techniques in taking the biopsy and handling of the specimen remain the greatest obstacles to achieving a correct diagnosis. Lymph nodes should be selected for biopsy on the likelihood that they reflect the pathological process. As multiple enlarged lymph nodes might be available for biopsy, it is preferable to remove the largest lymph node, even if less readily

A.S.-Y. Leong, *A Pattern Approach to Lymph Node Diagnosis*,
DOI 10.1007/978-1-4419-7176-0_3, © Springer Science+Business Media, LLC 2011

accessible, as this is generally more likely to yield a definitive diagnosis. Lymph nodes should be removed intact as far as possible and should not be squeezed or pulled during excision, as traction artifacts can result in significant architectural distortion. Small samples, extensive necrosis, and severe crush artifact also impede interpretation. The portion of the biopsy to be examined histologically, which in many cases is the entire node, should be placed in adequate volumes of 10% buffered formalin as soon as possible after removal. Delays in fixation and poor fixation due to insufficient time exposure to fixative or from inadequate quantities of fixative are common causes of the inability to arrive at a correct diagnosis. Inadequate fixation also impedes optimal use of certain ancillary investigations. Importantly, however, other techniques such as flow cytometry require fresh tissue, and the gross appearance or clinical suspicion may prompt submission of a portion of the node to the microbiology laboratory for bacterial culture.

Immunohistology

Immunohistology (or immunohistochemistry) is of particular diagnostic importance as it can be applied in routinely fixed, paraffin-embedded sections, enabling correlation of immunophenotypic expression with cytomorphologic features. The ability to work in the familiar medium of paraffin-embedded sections which allows good correlation with histomorphologic changes is one of the most important attributes of the technique; hence our preference for the term "immunohistology" over "immunohistochemistry." The large and increasing range of sensitive and specific antibodies immunoreactive in fixed tissue has contributed to the definition of many new entities among the lymphoproliferative disorders and has obviated the need to work with frozen sections, which have the major disadvantages of impermanence and poor morphologic preservation. Although the range of antibodies that react in frozen sections is larger and parallels that used in flow cytometry, there are now sufficient numbers of antibodies that are immunoreactive in paraffin-embedded sections to allow accurate diagnosis and prognosis. Only antibodies that are immunoreactive in formalin-fixed, paraffin-embedded sections will be discussed.

The reader is referred to specialized textbooks of immunohistology for details of antigen retrieval, staining procedures, detection systems, and relevant references. It should be noted that antigen retrieval has a pivotal role whatever the detection system employed. All staining protocols should be optimized to the tissue fixation and processing methods adopted by the individual laboratory, as differences in these procedures will affect the preservation of antigen in the tissues studied. It needs to be emphasized that optimization is not a simple titration of the primary antibody but more importantly optimization of the antigen retrieval protocol in respect of time, temperature, retrieval solution pH, and molarity to the requirements of the individual laboratory. Immunohistochemical stains can also be applied to cytological preparations of aspirated specimens and fluids, to cell blocks prepared from such samples, and to needle core biopsies. Staining protocols may have to be varied accordingly.

Before embarking on lymphocyte subset typing, confirmation of the lymphoid nature of the infiltrate should be firstly made. It is beyond the scope of this book to expand on the uses of immunohistochemistry to achieve this aim; instead, selected antibody panels to separate lymphomas and leukemias from their morphologic mimics in tissue sections are summarized in **Tables 3.1** and **3.2**. In this context, it cannot be overemphasized that antigens released by necrotic cells are often retained at the site of necrosis and it can be helpful to stain for such antigens particularly as the presence of a specific antigen may be indicative of the diagnosis. For example, the separation of carcinoma from lymphoma may be resolved if the necrotic lymph node tissue contains cytokeratins. Similarly, it is sometimes possible to subtype the lymphocyte population by the predominant lymphocyte antigen present at the necrotic site.

Aside from separating lymphoid infiltrates from mimics, immunohistology is employed to determine if a lymphoid infiltrate is benign or neoplastic; if neoplastic, whether it is a lymphoma; and, if so, whether it is non-Hodgkin or Hodgkin lymphoma.

In this chapter, only relevant diagnostic antibodies immunoreactive in routinely fixed, paraffin-embedded tissues will be discussed. It should be noted that relatively comprehensive panels of antibodies should be employed. The use of individual antibodies or extremely focused panels may produce misleading results, particularly if morphologic cues are not fully appreciated. For example, only staining for CD20, CD3, and Bcl2 to confirm a case of

Table 3.1
Antibody panel to differentiate round cell tumors in the lymph node

Differential diagnoses	Antibodies
Lymphoma/leukemia	CD45
Carcinoma	Broad spectrum cytokeratins: AE1/3, bovine keratin, MNF116, Mak6
Melanoma	S100, HMB45, Melan A, tyrosinase, microphthalmia transcription factor (MiTF)

Table 3.2
Antibodies to identify metastatic round cell tumors in the lymphnode

Diagnosis	Antibodies
GI tract	CK20+/CK7–, villin, CDX2, beta-catenin
Liver	HepPar1, glypican 3
Neuroendocrine carcinoma	Broad spectrum cytokeratin, synaptophysin, chromogranin
Thyroid	Thyroglobulin, thyroid transcription factor 1 (TTF1)
Germ cell	Placental alkaline phosphatase (PLAP), Oct4, CD117, D2-40
Prostate	Prostatic acid phosphatase, prostate specific antigen (PSA)
Breast	Gross cystic disease fluid protein 15 (GCDFP15), mammaglobin
Lung	Surfactant A, thyroid transcription factor 1 (TTF1)
Trophoblast	Human chorionic gonadotrophin, human placental lactogen
Skeletal muscle	Desmin, myogenin, MYOD1
Ewing's/PNET	CD99, FLI1
Angiosarcoma	CD34, CD31, D2-40, factor VIII-related protein
Renal	CD10, renal cell antigen (RCA), PAX-2

follicular lymphoma can be misleading as mantle cell lymphoma (MCL), like follicular lymphoma, is CD20+/CD3−/Bcl2+. On the other hand, indiscriminate use of antibodies is not only costly but can also increase the probability of misinterpretation because of unusual reactivity, false positivity, or unfamiliarity with the expected staining pattern.

Immunostaining can provide information that is not apparent morphologically, such as in the demonstration of immunoglobulin light chain restriction (especially in plasma cells). In both nodal and more so extranodal sites, the stains can draw attention to subtle morphological features that otherwise might be missed, including the highlighting small foci of lymphoma in markedly hyperplastic nodes, or in helping the identification of early or "in situ" involvement by MCL or follicular lymphoma.

B Cell Markers

Immunoglobulins

B lymphocytes are defined by their ability to synthesize immunoglobulins, as such this property should be a reliable marker of B cell lineage; however, plasma immunoglobulin diffuses into poorly fixed tissues, and there is passive uptake into lymphocyte cytoplasm, making interpretation difficult. Staining for immunoglobulin is thus capricious and is not widely employed. Synthesized immunoglobulin is granular as it occurs within endoplasmic reticulum. It also accumulates as cytoplasmic inclusions or in the Golgi as a paranuclear globule. Staining also occurs in the perinuclear endoplasmic reticulum, and occasionally surface immunoglobulin can be demonstrated in well-fixed tissues following a combination of heat-induced antigen retrieval in 4 Mol urea and proteolytic digestion, the protocol for demonstrating immunoglobulins in plasma cells being different to that for other lymphoid cells (**Figs. 3.1**, **3.2**, **3.3**, **3.4**, **3.5**, and **3.6**).

Immunoglobulins can also be used as clonality markers. Neoplastic B cell clones are monotypic, expressing only one light chain, although it should be emphasized that light-chain class restriction is not an absolute indicator of neoplasia and may be seen in some reactive conditions. In practice, the detection of monotypic populations can be capricious and not consistent

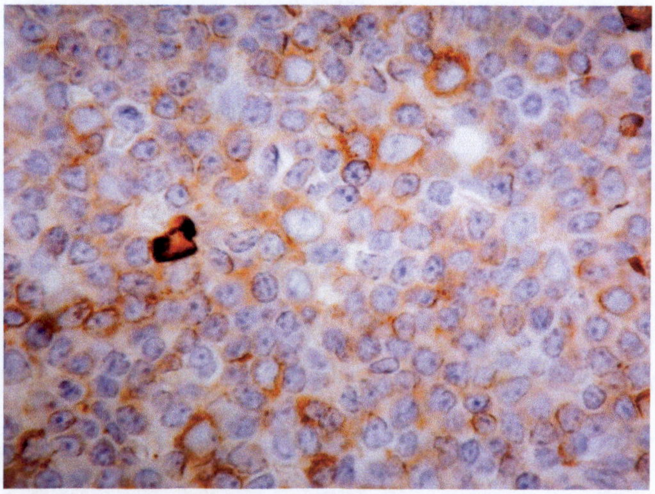

Fig. 3.1. CLL/SLL. There is cytoplasmic staining for Igλ in larger cells and many small cells show distinct staining of perinuclear endoplasmic reticulum.

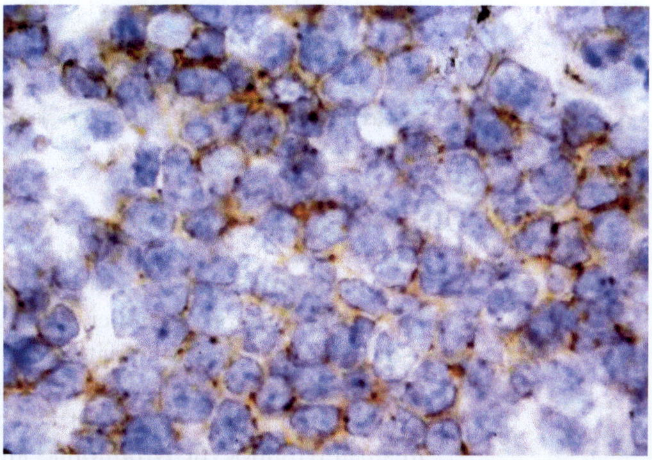

Fig. 3.2. Burkitt lymphoma. There is cIgκ restriction in both a dot-like and diffuse pattern. Igλ staining was negative (not shown).

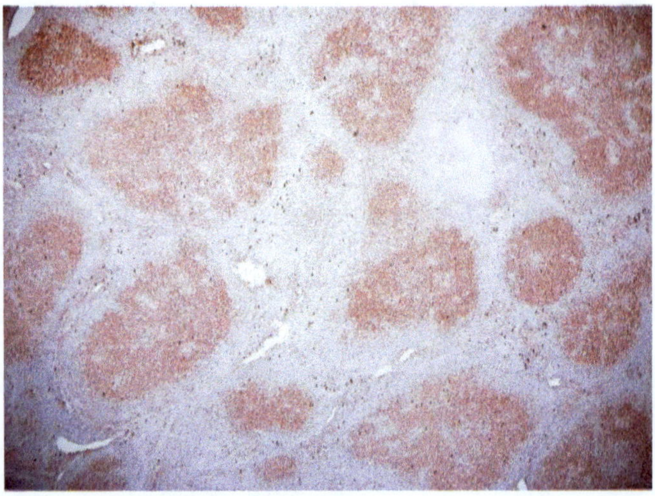

Fig. 3.3. Igκ light-chain restriction in a follicular lymphoma, grade 1. Corresponding staining for Igλ was negative (not shown).

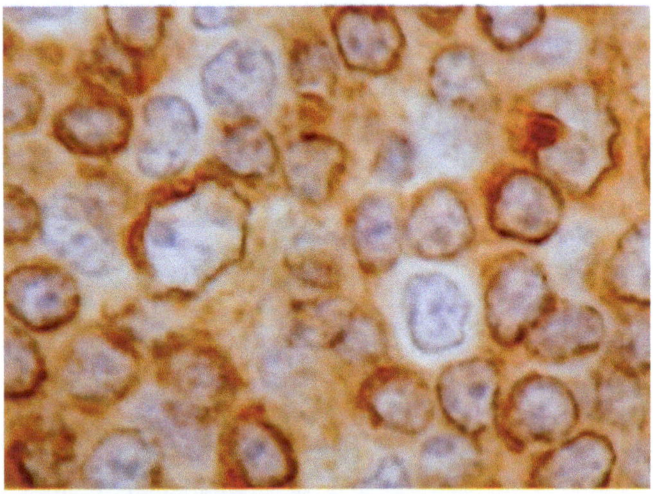

Fig. 3.4. There is distinct staining for Igκ in the perinuclear endoplasmic reticulum as well as cytoplasm. Golgi enhancement is also present (*arrow*).

except in well-fixed tissue, as background reactive lymphocytes generally stain even more strongly. Reactive lymphocytes express κ and λ light chains in a ratio of approximately 2:1. With respect to class or isotype, in general, IgM is the most readily detected as it is a larger molecule with relatively low concentration in the plasma; hence, diffusion artifacts are less frequent compared to other immunoglobulins. Surface IgD can also be demonstrated in small lymphocytic lymphomas and mantle cell lymphomas.

In situ hybridization identification of immunoglobulin light chains avoids some of the problems of non-specific staining but

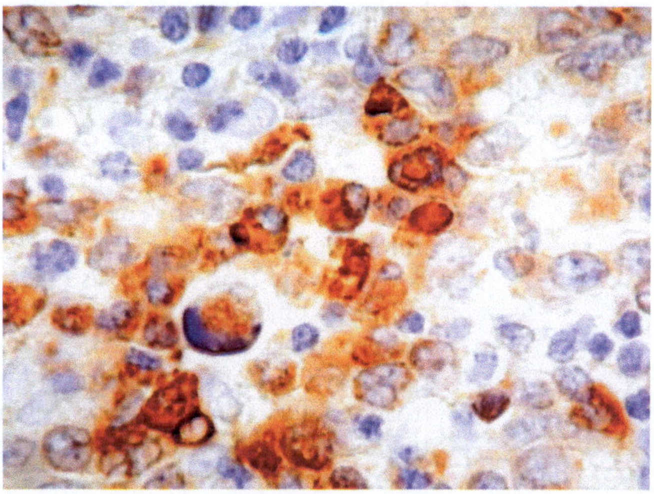

Fig. 3.5. Diffuse large cell lymphoma with globular cytoplasmic cIgκ light-chain restriction.

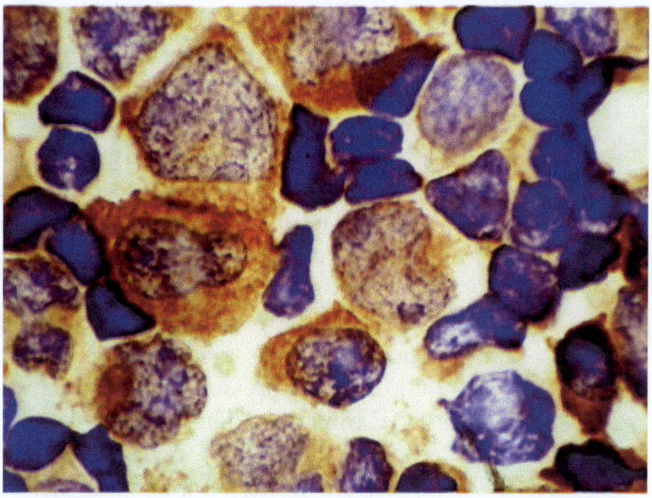

Fig. 3.6. Diffuse cytoplasmic staining for IgM in an imprint of the diffuse large B cell lymphoma as shown in the previous figure.

does not provide greater sensitivity. Flow cytometry is the easiest method to demonstrate light-chain restriction.

CD20

CD20 is a protein encoded by *MS4A1* on chromosome 11q12 that appears on the cell membrane after light-chain gene rearrangement but prior to expression of surface immunoglobulin. Expression is lost before plasma cell differentiation; consequently, while CD20 is an excellent marker of mature B cells, many B lymphoblastic and plasmacytic tumors lack CD20 expression. Staining for CD20 is usually weak in small lymphocytic lymphoma (CLL/SLL). CD20 has been observed rarely on T cell lymphomas and may be seen on thymic epithelial cells. Only membrane expression of CD20 is specific. Cytoplasmic, nuclear, and nucleolar staining should be disregarded.

CD79a

CD79a, also known as Igα, is encoded by a gene on chromosome 19q13.2. It is a subunit of the heterodimer that triggers intracellular signaling pathways upon antigen cross linking of membrane immunoglobulin molecules. CD79a is a more sensitive marker of B cell lineage than CD20, as it is strongly expressed throughout all stages of B cell differentiation and labels not only lesions of mature B cells but also precursor B-lymphoblastic lymphoma and plasmacytic lesions. Specificity is limited by clone-dependent positivity of subsets of precursor T-lymphoblastic lymphomas, acute myeloid leukemias, and normal megakaryocytes. Staining is cytoplasmic and membranous.

PAX5

PAX5, previously referred to as BSAP (B cell specific activator protein), is a transcription factor encoded on chromosome 9p13 and expressed in B cells but not in T cells. Staining for PAX5 shows positivity of most lymphomas of B cell lineage, including precursor B-lymphoblastic lymphoma and Hodgkin lymphoma, though intensity may be decreased in RS cells. Plasmacytic neoplasms are negative. Unfortunately, the rare large B cell lymphomas lacking CD20, e.g., primary effusion lymphoma, usually also lack PAX5. While T cell neoplasms do not show immunoreactivity, neuroendocrine carcinomas, including Merkel cell carcinoma, frequently express PAX5. Staining is nuclear.

CD23

CD23 is a glycoprotein that functions as a low-affinity receptor for IgE and is encoded by *FCER2* on chromosome 19p13.3. CD23 is expressed by activated B cells and is upregulated in EBV infection. The majority of CLL/SLL cases label for CD23, making it a useful marker to distinguish this lymphoma from other small cell lymphomas, including mantle cell and marginal zone lymphomas. The marker also labels follicular dendritic cells (FDC) and is useful in displaying proliferation and expansion of the FDC meshwork in mantle cell lymphoma and follicular lymphoma. Staining is membranous.

Cyclin D1 (Bcl1)

Cyclin D1, which is encoded by *CCND1* on chromosome 11q13, plays a role in control of the cell cycle by regulating cyclin-dependent kinases. In nearly all cases of mantle cell lymphoma, the gene is translocated to the immunoglobulin heavy chain (*IGH*) locus at 14q32, leading to overexpression of cyclin D1 protein. Cyclin D1 is the primary marker used to differentiate mantle cell lymphoma from other small B cell lymphomas. It may also stain some hairy cell leukemias and plasmacytomas, although generally weakly compared to MCL, as well as a variety of epithelial tumors. The antigen is localized to the nucleus, and cytoplasmic staining is false. Endothelial cells serve as internal controls.

Bcl2

The *BCL2* gene on chromosome 18q21.3 is involved in the t(14;18)(q32;q21) characteristic of follicular lymphomas, in which *BCL2* is juxtaposed with *IGH@* on chromosome 14q32. Bcl2 is an anti-apoptotic mitochondrial membrane protein; overexpression, as is associated with the t(14;18) translocation, results in a survival advantage. While most small B and T cells are positive for Bcl2, reactive germinal center B cells are negative. Follicular lymphomas, on the other hand, are usually Bcl2 positive; so staining with this marker is useful in distinguishing between reactive and neoplastic follicles. Positivity is also observed in CLL/SLL, mantle cell lymphoma, and a moderate number of marginal zone lymphomas, such that expression is not generally useful in the classification of small B cell lymphomas. Bcl2 expression in diffuse large B cell lymphomas may be an adverse prognostic marker, although data regarding this point are inconsistent across studies. Expression in Hodgkin and Reed–Sternberg cells is likely an adverse prognostic sign in cases of classical Hodgkin lymphoma. Bcl2 expression is not restricted to lymphoid cells, and it is detectable in a wide variety of epithelial and mesenchymal tumors.

Bcl6

The *BCL6* gene on chromosome 3q27 encodes a zinc finger transcription factor that is highly expressed in the nuclei of germinal center B cells and is also detectable in follicular helper T cells. Staining for Bcl6 shows positivity of neoplasms arising from such cells, namely, follicular lymphoma, Burkitt lymphoma, some diffuse large B cell lymphomas, nodular lymphocyte predominant Hodgkin lymphoma, and angioimmunoblastic T cell lymphoma. Expression may also be seen in ALK+ anaplastic large cell lymphoma. Mantle cell lymphomas are negative for the protein. Marginal zone lymphomas are Bcl6 negative, but some diffuse large B cell lymphomas arising from MALT lymphomas may express Bcl6. Together with CD10 and CDw75, Bcl6 is a reliable marker of follicle center derivation with a sensitivity approaching 100%.

CD10 (CALLA)

CD10, also known historically as the common acute lymphoblastic leukemia antigen (CALLA), is a neutral endopeptidase encoded by *MME* on chromosome 3q25 that is thought to inactivate regulatory peptides favoring cell differentiation. CD10 is expressed by germinal center B cells and most follicular lymphomas; staining is stronger in the latter, allowing another method of distinguishing between the two forms of follicles. It is also expressed in most precursor B-lymphoblastic lymphomas, a subset of precursor T-lymphoblastic lymphomas, Burkitt lymphoma, and angioimmunoblastic T cell lymphoma. Positivity of at least 30% of the neoplastic cells in cases of diffuse large B cell lymphoma (DLBCL) fits with the germinal-center-like subtype as defined by gene expression profiling. A range of non-lymphoid tissues and tumors, including endometrial stromal sarcoma and certain types of renal cell carcinoma, also express CD10. Expression is on the cell membrane.

MUM1/IRF4

Interferon regulatory factor 4, commonly referred to as IRF4 or MUM1, is a transcription regulatory factor encoded by *IRF* on chromosome 6p25. While expression is seen in B cells and activated T cells, normal Bcl6+ germinal center B cells are negative for MUM1/IRF4. In contrast, coexpression of these proteins may be seen in some cases of DLBCL; the detection of MUM1/IRF4 by immunohistology in DLBCL is associated with the non-germinal-center-like subtype.

CD45RA (4KB5, MB1, KiB3, MT2)

The CD45RA group of antibodies recognize isoforms of CD45 that are expressed on the surface of most B cells as well as post-thymic naïve T cells and some medullary thymocytes. These isoforms of the protein tyrosine phosphatase, like all variants of CD45, are encoded by *PTPRC* on chromosome 1q31–q32. The CD45RA antibodies were used as B cell markers but have largely been superseded by other more reliable markers such as CD20 and CD79a. MT2 may be of assistance in distinguishing reactive from neoplastic follicles, the latter being positive in many cases, although the occasional reactive follicle may stain with this marker; consequently, Bcl2 remains a more reliable marker in distinguishing follicular lymphoma from hyperplasia.

CDw75 (LN1)

Antibodies to CDw75 (also referred to as CD75 s) stain a sialylated carbohydrate determinant present on the surface of germinal center B cells but not on T cells. This antigen is also expressed by a variety of epithelial cells, including those lining distal renal tubules, mammary glands, bronchi, and prostatic glands. While there are other more specific markers of follicle center cells, antibodies to CDw75 may be used for identification of follicular lymphomas, as no immunoreactivity is seen in small lymphocytic lymphomas or T cell lymphomas. Staining is membranous with a distinct paranuclear dot representing staining of the Golgi.

CD38

The *CD38* gene on chromosome 4p15 encodes a 46-kD protein expressed by precursor cells of myeloid and lymphoid lineages, monocytes, activated T cells and B cells, and plasma cells. This transmembrane glycoprotein is multifunctional and has roles in signal transduction, cell adhesion, and cyclic adenosine diphosphatate–ribose synthesis. Besides being expressed on plasma cells and their tumors, CD38 has been found on pyramidal neurons and astrocytes and in benign prostatic basal and epithelial secretory cells. Expression of CD38 by >30% of the neoplastic B cells in chronic lymphocytic leukemia is regarded as an adverse prognostic sign associated not only with an unmutated immunoglobulin heavy-chain variable region gene (*IGHV@*) but also with nodal involvement by small lymphocytic lymphoma.

CD138

CD138 (syndecan-1) is a transmembrane heparan sulfate proteoglycan encoded by *SDC1* on chromosome 2p24.1 that has roles in cell proliferation, migration and interactions with extracellular matrix proteins, and it is associated with late-stage B cell differentiation. While it may be detected on B cell precursors, staining for CD138 is used more frequently to highlight plasma cells and their neoplastic counterparts. Staining occurs in primary effusion lymphoma, plasmablastic lymphoma, and DLBCL associated with chronic inflammation. CD138 expression in DLBCL, NOS is associated with the non-germinal-center-like subtype. It is also expressed on stratified variety of epithelial tumors, and loss of expression is associated with tumor aggressiveness in squamous cell carcinoma of head and neck. Staining is membranous.

ZAP-70

Zeta chain-associated protein kinase 70 kD (ZAP-70) is a protein tyrosine kinase that plays an essential role in signal transduction during T cell activation. The *ZAP70* gene is on chromosome 2q12. ZAP-70 is expressed in T cells, NK cells, and neoplasms of T cell lineage as well as in a subgroup of chronic lymphocytic leukemias. It is employed as a prognostic marker in CLL and has been shown to be a stronger predictor of aggressive CLL/SLL than unmutated immunoglobulin heavy-chain variable region gene (*IGHV@*) (**Table 3.3**).

T Cell Markers

T lymphocytes may make up a large proportion of reactive lymphocytic proliferations, and many B cell lymphomas may contain large numbers of T cells, including some follicular lymphomas and T cell-rich B cell lymphomas. Unlike B cells, T lymphocytes do not express a mutually exclusive pair of molecules analogous to Ig light chains; as such, there are no easily accessible immunohistochemical markers to identify clonal populations of T lymphocytes. Antibodies specific for most of the variable regions of the T cell receptor β-chain gene have recently been developed and can be employed to assess T cell clonality but currently are used only in flow cytometry. T cell lymphomas are generally characterized by immunophenotypic aberrancy, such as loss of expression of one or more pan-T cell markers (CD2, CD3, CD5, CD7) and predominance of either the CD4 or CD8 subset, but such aberrancy may be difficult to detect, as there is often an admixture of reactive T cells with the neoplastic cells in T cell lymphomas.

Table 3.3
Markers of B cell neoplasms

Immunoglobulins
Immunoglobulin light chain restriction – clonality
CD20 – B cell lymphomas *excluding* pre-B and plasmacytic lymphomas
CD79a – B cell lymphomas *including* pre-B and plasmacytic lymphomas
PAX5 – B cell lymphomas including pre-B, but not plasmacytic, lymphomas
CD23 – CLL/SLL (also FDC sarcoma)
Cyclin D1 – Mantle cell lymphoma; weaker staining in HCL and some plasmacytomas
Bcl2 – Neoplastic follicles, also CLL/SLL, mantle cell and marginal zone lymphomas
Bcl6 – Follicular lymphoma, Burkitt lymphoma, NLPHL, AITL, some DLBCL CD10 (CALLA) – fFollicular lymphomas; reactive follicles also express CD10 but weakly
MUM1/IRF4 – Non-germinal-center-like DLBCL; used with CD10, Bcl6
CD45RA – Neoplastic follicles
CDw75 – Follicular lymphomas
CD38 – Plasmacytic lymphoma and plasmacytoma
CD138 – Plasmacytic lymphoma and plasmacytoma
ZAP-70 – Predictor of aggressive CLL/SLL

T Cell Receptor

The defining marker of T cells should be the T cell receptor molecule (TCR), either TCRαβ or TCRγδ, but the only antibodies available that are immunoreactive in paraffin-embedded tissues are to the TCRβ chain (clone βF1) that recognize T cells with the αβ receptor. For a number of reasons, including low sensitivity, these antibodies are not widely used.

CD1a

The *CD1A* gene on chromosome 1q22-q23 encodes a glycoprotein that participates in antigen presentation, and while CD1a is expressed on cortical thymocytes, its clinical utility is greatest in the identification of Langerhans cells and the classification of thymomas. Along with some precursor T-lymphoblastic lymphomas, myeloid leukemias and some B cell neoplasms may be positive for CD1a. Expression is both membranous and cytoplasmic.

CD2

The CD2 molecule is a glycosylated transmembrane receptor that is responsible for the spontaneous E-rosetting of human T lymphocytes with sheep red blood cells. Encoded by a gene on chromosome 1p13.1, CD2 is one of the earliest T cell lineage restricted antigens to appear and is expressed by all T lymphocytes and natural killer cells but not by B cells or other cell types. CD2 appears after CD7 and before CD1, but its temporal relationship with CD3 is less well characterized. A few antibody clones to CD2 that are immunoreactive in formalin-fixed paraffin-embedded sections are now available. Prior to the development of antibodies to CD2, spontaneous rosetting with sheep erythrocytes was one of the more reliable methods of establishing T cell lineage.

CD3

The CD3 γ, δ, and ϵ proteins are encoded by *CD3G, CD3D,* and *CD3E* on chromosome 11q23 and are closely associated (in the form of ε and δε heterodimers) with the T cell receptor (TCR) heterodimer. CD3 is detectable in the cytoplasm before the TCR complex is fully assembled and inserted into the cell membrane. Binding of antigen to the TCR results in T cell activation and proliferation via signal transduction by CD3 with release of cytokines and display of non-specific cytotoxicity, properties requiring the participation of accessory cells. Expression of CD3 is restricted to the T cell lineage and occurs virtually throughout T cell differentiation; consequently, CD3 is the most sensitive and specific marker of T cell lineage available for the immunophenotyping of lymphoproliferative disorders. Most monoclonal antibodies label only the membranous and not the cytoplasmic antigen.

CD4

CD4 is a glycoprotein that functions as a co-receptor with TCR, binding with class II MHC molecules, and is used by HIV to infect T cells. Encoded by a gene on chromosome 12pter-p12, CD4 appears at the common thymocyte stage of T cell differentiation and is generally a marker of helper T cells, labeling a majority of mature peripheral T cells. The phenotype/function association of CD4 to helper and CD8 to suppressor/cytotoxic function is not universal, and subpopulations of suppressor/cytotoxic T cells can be identified among CD4+ T cells. B cells do not express CD4, but the antigen is expressed by histiocytes, monocytes, Langerhans cells, and other dendritic cells. Expression of CD4 by neoplastic T cells is seen in most cases of adult T cell leukemia/lymphoma, mycosis fungoides, and angioimmunoblastic T cell lymphoma, as well as in many cases of anaplastic large cell lymphoma and peripheral T cell lymphoma, NOS.

CD5

The CD5 molecule is a transmembrane glycoprotein involved in signal transduction. It is encoded on chromosome 11q13, first seen in intrathymic T cell progenitors, and serves as an excellent marker of reactive and neoplastic T cells. A minority of B lymphocytes are positive for CD5, but expression is much weaker than that seen on T cells. Similarly, the weak expression of CD5 by CLL/SLL and mantle cell lymphoma does not create major confusion with T cell lymphomas, as the B cell lymphomas also express CD20 and CD79a.

CD7

CD7 is a surface glycoprotein expressed by NK cells and T cells (mature and immature) and encoded on chromosome 17q25.2-q25.3. Being the first of the pan-T cell markers expressed in

T cell development, it is consistently detectable in precursor T-lymphoblastic lymphomas, but the pan-T cell antigen is most likely to be absent from mature post-thymic T cell neoplasms. CD7 is conspicuously absent in adult T cell leukemia/lymphoma and is not expressed in mycosis fungoides/Sezary syndrome.

CD8

CD8 is the designation given to glycoproteins encoded by *CD8A* and *CD8B* on chromosome 2p12 and expressed in the forms of αα homodimers and αβ heterodimers on the surface of T cells. CD8 functions as a TCR co-receptor on suppressor/cytotoxic T cells, binding to class I MHC molecules. Like CD4, CD8 appears during the common thymocyte stage of T cell differentiation. Expression of CD4 and CD8 becomes mutually exclusive with T cell maturation, however, and only a minority of mature peripheral T cells are CD8+. Lower levels of CD8 expression are detectable in a minority of NK cells. The CD8 antigen may be expressed by precursor T-lymphoblastic lymphomas, but like CD4, CD8 may be aberrantly deleted from neoplastic T cells.

CD43 (Mt1)

MT1 recognizes a sialoglycoprotein encoded by *SPN* on chromosome 16p11.2 and present on the membranes of normal T cells, myeloid cells, and macrophages, with variable positivity in megakaryocytes. CD43 antibodies react with most lymphomas of T cell lineage, whether mature or lymphoblastic; however, positivity in significant numbers of B cell lymphomas and in nearly all myeloid sarcomas precludes its use as a lineage specific T cell marker. The expression of CD43 in a large B cell lymphoma may reflect dedifferentiation from a small cell lymphoma. Among the small B cell neoplasms, expression of CD43 is consistently detected in small lymphocytic lymphoma and mantle cell lymphoma, sporadically detectable in marginal zone lymphoma, and generally absent in follicular lymphoma.

CD45RO (UCHl1, OPD4)

CD45RO antibodies detect an isoform of CD45 that is expressed on the surface of most cortical thymocytes, in about one-half of medullary thymocytes, and in a majority of lymph node T cells. Mature monocytes/macrophages and granulocytes are generally CD45RO-positive. The antigen is expressed by most mature T cell lymphomas, with variable expression by T-lymphoblastic lymphoma. A proportion of diffuse large B cell lymphomas also expresses the antigen, reducing its value as a marker of T cell lineage in large cell lymphoma.

Cytotoxic Molecules (TIA-1, Granzyme B, Perforin)

Cytotoxic T cells and NK cells are characterized by the presence of cytoplasmic granules that are released in response to target cell recognition, and these granules contain proteins such as granzymes and perforin. Perforin allows for the entry of granzyme molecules into targeted cells, where they induce apoptosis. TIA-1 is an RNA-binding protein, but its exact role in cytotoxicity is not well understood. These antigens are expressed by NK cell neoplasms and by some T cell lymphomas, such as anaplastic large cell lymphoma and enteropathy-associated T cell lymphoma.

PD-1 (CD279, CXCR5)

Programmed cell death-1 (PD-1), encoded by *PDCD1* on chromosome 2q37.3, is a surface protein structurally related to CD28. It is expressed by germinal-center-associated helper T cells in reactive tissues and activated B cells. PD-1, in contrast to CD28, appears to have a role in inhibiting cellular activation. Expression of PD-1 is observed in angioimmunoblastic T cell lymphoma, and the T cells that form rosettes around the L&H cells of NLPHL. The latter coexpress CD3, CD4, Bcl6, CD57, and CXCL13. PD-1 may also be expressed by CLL/SLL and can potentially be employed in the panel for classifying small cell lymphomas.

CXCL13

CXCL13, a chemokine that is specifically expressed in lymphoid follicles and required for B cell entry into germinal centers, is one of the most highly up-regulated genes in follicular helper T cells. Like PD-1, it has been shown to be expressed by angioimmunoblastic T cell lymphoma and to facilitate its distinction from other peripheral T cell lymphomas. CXCL13 is localized to the cytoplasm with paranuclear dot enhancement (**Table 3.4**).

Table 3.4
Markers of T cell neoplasms

TCRβ – T cells with αβ TCR
CD1a – Precursor T lymphoblastic lymphoma, (also Langerhans cell histiocytosis, thymoma)
CD2 – Pan T
CD3 – Pan T
CD4 – Helper/inducer T cells
CD5 – Pan T, also mantle cell lymphoma and CLL/SLL
CD7 – Pan T, often lost in T cell lymphoma
CD8 – Supressor/cytotoxic T cells
CD43 – T cell lymphoma, ALCL, B cell lymphoma, granulocytic sarcoma
CD45RO – T cell lymphoma, large B cell lymphoma
Cytotoxic molecules – Cytotoxic T cells, NK cell tumor, ALCL, enteropathy-associated T cell lymphoma
TdT – Precursor T cell tumor
PD-1 – Angioimmunoblastic T cell lymphoma; rosetting T cells in NLPHL
CXCL13 – Angioimmunoblastic T cell lymphoma; rosetting T cells in NLPHL

Natural Killer and T/NK Cell Markers

CD56 (Neural Cell Adhesion Molecule 1)

CD56 is also known as neural cell adhesion molecule 1 and is encoded by *NCAM1* on chromosome 11q23.1. While it can be found on a variety of epithelial and neural tissues and their corresponding neoplasms, the current major application of CD56 in lymphoid tissue is for the diagnosis of NK and NK-like T cell lymphomas. CD56+ lymphomas are heterogenous and encompass nasal NK/T cell lymphoma, aggressive NK cell leukemia/lymphoma, and most cases of hepatosplenic T cell lymphoma. Plasmacytoid dendritic cell tumors are also recognized to have a CD56+CD4+ phenotype, and a proportion of acute myeloid leukemias express CD56. Lastly, microvillous B cell lymphomas that are CD20+, CDw75+, and CD74+ with clonal heavy-chain immunoglobulin are positive for CD56 in about 50% of reported cases.

CD57

CD57 antibodies bind a carbohydrate epitope expressed on a variable proportion of peripheral blood lymphocytes but not on other hematopoietic cells. The CD57+ population of lymphocytes includes a subset of CD8+ T cells as well as NK cells. Some T and NK cell lymphomas express this marker, though less than 10% of CD56+ nasal-type T/NK cell neoplasms are CD57+. Many of the CD4+ T cells found in germinal centers express CD57. CD4+/CD57+ T cells produce spontaneous rosettes with the multilobated cells of NLPHL, a helpful feature to separate this lymphoma from its mimics. CD57 is also expressed in a wide range of non-hematopoietic neoplasms and tissues including neural tissue, neuroendocrine cells, and epithelial cells (**Table 3.5**).

Table 3.5
Markers of NK and T/NK cell tumors

CD56 –	Nasal NK/T cell tumor, aggressive NK cell lymphoma, hepatosplenic T cell lymphoma, plasmacytoid dendritic cell tumor, microvillous B cell lymphoma
CD57 –	Nasal NK/T cell tumor, rosettes around LP cells of NLPHL, non-hematopoietic neuroendocrine and epithelial tumors

Precursor B- and T Cell Markers

Terminal Deoxynucleotidyl Transferase (TdT)

Terminal deoxynucleotidyl transferase (TdT), a 58-kD intranuclear DNA polymerase encoded by *DNTT* on chromosome 10q23-q24, catalyzes the random addition of deoxynucleotidyl residues to DNA. TdT expression is restricted to a proportion of multipotent cell precursors and to immature B- and T cell precursors. In the bone marrow, TdT+ lymphocytes are interspersed in interstitial spaces, and in the thymus, cortical thymocytes are positive for the polymerase. TdT expression is a marker of precursor B and T cell lymphoblastic lymphomas and may also be expressed in cases of chronic myelogenous leukemia in blast phase. Staining is nuclear, and cytoplasmic staining should be disregarded.

CD34

CD34, a glycosylated membrane protein encoded on chromosome 1q32, is expressed by hematopoietic progenitor cells and by endothelial cells. Expression is a specific, but not sensitive, marker of immaturity in hematopoietic neoplasms such as lymphoblastic lymphoma and myeloid sarcoma. Immunoreactivity is also seen in vascular tumors and a variety of other tumors, including solitary fibrous tumor and dermatofibrosarcoma protuberans (**Table 3.6**).

Table 3.6
Markers of precursor B and T cell lesions

TdT –	Lymphoblastic lymphoma (precursor B and precursor T)
CD34 –	Lymphoblastic lymphoma (precursor B and precursor T), myeloid sarcoma, vascular tumors, other mesenchymal lesions

Monocyte/ Macrophage Markers

Most markers of monocytes/macrophages also stain myeloid cells and precursors. Monocytes/macrophages express CD45, although this may be weaker compared to cells of the lymphoid series.

CD68

CD68, a 110-kD protein encoded on chromosome 17p13, is a member of a family of highly glycosylated lysosomal glycoproteins expressed by monocytes and macrophages in a wide range of tissues, such as the lung, lymph node, and liver (Kupffer cells). Osteoclasts and myeloid precursors in the bone marrow are strongly labeled, and there is also labeling of neutrophils and basophils. Histiocytic sarcomas express CD68, as do acute myeloid leukemias with monocytic differentiation and myeloid sarcoma. Plasmacytoid monocytes and mast cells show scattered granules of CD68 positivity, and dendritic cells and their corresponding tumors can also be positive. Melanomas may be positive for CD68, as are other cells that are rich in lysosomes.

CD163

CD163 is a hemoglobin scavenger receptor encoded on chromosome 12p13.3 and expressed on the surface of monocytes and macrophages, where it mediates endocytosis of haptoglobin–

hemoglobin complexes. CD163 is a sensitive marker of lesions with monocytic/histiocytic differentiation, including sinus histiocytosis with massive lymphadenopathy (Rosai–Dorfman disease), Langerhans cell histiocytosis, histiocytic sarcoma, and monoblastic sarcoma. It is currently the most specific marker of histiocytes/macrophages and, unlike CD68, does not label cells that are lysozyme-rich.

Mac387

Mac387 antibodies recognize calprotectin, a member of the S100 family of calcium-binding proteins that is encoded by *S100A9* on chromosome 1q21. Immunoreactivity is observed on many myelomonocytic cells and is seen in several histiocytic lesions, including Rosai–Dorfman disease, Langerhans cell histiocytosis, and a small number of anaplastic large cell lymphomas. Mac387 is also positive in a variety of epithelial tumors and as such is not specific with respect to histiocytic differentiation.

Ham56

HAM56 was raised against human alveolar macrophages and can be used with the other conventional markers of monocytes/macrophages, which should include CD163, CD68, and Mac387; its expression is not specific to macrophages, however, as immunoreactivity has been reported in lymphoid and endothelial cells and in adenocarcinomas.

Lysozyme (Muramidase)

Lysozyme is a mucolytic enzyme found in saliva, gastrointestinal secretions, tears, urine, and serum. Encoded by *LYZ* on chromosome 12q15, lysozyme is expressed not only by histiocytes but is also seen in granulocytes, the secretory granules of Paneth cells, and in the brush border of mucus cells of the small intestine. Lysozyme is present in tingible body macrophages of the germinal center and is a useful marker of histiocytic and myeloid cells. Lysozyme is not a specific marker and should be used in the context of a panel that includes other macrophage markers; moreover, diffusion of this enzyme causes artifactual staining.

α-1-Antitrypsin and α-1-Antichymotrypsin

α-1-Antitrypsin (AAT) and α-1-antichymotrypsin (AACT) are serine protease inhibitors that are synthesized by monocytes and encoded by *SERPINA1* and *SERPINA3*, respectively, on chromosome 14q32. Their popularity as markers of monocytes/macrophages came about when they were employed to distinguish histiocytic from lymphoid neoplasms. However, when it was shown that AAT and AACT (and lysozyme) immunoreactivity was common in a large variety of both epithelial and mesenchymal tumors, including neuroendocrine tumors, melanomas, and uterine sarcomas, enthusiasm for these markers rapidly fell off (**Table 3.7**).

Table 3.7
Markers of Monocyte/Macrophage Tumors

CD45 – Weaker staining than in lymphoid cells
CD68 – Stains lysosomal bodies in histiocytic cells; also stains myeloid tumors, dendritic cells, and other lysozyme-rich tumors
CD163 – Most specific marker of monocytic/histiocytic differentiation; stains leukemias with monocytic differentiation, Langerhans cell histiocytosis, histiocytic sarcoma, Rosai–Dorfman disease
Mac387 – Histiocytic tumors; less specific marker
HAM56 – Histiocytic tumors; less specific marker
Lysozyme – Less specific marker of histiocytic cells
AAT and AACT – Less specific markers of histiocytic cells; also stain many epithelial and mesenchymal tumorsCD163 – most specific marker of monocyte/histiocytic differentiation, stains leukemias with monocytic differentiation, dendritic cell tumors, Langerhans histiocytosis, histiocytic sarcoma, Rosai–Dorfman disease

Langerhans Cell, Follicular Dendritic Cell, and Interdigitating Dendritic Reticulum Cell Markers

CD21

CD21, a 145-kD glycoprotein, is a receptor for the C3d fragment of complement and transduces growth promoting signals for B lymphocytes. Encoded by *CR2* on chromosome 1q32, CD21 also functions as a receptor for the Epstein–Barr virus. While the antibody stains a range of B cells, much stronger staining is seen in follicular dendritic cells (FDC). Staining for CD21 is thus used to demonstrate the meshwork of FDC in follicular lymphoma, mantle cell lymphoma and marginal zone lymphomas. FDC proliferation is also seen in Castleman disease and in angioimmunoblastic T cell lymphoma, in the latter, typically around high endothelial venules. CD21 also stains FDC sarcoma.

CD23

See above (B Cell Markers).

CD35

CD35 is an epitope of the receptor for C3b and C4b fragments of human complement. This single glycoprotein chain of about 220 kD, encoded by *CR1* on chromosome 1q32, is expressed on FDC and is also demonstrable on renal podocytes. Its applications are largely for the demonstration of FDC meshwork and FDC tumors, similar to those for CD21 (*see* above).

D2-40 (Podoplanin)

Podoplanin is a membrane glycoprotein encoded by *PDPN* on chromosome 1p36.21 and expressed by endothelial cells (especially those of lymphatics) as well as a variety of other cell types. More recently, podoplanin demonstrated by the antibody D2-40 has been shown to have sensitivity for FDC at least equal to that of other markers including CD21, CD35, and clusterin. Staining for D2-40 is membranous and cytoplasmic. With respect to neoplasms, D2-40 stains not only FDC sarcomas and lymphovascular neoplasms but also a variety of non-vascular tumors including mesothelioma, rendering it less specific than other FDC markers.

Clusterin

Clusterin is a glycoprotein expressed by follicular dendritic cells and by cells in a variety of organs, including liver and brain. Encoded by *CLU* on chromosome 8p21-p12, this protein's function has not yet been clearly delineated. Expression of clusterin has been demonstrated in anaplastic large cell lymphoma, rarely in other lymphoid neoplasms, and in carcinomas arising in a variety of sites. Clusterin appears to be a sensitive marker of follicular dendritic cells, and strong immunoreactivity appears to distinguish neoplasms of FDC from interdigitating dendritic cell tumors and Langerhans cell histiocytosis.

Langerin (CD207)

Langerin, a lectin with mannose-binding specificity encoded by *CD207* on chromosome 2p13, is found on the surface and in the Birbeck granules of Langerhans cells. Langerin mediates endocytosis of mannose-containing ligands for antigen processing by Langerhans cells. Antibodies to langerin show consistent immunoreactivity in Langerhans cell histiocytosis but only rare positivity in other histiocytic lesions.

S100 Proteins

The S100 proteins, so named because they are soluble in a 100% saturated ammonium sulfate solution, are calcium-binding proteins expressed by a large range of tissues and neoplasms, including malignant melanoma and schwannoma. Multiple genes clustered on chromosome 1q21 encode S100 proteins. The main use of S100 antibodies in hematopathology is that it is used as a marker for Langerhans cells and interdigitating dendritic cells; variable positivity is seen in histiocytic sarcoma and FDC tumors.

HLA-DR

HLA-DR is a heterodimeric class II MHC molecule with a single binding site for immunogenic peptides. The α and β chains are encoded by genes in the HLA locus on chromosome 6p21.3. HLA-DR is expressed on antigen-presenting cells such as dendritic cells, monocytes, macrophages, and B cells of the germinal center and mantle cells. Activated T cells may also express HLA-DR, as may endothelial and epithelial cells (**Table 3.8**).

Markers of Reed–Sternberg Cells in Hodgkin Lymphoma

While Reed–Sternberg (RS) cells express several distinguishing markers including CD15, CD30 and LMP1, none is specific and

Table 3.8
Markers of langerhans cells, FDC and IDRC

CD1a – Precursor T lymphoblastic lymphoma, thymoma, Langerhans cell histiocytosis
CD21 – FDC sarcoma
CD23 – FDC sarcoma; CLL/SLL
CD35 – FDC sarcoma
D2-40 – FDC sarcoma, but a less specific than others; lymphovascular and other non-hematopoietic tumors
Clusterin – Strongly positive in FDC tumors but not in IDC tumors; ALCL; a wide variety of carcinomas
Langerin – Langerhans cell histiocytosis
S100 – Langerhans cell histiocytosis, IDC sarcoma
HLA-DR – Histiocytic and dendritic cell lesions

when used for diagnostic purposes, should be employed with other markers that are negative in these cells. The RS cells of classical Hodgkin lymphoma are very often negative for CD45, ALK, CD3, and CD20. In contrast, the multilobated cells of nodular lymphocyte predominant Hodgkin lymphoma (NLPHL) often display markers of B cells such as CD20, CD79a, OCT2, and BOB.1; express J chain; and are CD45 positive.

CD15

CD15 antibodies recognize a sugar sequence referred to as Lewis X, which is expressed in the later stages of myeloid differentiation. The RS cells in most cases of classical Hodgkin lymphoma show staining for the antigen in a membranous pattern and/or as a paranuclear Golgi dot; in contrast, the L&H cells of NLPHL are negative, as are the neoplastic B cells in DLBCL. Neutrophils and eosinophils serve well as positive internal controls in cases of classical Hodgkin lymphoma. Weaker staining may be seen in some small B and T cell lymphomas and in anaplastic large cell lymphoma. Many epithelial cells and carcinomas express CD15.

CD30

CD30 is a membrane-bound glycoprotein encoded by *TNFRSF8* on chromosome 1p36. A member of the tumor necrosis factor receptor superfamily, CD30 is expressed by activated B and T lymphocytes. In reactive nodes, scattered parafollicular immunoblasts express the antigen; such cells may be quite numerous in the setting of viral infection, as with EBV. Expression is seen in a variable proportion of large B and T cell lymphomas. Strong positivity is seen in anaplastic large cell lymphoma, and the majority of RS cells in classical Hodgkin lymphoma expresses CD30. Staining is membranous with or without a paranuclear

Golgi dot. Cytoplasmic staining in the absence of membrane and Golgi staining is false.

CD40

CD40, like CD30, is a member of the tumor necrosis factor receptor superfamily. A 48-kD integral membrane protein encoded by *CD40* on chromosome 20q12-q13.2, it plays an important role in B cell activation by helper T cells. CD40 is expressed not only by B lymphocytes but also by dendritic cells, monocytes, epithelial cells, and endothelial cells. Immunoreactivity has been observed in a variety of epithelial tumors, most B cell lymphomas, and the RS cells of all subtypes of Hodgkin lymphoma regardless of their antigenic phenotype. It is generally not expressed in anaplastic large cell lymphoma. Staining is membranous with a paranuclear Golgi dot.

OCT2 and BOB.1

OCT2 and BOB.1 are markers of B cells that are employed largely to differentiate lymphocyte predominant Hodgkin lymphoma from classical Hodgkin lymphoma, both markers being down-regulated in the latter.

OCT2, encoded by *POU2F2* on chromosome 19q13.2, is a transcription factor in B lymphocytes that targets the octomer motifs in the immunoglobulin promoter in conjunction with co-activator BOB.1 to activate immunoglobulin gene transcription. It is thought to play a role in germinal center formation and in the differentiation of B cells into plasma cells. While usually not detectable in RS cells of classical Hodgkin lymphoma, immunoreactivity may be seen in a small proportion of cases.

BOB.1 is a transcription factor that is required for germinal center formation and immunoglobulin production. Encoded by *POU2AF1* on chromosome 11q23.1, it acts as a co-activator with OCT2. It is less lineage specific than OCT2, being expressed in T cell as well as B cell lymphomas. BOB.1 is strongly positive in a range of non-Hodgkin lymphomas and nodular lymphocyte predominant Hodgkin lymphoma. It is generally not expressed in classical Hodgkin lymphoma; however, weak expression has been reported, making interpretation confusing.

Staining for both OCT2 and BOB.1 is nuclear.

Latent Membrane Protein 1 (LMP1)

LMP1 is a membrane protein expressed by Epstein–Barr virus (EBV) in latent infection (latency gene expression programs II and III). Immunohistochemical detection of LMP1 correlates well with the results of EBV-encoded RNA (EBER) in situ hybridization in classical Hodgkin lymphoma, with both methods showing positivity of RS cells most frequently in the mixed cellularity type. Sensitivity is also high in infectious mononucleosis, and AIDS-related non-Hodgkin lymphomas. LMP1 staining has less sensitivity in other types of EBV-associated neoplasms, such as nasopharyngeal carcinoma, NK/T cell lymphoma, and angioim-

Table 3.9
Markers of Reed–Sternberg cells in Hodgkin lymphoma

CD15 –	Also stains neutrophils
CD30 –	Also stains activated lymphoid cells and epithelial cells
CD40 –	Stains all subtypes of Hodgkin lymphoma, most B cell lymphomas and many carcinomas
OCT2 –	Stains NLPHL
BOB.1 –	Stains NLPHL but may stain classical Hodgkin lymphoma
LMP1 –	Stains classical Hodgkin lymphoma, most of mixed cellularity type, also stain other EBV-associated lymphomas

munoblastic T cell lymphoma, the differences being dependent on the latency pattern expressed by the EBV-associated malignancy. Despite its name, staining for LMP1 is mainly cytoplasmic with paranuclear Golgi enhancement, although membrane staining may be present (**Table 3.9**).

Miscellaneous Markers

Ki-67

Ki-67 is a nuclear protein encoded by *MKI67* on chromosome 10q25-qter, and it is closely associated with cell proliferation. It is expressed through all phases of the cell cycle except G0. Intensity of staining is variable, as expression begins at G1 and is maximal at the mitotic phase of the cycle. The percentage of neoplastic cells positive for Ki-67 (the proliferation index) may have prognostic significance in certain lymphomas, and the pattern of expression is diagnostically useful in distinguishing reactive follicles from follicular lymphoma. Ki-67 staining also has roles in the separation of low-grade small-cell lymphomas with low proliferation indexes from higher grade lesions and in the recognition of Burkitt lymphoma, which has a proliferation index approaching 100%.

ALK (CD246)

ALK is closely related to leucocyte receptor tyrosine kinase but is not expressed in normal lymphoid cells. ALK-positive anaplastic large cell lymphoma (ALCL) is characterized by chromosomal translocations involving the anaplastic lymphoma kinase (*ALK*) gene located on chromosome 2p23, the most common of which is t(2;5)(p23;q35) and involves the *NPM* (nucleophosmin) gene. The chimeric protein consists of the N-terminal portion of the NPM protein joined to the entire cytoplasmic domain of the ALK protein. Cases of ALCL with t(2;5) show cytoplasmic, nuclear, and nucleolar staining for ALK, while variant translocations display cytoplasmic and/or membrane staining depending on the translocation partner. ALK staining is highly restricted in lymphomas, being observed in ALCL and in a rare group of ALK-positive large B cell lymphomas. The latter usually display immunoblastic or plasmablastic features and are CD20−, CD79a^{-}, and CD30^{-}, and they may have a t(2;17) translocation involving the clathrin gene; ALK staining in these cases is cytoplasmic and granular. Inflammatory myofibroblastic tumors may have translocations of the *ALK* gene and express cytoplasmic ALK. With the exception of occasional cells in the central nervous system, normal cells consistently lack ALK expression. Polyclonal antibodies can produce false-positive staining, and hence monoclonal antibodies are preferred.

CD72 (DBA.44)

CD72, which is encoded on chromosome 9p13.3 and involved in the regulation of B cell differentiation, is expressed on mantle cells, reactive immunoblasts, monocytoid B cells and their corresponding neoplasms, as well as in a small proportion of low- and high-grade lymphomas. Among the low-grade B cell neoplasms, CD72 is expressed by essentially all hairy cell leukemias (HCL) and appears to be more sensitive for this tumor when compared with tartrate-resistant acid phosphatase. In contrast to its high sensitivity for HCL, the specificity of CD72 is limited, as expression is demonstrable in a significant subset of splenic marginal zone lymphomas.

Myeloid Cell Markers

In the context of leukemic infiltration of the lymph nodes and granulocytic sarcoma, it may be necessary to employ markers of myeloid cells for diagnosis. Myeloperoxidase is expressed in both early (immature) and mature myeloid cells, and its appearance precedes that of neutrophil elastase. CD34 (described above under Precursor B- and T Cell Markers) is expressed in hematopoietic precursors, including cells committed to the myeloid lineage. It is thus not a lineage specific marker and also labels endothelial cells, stromal dendrocytes, and a number of mesenchymal tumors. Other markers such as CD15, Mac387, CD68, CD43, CD45RO, CD99, CD117, lysozyme, AAT, and AACT label myeloid cells but are not specific (**Table 3.10**).

Table 3.10
Myeloid cell markers

Myeloperoxidase – Immature and mature myeloid cells
CD34 – Hematopoietic precursors, including myeloid precursors
Neutrophil elastase – Mature granulocytes
Other less specific markers – CD43, CD15, Mac387, CD68, CD45RO, CD99, CD117, lysozyme, AAT, AACT

Mast Cell Markers

Mastocytosis should always be kept in mind when atypical infiltrates are observed, mimicking lymphoma and leukemia so that their definitive identification is required. Mast cell granules are metachromatic in stains like Giemsa and toluidine blue, but such granules may be sparse, and immunohistochemistry is a more definitive tool for identification. In the context of the differential diagnoses, mast cell tryptase, CD25, and MiTF (microphthalmia transcription factor) are specific. CD117, CD43, myeloperoxidase, CD68, and CD2 also stain mast cells to a lesser extent but label myeloid leukemia and lymphoma cells, rendering positivity for these markers less specific with respect to lineage (**Table 3.11**).

Table 3.11
Mast cell markers

Mast cell tryptase – Sensitive and specific
CD25 – Sensitive but not specific, stains myeloid and T cells
MiTF – Sensitive and specific in the appropriate context
Other less specific markers – CD117, CD43, CD68, myeloperoxidase, CD2

Diagnostic Approach with Immunohistochemical Stains

Clearly, with the vast number of lymphocyte markers now available, it would be prudent to adopt a diagnostic approach with the application of immunohistochemistry. As mentioned previously, using a highly focused panel can be misleading, whereas the indiscriminate use of antibodies is not only expensive but can also produce misleading and even confusing results. A diagnostic algorithm would be ideal, and this should parallel the morphologic algorithm, but such an approach is often too expansive to be of practical value. An alternative practical and more restricted approach with immunohistochemical stains would be to address specific questions raised by the morphologic pattern and differential diagnoses.

Staining for Follicular Dendritic Cells

Highlighting the distribution of follicular dendritic cells (FDC) is often very helpful, as it provides insights into the architecture of the node. The architecture may be distorted by lymphoid proliferation, particularly when the expanded compartment is the paracortex and the B cell compartment is compressed or obliterated. Some situations in which the demonstration of FDC is of diagnostic relevance are discussed briefly below, and detailed discussion is provided with the specific entities elsewhere in this book.

FDC are stained by CD21, CD35, CD23, and D2-40. Other markers like clusterin, HLA-DR, and CD40 can also stain FDC but with less specificity.

Follicular Dendritic Cells in Angioimmunoblastic T Cell Lymphoma

In the specific example of angioimmunoblastic T cell lymphoma, a marked proliferation of FDC replacing regressed germinal centers and ensheathing prominent arborizing vessels in the paracortex is a diagnostic feature of the disease.

Follicular Lymphoma Versus Reactive Follicles

Follicles and lymphoid nodules are the most striking features of lymph nodes, and it is often useful to examine the location and detailed composition of these structures by staining for FDC. In the neoplastic follicles of follicular lymphoma (FL), FDC proliferates and displays thick branching and sometimes fragmented processes in expanded meshworks. Neoplastic follicles stain for Bcl2 and CD45RA (MT2), whereas reactive follicles do not. Reactive germinal centers show polarization with a denser network of FDC in the light zone compared to the dark zone. Light-chain restriction may be demonstrable in neoplastic follicles. CD3 may reveal a diffuse distribution of scattered T cells within neoplastic follicles, as opposed to the pattern of localization of T cells in the periphery of reactive germinal centers.

The demonstration of expanded and confluent FDC meshworks is essential to separate FL from areas of transformation to DLBCL; the latter does not display a FDC meshwork.

The large nodules of progressively transformed germinal centers display partially preserved mantle zones with migration of mantle cells into the germinal center as demonstrated with CD20. Staining for FDC shows an expanded network fragmented by groups of mantle cells within the germinal centers.

A proliferation of FDC is also observed in the follicles of Castleman disease, and conversion to an FDC tumor is a rare occurrence.

Other Lymphoid Nodules

The neoplastic B cells comprising nodules of mantle cell lymphoma (MCL) stain for cyclin D1. This marker is not expressed in other nodular proliferations in the lymph node. Bcl2 is also found in MCL, but unlike follicular lymphomas, the nodules of small cells stain homogenously, and there is a marked proliferation of the FDC network which is fragmented but often with confluence of adjacent nodules to produce irregular outlines. In addition, the nodules of MCL stain for CD5 but not for Bcl6 or CD10, the latter labeling neoplastic follicles in FL. MCL may show a high proliferative index with Ki-67.

The nodules of Hodgkin lymphoma can also show proliferation of FDC, especially in the nodular lymphocyte predominant type, where the expanded FDC meshworks overlap expanded mantle zones. Unstained lymphocytic and histiocytic (L&H) cells and their accompanying T cell rosettes are sharply demarcated by the stained dendritic processes. L&H cells are CD20+ and rosetting T cells are CD3+CD57+. The nodular sclerosing subtype of classical Hodgkin lymphoma shows sharply defined, sometimes irregular FDC meshworks surrounding negative Reed–Sternberg cells (CD15+, CD30+, CD45−), but FDC may also be sometimes reduced or sparse.

Pseudonodular proliferations of lymphoblastic lymphoma are TdT positive, show a high proliferative index with Ki-67, and display T or B cell markers. They do not stain for Bcl6 or CD10 and do not contain FDC.

Proliferation centers of small lymphocytic lymphoma/chronic lymphocytic leukemia do not contain FDC and do not stain for Bcl6 or CD10. The neoplastic cells are CD5+ and CD23+ (**Table 3.12**).

Table 3.12
Markers to distinguish follicular and nodular lymph node proliferations

Neoplastic follicles (follicular lymphoma)	Bcl2+, CD45RA+, Bcl6+, CD10+, expanded FDC meshwork (CD21, CD35, D2-40), Ig light-chain restriction
Progressive transformation of germinal centers	Expanded FDC meshwork (CD21, CD35, D2-40), irregular thinned mantle zone, mantle cells in germinal center (Bcl2+)
Mantle cell lymphoma	cyclinD1+, Bcl6−, CD10−, often a higher proliferative index (Ki-67), expanded FDC meshwork
Hodgkin lymphoma	Expanded FDC meshwork with negative neoplastic cells, neoplastic cells CD20+ or CD15+ and CD30+
Acute lymphoblastic lymphoma	Tdt+, T cell or B cell makers, Bcl6−, CD21−, CD35−
CLL/SLL	CD23+, Bcl2−, CD21−, CD35−

Immunohistological Identification of Diffuse Lymphoid Infiltrates

The identification of diffuse infiltrates based on immunophenotypic markers is much more difficult and often cannot be done in isolation from the morphological changes, largely because diffuse infiltrates tend to be heterogenous. It can be helpful, however, to identify the different cell types making up the infiltrate, in particular if one cell type is clearly morphologically atypical. The identification of residual benign follicles by staining for FDC may also contribute, as they can reveal colonization of the follicles by a diffuse neoplastic population.

In diffuse infiltrates, immunohistological stains are directed at the cells of interest. In small lymphocytic infiltrates, the question usually raised is “Is the infiltrate neoplastic?” To this end, pan-B and pan-T cell markers like CD79a and CD3, respectively, will give an insight to the distribution of these cells, especially in extranodal tissues. If one population strongly predominates almost to the exclusion of the other, the diagnosis of a neoplastic process is supported. It should be noted that in some reactive conditions and in some sites such as the skin, T cells may predominate and further labeling with CD4 and CD8 may be helpful. While these markers do not indicate clonality, marked predominance of one subtype may be indicative of a neoplastic population of T cells. The diagnosis of a T cell lymphoma is often based on the loss of a pan-T cell antigen such as CD2, CD3, CD5, or CD7 and on the molecular studies for T cell receptor gene rearrangement.

Diffuse Small Cell Infiltrates

A panel of antibodies can be employed to distinguish diffuse small lymphocytic infiltrates that include small lymphocytic lymphoma, mantle cell lymphoma, marginal zone lymphoma, lymphoplasmacytic lymphoma, and follicular lymphoma. Markers for small lymphocytic lymphoma/chronic lymphocytic leukemia are CD23+, CD5+, and CD43+; for mantle cell lymphoma cyclin D1+, CD5+, CD43+; for lymphoplasmacytic lymphoma CD38+, CD43+; and for follicular lymphoma Bcl6+, CD10+; marginal zone lymphoma is frequently negative for all these markers (**Table 3.13**).

Table 3.13
Panel for small B cell lymphomas

	CD43	CD5	CD23	Cyclin D1	CD10	Bcl6	CD38
SLL/CLL	+	+	+	–	–	–	–
MCL	+	+	–	+	–	–	–
MZL	+/–	–	–	–	–	–	–
LPL	+	–	–	–	–	–	+
FL	–	–	–	–	+	+	–

Note: SLL/CLL, small lymphocytic lymphoma/chronic lymphocytic leukemia; MCL, mantle cell lymphoma; MZL, marginal zone lymphoma; LPL, lymphoplasmacytic lymphoma; FL, follicular lymphoma.

Diffuse Large Cell Infiltrates

In the case of a diffuse large cell infiltrate, the initial process is to exclude mimics of large cell lymphoma such as carcinoma and melanoma. Often this can be done on the basis of morphology alone. Once confirmed to be lymphoma, the diffuse large cell lymphoma should be typed as a B or T cell lymphoma. This can be done simply by using the pan-B and pan-T cell markers CD79a and CD3. Demonstration of CD20 on B cell lesions is helpful in establishing the case for targeted anti-CD20 therapy; if the patient has been receiving rituximab, staining with multiple markers of B cell lineage such as CD79a and PAX5 may be necessary to characterize a large cell infiltrate.

Diffuse Mixed Cell Infiltrates

It may be necessary to identify the nature of large cells in a diffuse mixed cell infiltrate. The approach described above for diffuse large cell infiltrates is applicable, though the presence of non-lymphoid cells should also be considered. Histiocytes/macrophages are identified by CD68 which is currently the most specific and sensitive marker of the markers shown in **Table 3.7**. Of the markers of Langerhans cells and dendritic cells listed in **Table 3.8**, langerin, CD68, and CD1a are best for Langerhans cells and their neoplasms, and CD21, CD35, and D2-40 label FDC. Markers for the identification of Reed–Sternberg cells include CD15 and CD30 (**Table 3.9**). In addition, large cells in a heterogenous diffuse infiltrate may represent those of an anaplastic large cell lymphoma and can be identified by CD30 and ALK protein, often accompanied by EMA positivity and an absence of CD45 staining. Metastatic carcinoma and melanoma should be excluded with markers listed in **Tables 3.1** and **3.2**.

Immunophenotype Subgrouping

Among diffuse infiltrates shown to represent neoplastic B cell proliferations, it may be of use conceptually to distinguish cases with germinal-center-like immunophenotype from those with a non-germinal-center-like immunophenotype or a naïve B cell immunophenotype. A germinal-center-like phenotype is defined by the expression of Bcl6 and/or CD10, while the post- or non-germinal-center-like phenotype displays proteins ushering B cells into plasmacytic differentiation including IRF4/MUM1 and CD138. DLBCL cases may fall into either the GC-like or the non-GC-like categories; Burkitt lymphoma is GC-like, as is follicular lymphoma, while lesions with plasmacytic differentiation fall into the post- or non-GC-like category. Separate from each of these is the naïve B cell immunophenotype associated with positivity for CD5 and coexpression of sIgM and sIgD, which can be seen in mantle cell lymphoma.

Histochemical Stains

Various biochemical and enzymatic cell markers may be useful in lymph node diagnosis, although many have been superseded by immunohistological markers.

Periodic Acid–Schiff (PAS) Stain

Used much more frequently in general surgical pathology than in hematopathology, staining by the periodic acid–Schiff (PAS) reaction highlights the amorphous material deposited between cells in angioimmunoblastic T cell lymphoma. Additionally, diastase-resistant PAS positivity may be observed in plasmacytoid lymphocytes and plasma cells that contain abundant immunoglobulins in their cytoplasm particularly IgA because of its high carbohydrate content. PAS–diastase also stains deposits of immunoglobulin in Dutcher bodies and Russell bodies and in amorphous interstitial deposits seen in reactive germinal centers and in a variety of lymphomas.

PAS stains glycogen present as large intracytoplasmic aggregates in acute lymphoblastic leukemia/lymphoma.

Silver Impregnation for Reticulin

Staining by silver impregnation techniques highlights the network of fine reticulin (type III collagen) fibers underlying normal lymph node structure. An intact reticulin framework of normal sinusoids distinguishes a reactive process from lymphoma. The presence of an abnormal cellular infiltrate, whether lymphoid or non-lymphoid, can produce disruption of the normal reticulin framework. Metastatic tumors tend to destroy the normal reticulin framework of lymph nodes compared to lymphomas which have a well-developed, fine, branching reticulin network with pericellular fibrils.

Methyl Green Pyronin Stain

Methyl green pyronin stains ribonucleic acid (RNA) and identifies cells rich in RNA, such cells commonly being plasma cells, plasmacytoid cells, and Burkitt lymphoma cells, allowing distinction from mature B lymphocytes and lymphoblasts.

Non-specific Esterases

Non-specific esterases are characteristic of monocytes/histiocytes. With substrates such as α-naphthyl acetate (ANA) or α-naphthyl butyrate (ANB), monocytes/histiocytes show a strong diffuse orange–brown stain that is inhibited by sodium fluoride in monocytes/histiocytes. This is not observed in myeloid cells, which have a fluoride-resistant isoenzyme. T lymphocytes exhibit a dot-like pattern of staining with ANA esterase. Platelets and megakaryocytes stain with ANA but not with ANB.

Specific Naphthol AS-D Chloroacetate Esterase

The substrate in this stain is naphthol AS-D chloroacetate, which produces a red reaction product in myeloid and mast cells, and is negative in monocytes and histiocytes.

Peroxidase Reaction

The peroxidase reaction is positive in neutrophils and eosinophils, and weakly positive in monocytes, but there is no reaction with lymphoid and erythroid cells.

Sudan Black B

Sudan black B stains phospholipids in cells of acute myeloid, lymphoid, and myelomonocytic leukemias. This stain parallels the peroxidase reaction, staining progressively more strongly as myeloid cells differentiate and increase their content of cytoplasmic granules. Auer bodies stain intensely. There is weak staining of monocytes but no staining in lymphoid cells. Unlike the peroxidase reaction, sudanophilia does not diminish with time or exposure to light.

Tartrate-Resistant Acid Phosphatase

Tartrate-resistant acid phosphatase (TRAP) is an isoenzyme that is almost exclusively expressed in hairy cell leukemia and is absent from other lymphoid neoplasms (**Table 3.14**).

Table 3.14
Useful histochemical stains for cell identification

Periodic acid–Schiff-diastase – Plasma cells
Silver reticulin – Reticulin framework of lymph node for assessment of architecture especially sinuses
Methyl green pyronine – Plasma cells, plasmacytic cells, immunoblasts
Non-specific esterase – Myeloid cells, monocytes, megakaryocytes, T lymphocytes (dot-like)
Chloroacetate esterase – Myeloid cells, mast cells
Peroxidase – Myeloid cells, eosinophils, monocytes
Sudan black B – Myeloid cells, monocytes
Tartrate-resistant acid phosphatase – Hair cell leukemia
Giemsa and toluidine blue – Metachromatic granules of mast cells

Flow Cytometry

In contrast to immunohistology, flow cytometry permits rapid, simultaneous assessment of multiple markers on cells of interest. Of particular use is the ability to assess B cells for the expression of monotypic (monoclonal) immunoglobulin light chains, which is more readily detected by this method than by immunohistochemical staining. While no analogous marker of T cell clonality is in common clinical use, abnormal levels of expression of pan-T cell markers (CD2, CD3, CD5, and CD7) are more easily detected using flow cytometry than immunohistology, as the former permits quantitative assessment of marker expression. Additionally, specific patterns of marker expression may be of great assistance in the recognition of abnormal cells, even when present in only small numbers, as may be the case due to sampling or due to effects of chemotherapy. As noted in **Chapter** 2, however, fresh tissue is required for flow cytometric immunophenotyping; additionally, due to the need for the tissue to be disaggregated into a single cell suspension, a major disadvantage in comparison to immunohistology is the inability to assess the immunoarchitecture of the lymph node. Nonetheless, flow cytometry has proven to be a valuable adjunct in the evaluation of abnormal lymphoid tissue.

While a detailed discussion of flow cytometric instrumentation is beyond the scope of this text, basic familiarity with the graphical output of cytometric studies is readily achievable if the underlying principles are understood. Antibodies directed against antigens of interest are tagged with fluorochromes having emission maxima at differing wavelengths. Each time a cell passes through the instrument's laser beam, any fluorochrome molecules present on or in the cell emit photons that are detected and converted to current that is measured by the instrument. The greater the number of targeted antigen molecules on a cell, the more antibody will bind, resulting in the presence of more fluorochrome and in the detection of a greater signal; the instrument's optics discriminate among emissions from the various fluorochromes, resulting a separate measurement for each antigen's expression on each cell tested.

A typical clinical flow cytometry study involves the assessment of at least 5,000 lymphocytes in each of several tubes; with data for each of the fluorochromes plus light scatter properties for each cell, even one study generates a large array of data that are not easily interpreted if left in a tabular format. If the values for any two antigens/fluorochromes are used as Cartesian coordinates, with each cell's values being plotted as a point, clusters of dots corresponding to normal populations (e.g., helper T cells) and abnormal populations (e.g., large B cells with monotypic lambda light chains) can emerge. For example, the following scatterplot shows results for CD3 and CD4 detection on a mixed lymphoid population (**Fig. 3.7**).

In **Fig. 3.8**, each dot corresponds to a cell, and the readily apparent clustering of the dots indicates the relative homogeneity of the various lymphoid subsets in this specimen with respect to expression of these two antigens. The cells represented by dots in

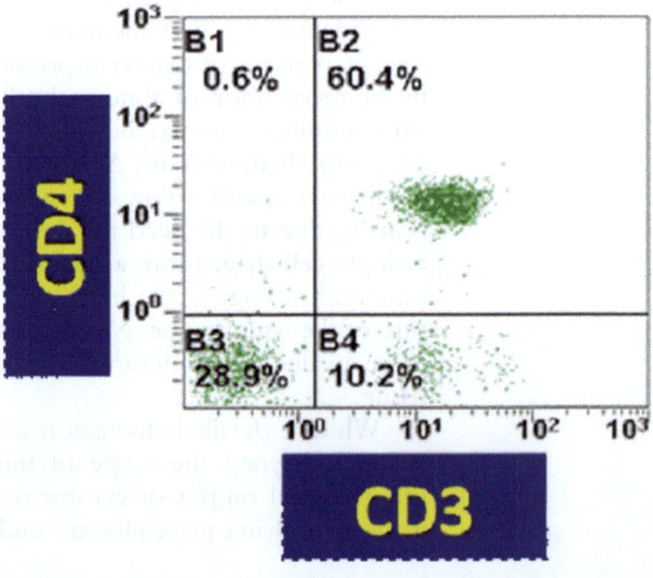

Fig. 3.7. Scatterplot showing CD3 and CD4 values for various lymphoid populations in one sample.

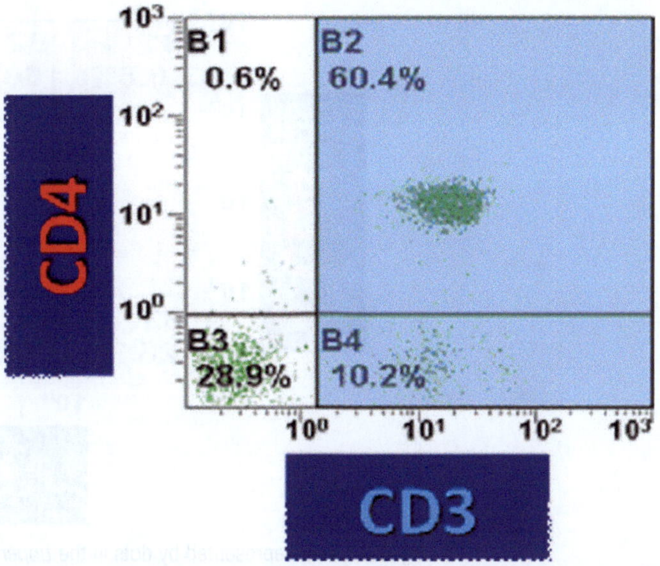

Fig. 3.8. Cells represented by dots in the right-hand quadrants (*shaded blue*) are positive for CD3, while those in the left-hand quadrants are negative.

the two left-hand quadrants (B1 and B3) show values for CD3 that are similar to the non-specific fluorescence that would be detected if the anti-CD3 antibody had not been added, and such cells are regarded as negative for CD3. Among these cells are B cells and NK cells. In contrast, the dots in the right-hand quadrants (B2 and B4) represent cells expressing CD3 (CD3+ cells, i.e., T cells).

Similarly, in **Fig. 3.9**, the dots in the lower two quadrants represent cells lacking CD4 expression, while those in the upper quadrants correspond to CD4+ cells.

Combining this information regarding CD3 and CD4 expression with the percentages provided with the scatterplots enables us to deduce that 60.4% of the lymphocytes in this specimen are helper T cells coexpressing CD3 and CD4. 10.2% are CD3+ T cells lacking CD4 expression, and these cells form not one cluster, but rather two, in the lower right-hand quadrant, and the cells comprising these clusters exhibit differing levels of CD3 expression. The cluster to the left, comprised a majority of the dots in this quadrant, expresses less CD3 than do the cells represented by the smaller cluster to the right. The small cluster probably represents a gamma–delta T cell population, as such cells are known to express CD3 more "brightly" than the CD8+ cytotoxic T cells comprising the cluster to the left (**Fig. 3.10**).

The principles illustrated in this example are used to interpret findings with respect to each combination of antibodies in a flow cytometric study. Familiarity with normal cell populations is requisite for recognition of immunophenotypically abnormal clus-

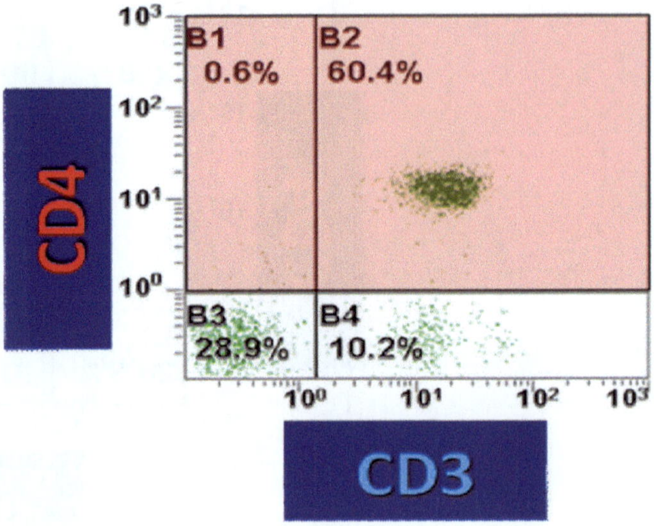

Fig. 3.9. Cells represented by dots in the *upper* quadrants (*shaded red*) are positive for CD4, while those in the lower quadrants are negative.

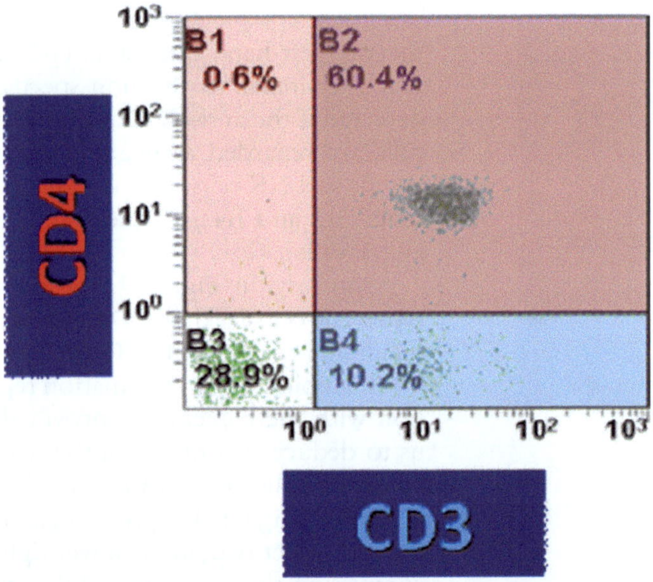

Fig. 3.10. Cells in the *upper right* quadrant (*shaded purple*) are helper T cells (CD3+CD4+). In the *lower right* quadrant (*shaded blue*) are CD8+ T cells and gamma–delta T cells, with the latter comprising the smaller cluster with "brighter" CD3 expression.

ters, and correlation of flow cytometric findings with morphologic findings is essential to ensure proper interpretation. If, for example, the sections show a population of abnormal large cells, the flow cytometry scatterplots must be scrutinized for a corresponding population with increased forward light scatter. On occasion, such cells may not have properties (e.g., bright CD45 expression, low orthogonal light scatter) typical of small benign lymphocytes; consequently, it is important to examine the properties of all of the cellular populations and not just the one found in the usual lymphocyte "gate." Additionally, caution is necessary to avoid overlooking a small neoplastic population present amidst numerous reactive lymphocytes, as may be seen with partial nodal involvement by lymphoma.

The reader is referred to specialized textbooks for details of flow cytometry instrumentation, applications, and methodology.

Molecular Diagnostics

Immunohistology and flow cytometry identify protein expression. Molecular techniques directly analyze the DNA of genes encoding immunoglobulins (Igs) and T cell receptors (TCRs) that rearrange during B- and T cell development. The DNA of oncogenes and supressor genes can also be analyzed by molecular techniques. Only general principles and the advantages and disadvantages of each technique will be discussed.

Detection of Clonality

Molecular analysis is currently the gold standard for the detection of B- and T cell clonality. Only lymphoid cells that rearrange their genes can be assessed for gene rearrangements. Natural killer (NK) cells maintain their antigen receptor gene segments in a germline configuration; as such, their corresponding neoplasms do not carry antigen receptor gene rearrangements. It is also important to note that a variety of reactive conditions may contain detectable clones and that clonality of lymphoid cells is not synonymous with malignancy. Results of molecular analyses must therefore be correlated with clinical, morphological, and immunophenotypic information.

Southern blot hybridization and the polymerase chain reaction (PCR) are the most useful methods for determining clonality in the diagnostic laboratory.

Analysis of Antigen Receptor Genes – Southern Blot

Immunoglobulin Heavy- and Light-Chain Genes

Probes to both the joining region (JH) and constant region (Cμ) probes are commonly used in Southern blot analysis of the IgH genes. JH probes are more reliable for the detection of IgH gene rearrangements as the Cμ region is deleted when Ig heavy-chain class switching occurs. Igκ light-chain gene rearrangements are analyzed with Jκ probes. In the case of the Igλ light-chain gene, the number of Cλ regions and the polymorphic nature of this region yield a number of germline bands so that recognition of a true gene rearrangement is difficult and the Igλ light-chain gene is not usually evaluated by this method.

T Cell Receptor Chain Genes

Analysis of the TCRβ gene by Southern blot is a reliable method of assessing T cell clonality and can detect 90–95% of T cell lymphomas and leukemias.

Analysis of TCRγ gene is better done by PCR than Southern blot hybridization, with a sensitivity of 1–5%.

Southern blot analysis is not suitable for the analysis of TCRα gene because of its large size which is best evaluated in the research setting with pulsed field gel electrophoresis.

The TCRδ is relatively small and can be evaluated with Jδ probe using Southern blot analysis.

Analysis of Antigen Receptor Genes – Polymerase Chain Reaction (PCR)

The polymerase chain reaction (PCR) is useful for the assessment of clonality, chromosome aberrations, minimal residual disease, and gene mutations. The technique has the strong advantage of being applicable to specimens that are fresh, frozen, stored in buffer, or formalin-fixed, and routinely processed. Both genomic DNA and messenger RNA, the latter converted to complementary DNA by reverse transcriptase (RT-PCR), can be detected by application of standard PCR.

For effective molecular analysis, the DNA target should span 2000 bp or less. Targets of less than 200 bp are optimal in fixed, paraffin-embedded tissues. To synthesize the primers of short, complementary oligonucleotides of 20–30 bp, the sequences upstream (5′) and downstream (3′) of the target should be known. These primers specifically anneal to the template DNA to provide the initial sequences for *Taq* DNA polymerase extension. With completion of the amplification, the PCR products can be detected by electrophoretic separation according to size, with monoclonal populations yielding one or two distinct homogenous bands. Alternative gel systems such as single stranded conformational polymorphism gel electrophoresis and denaturing gradient gel electrophoresis may be used. Fluorescent dyes are now incorporated into primers so that the PCR amplicons are fluorescent. The products are subsequently separated by capillary electrophoresis and analyzed by genetic analyzers with powerful software, providing a more sensitive method and faster turnaround. The concomitant reduction in steps reduces errors and represents a more reliable measurement of the amplicon size. These properties have made PCR-based methods the preferred technology over Southern blot analysis in the routine assessment of Ig and TCR antigen receptor gene rearrangements. PCR-based methods are also less laborious and can be used for small samples and formalin-fixed, paraffin-embedded material. Unlike Southern blot, which analyses a homogenized sample of all cells contained in the biopsy, PCR recognizes specific cells of interest. One caveat of the high sensitivity of PCR assays is that very small monoclonal B- and T cell populations may be detected in histologically and immunophenotypically benign specimens. Such monoclonal populations are real but their clinical and biological significance is unknown. All PCR results should thus be viewed in the context of the clinical, pathological, and immunophenotypic information. A positive PCR result may therefore be of less significance than a positive result from Southern blot analysis, as the latter is less sensitive and detects a larger monoclonal population of cells.

False-negative results may be obtained with PCR because of failure of the primers to anneal. The frequency of such results can be reduced by using multiple primers and by analysis of both IgH and Igκ or TCRγ and TCRβ genes for clonality. Despite such measures, depending on the morphological subtype of T cell lymphoma, clonality in a percentage of cases will remain undetected.

Molecular Diagnosis of Chromosomal Translocations

The pathogenesis of malignant lymphomas often involves activation of oncogenes via a number of mechanisms, the most common of which is chromosomal translocation. Translocations generally juxtapose an oncogene with either an Ig or TCR gene with no disruption of the reading frame of the oncogene. This form of translocation results in overexpression of a qualitatively normal oncogene protein, such as when *IgH* juxtaposes with *MYC* in Burkitt lymphoma or with *CCND1* in mantle cell lymphoma. In another common type of translocation, the antigen receptor gene locus is not involved but a gene on each partner chromosome is disrupted. The disrupted genes are recombined to create a novel protein such as in anaplastic large cell lymphoma where there is translocation of the *ALK* gene and in the t(11;18)(q21;q21) of extranodal marginal zone B cell lymphoma of mucosal-associated lymphoid tissue (MALT). There is currently poor understanding of mechanisms involved in the genesis of this type of translocation.

Conventional cytogenetics, FISH, Southern blot analysis, and PCR-based techniques can be employed to detect chromosomal translocations; the choice of method is determined by the type of sample available, anatomy of the genes involved, number and location of the breakpoints, and aims of the analysis.

Genotype Subgroups

Similar to immunophenotypic subgrouping, genotyping can be employed to divide B cell lymphoma into GC, post-GC, and naïve subgroups. A GC genotype is defined by the presence of ongoing somatic hypermutations (SHM) in the variable regions of immunoglobulin (*IgV*) genes. A post-GC genotype is defined by the presence of static and not ongoing SHM in *IgV* genes.

Naïve B cells are cells that have not been processed through the GC and lack mutation in the *IgV* genes.

Conventional Cytogenetics

Conventional cytogenetics has the major advantage of allowing assessment of all 46 chromosomes for visual abnormalities. It can detect involvement of specific oncogenes with multiple partner genes, and when breakpoints involving a chromosomal translocation are highly variable, it can detect the variations. Other molecular techniques including FISH are more focused on specific abnormalities and do not allow the assessment of all partner genes, and some methods, particularly those that are PCR-based, are compromised by multiple or widely spaced breakpoints.

The disadvantages of conventional cytogenetics include the requirement for fresh, viable tissue, the necessity for the cells to grow in cell cultures, and a slow turnaround time. In addition, the resolution of band patterns in Giemsa-stained metaphase spreads is limited, so that some deletions, insertions, or inversions can be too small to be visualized, and specific gene mutations cannot be identified.

Fluorescence In Situ Hybridization (FISH)

Fluorescence in situ hybridization (FISH) can identify both numerical and structural abnormalities and is useful for localizing and enumerating specific genetic loci within intact cells. The probes, when conjugated to fluorochromes, are large and well suited for the analysis of widely dispersed chromosomal breakpoints. FISH does not require cells growing in culture and can be performed on cells in interphase as well as in metaphase. A variety of materials can be studied, including smears of bone marrow, peripheral blood, fine-needle aspirates, touch or scrape preparations from lymph nodes or other tissues, and fixed, paraffin-embedded tissue sections. FISH is also a much less labor intensive compared to routine karyotype analysis. It has the disadvantage of being highly focused, so that a prior selection of the genetic lesion of interest needs to be made. Another disadvantage is the need for manual counting when used to assess minimal residual disease.

Southern Blot Analysis

Southern blot analysis for chromosomal translocations is more laborious than FISH and PCR-related methods and yields less information than conventional cytogenetics. It requires fresh or frozen tissue; furthermore, the partner gene will not be identified. For these reasons, Southern blot analysis is not used to determine chromosomal translocations.

Polymerase Chain Reaction (PCR)

Polymerase chain reaction (PCR) is an extremely useful method to study chromosomal translocations, as it can be used on a variety of materials, including fixed, paraffin-embedded tissues. It is extremely sensitive and can detect one abnormal cell in 100,000 normal cells. There are three requirements for its successful application, viz, the number of partner genes involved in the translocation must be limited, preferably to one, the DNA sequences surrounding the breakpoint must be known, and the breakpoints on each chromosome must be clustered. If these criteria are not satisfied, as in the case of the t(11;14) associated with mantle cell lymphoma, wherein the 11q13 breakpoints are not clustered, sensitivity of PCR may be markedly inferior to that of FISH for translocation detection.

Gene Expression Profiling

Gene expression profiling using DNA microarrays has contributed to our understanding of lymphoma pathogenesis and revealed new molecular markers and signatures useful for diagnosis and prognostication. This new technology is still largely in the research domain, and many challenges related to standardization of data analysis and quality control need to be overcome before it establishes a role in routine diagnosis, prognostication, and treatment. However, data generated using this technique have already guided the development of immunohistologic approaches to diagnosing and subtyping lymphomas; examples include staining for CXCL13 in suspected cases of angioimmunoblastic T cell lymphoma and the use of antibody panels to distinguish germinal-center-like and non-germinal-center-like subgroups of diffuse large B cell lymphoma.

Chapter 4

Anatomical and Functional Compartments

Key words: B cell differentiation, T cell differentiation, immunohistology, markers.

There is some variation in the structure of lymph nodes at different anatomical sites, but the histological compartments are the same and the variation is largely in their size. The typical lymph node structure is exhibited by cervical nodes which show the pattern of follicles, cortex, paracortex, medulla, and sinuses. These anatomical divisions also represent functional compartments in that the cortex, with its primary and secondary lymphoid follicles, is composed largely of B cells, whereas the paracortex comprises mostly T cells. The medullary sinuses are traversed by small vessels and represent the domain of histiocytes and plasma cells. Secondary follicles are identified by the presence of germinal centers with their larger and paler cells and are surrounded by an eccentric rim of small dark mantle cells. While the marginal zone is not visible in the resting lymph node, when hyperplastic, a marginal zone of post-germinal center B cells may be seen peripheral to the dark rim of mantle cells. The marginal zone cells are slightly larger than mantle cells and have more and paler cytoplasm. Unlike peripheral nodes, mesenteric nodes have more prominent sinuses with less conspicuous follicles and paracortex, and unstimulated axillary nodes have a rim of lymphoid tissue around a hilum of adipose tissue.

The lymph node is in a dynamic state and the relative proportion of each compartment changes with antigenic stimulation (**Fig. 4.1**).

It is important to have an understanding of normal lymphocyte differentiation, especially of B cells as their neoplasms tend to reflect stages of normal B cell differentiation with corresponding immunophenotypic and molecular characteristics that represent the major basis for their classification.

A.S.-Y. Leong, *A Pattern Approach to Lymph Node Diagnosis*,
DOI 10.1007/978-1-4419-7176-0_4, © Springer Science+Business Media, LLC 2011

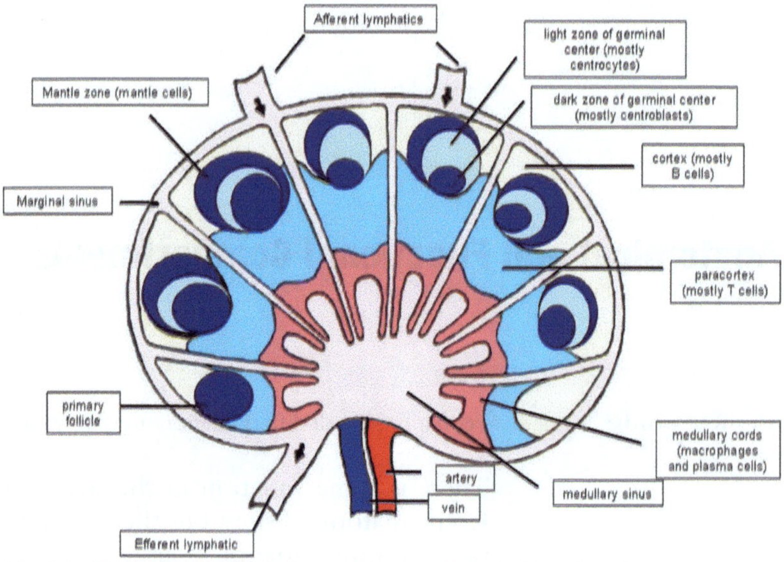

Fig. 4.1. Diagram of anatomical compartments of cervical lymph node.

B Cell Differentiation and Corresponding B Cell Lymphomas

B cell neoplasms tend to correspond to the stages of normal B cell differentiation, and this resemblance forms the basis of a conceptual understanding of B cell neoplasms and a convenient and relevant method of classification and nomenclature.

The Cortex

The cortex of the lymph node is largely populated by B cells which occupy the follicles, germinal centers, and also the interfollicular areas.

Progenitor B cells or B lymphoblasts arise in the bone marrow and are the precursor cells of the entire B cell line. They undergo immunoglobulin *VDJ* gene rearrangement and differentiate into mature surface immunoglobulin (sIg)-positive naïve B cells (IgM+/D+) via pre-B cells and immature B cells (both expressing cytoplasmic IgM+). Naïve B cells express CD23, CD43, and show weak expression of CD21 and CD35. Naïve B cells are also often CD5+ and circulate in the peripheral blood, localizing to the primary lymphoid follicle and mantle zone. The primary follicle is composed of small sIgM+/D+ B cells and follicular dendritic cells (FDC).

The Lymphoid Follicle

When stimulated by the appropriate antigen that fits their surface immunoglobulin receptors, naïve B cells undergo transformation, proliferation, and ultimately mature into antibody secreting plasma cells and memory B cells. These changes occur mostly in the germinal center of the secondary follicle where the centroblasts express low levels of sIg and switch off expression of Bcl2 (an anti-apoptotic protein) so that they and their progeny are susceptible to apoptosis. Only those B cells selected for good affinity re-express Bcl2 and survive; a large proportion undergo apoptosis and are taken up by macrophages to form tingible body macrophages within the germinal center.

In the germinal center, somatic hypermutation occurs in the immunoglobulin heavy- and light-chain variable (*IGV*) region genes and there is also a switch from IgM to IgG or IgA production, giving rise to higher affinity IgG or IgA antibodies of late primary or secondary immune response. Centroblasts and centrocytes express CD10 and Bcl6. Bcl6 is not expressed in naïve B cells and is switched off in memory B cells and plasma cells. The *Bcl6* gene undergoes somatic mutation in the germinal center but at a lower frequency than the *IG* genes. Ongoing *IGV* region gene mutation with intraclonal diversity is a hallmark of germinal center cells, and this and the *Bcl6* mutation serve as molecular hallmarks of cells that have been processed through the germinal center.

Secondary follicles show distinct polarity or zonification, although this may not always be demonstrable because of the plane of sectioning. Polarity is most prominent in the tonsil, with centroblasts forming a basal dark zone because of cytoplasmic basophilia. Their progeny, the centrocytes, form the light zone. Centrocytes express sIg that has an altered antibody combining site as compared with that of their progenitors, based both on somatic mutations and heavy-chain class switching. Those centrocytes with mutations that result in increased affinity are rescued from apoptosis by the re-expression of Bcl2 protein. Their interaction with FDC and small helper T cells, which also populate the germinal center, allows centrocytes to switch off Bcl6 protein expression and differentiate into memory B cells or plasma cells. MUM1 plays an important role in down-regulation of Bcl6 and the two proteins are reciprocally expressed, MUM1 being expressed in late centrocytes and plasma cells (**Figs. 4.2**, **4.3**, and **4.5**).

Germinal centers are surrounded by a mantle zone of small angulated B lymphocytes of the same phenotype as cells in the primary follicles. Mantle cells correspond to CD5+ naïve B cells that express relatively intense sIgM and sIgD and are CD43+ but lack CD10 and Bcl6. CD23 is negative or staining is weak. Cyclin D1, an important distinguishing antigen, is positive in corresponding mantle cell lymphomas. The marginal zone is generally absent or inconspicuous.

Monocytoid B cells are generally not seen in the resting lymph node, but in hyperplastic nodes they may be seen as bands or arcs in the marginal zone around reactive follicles. These cells

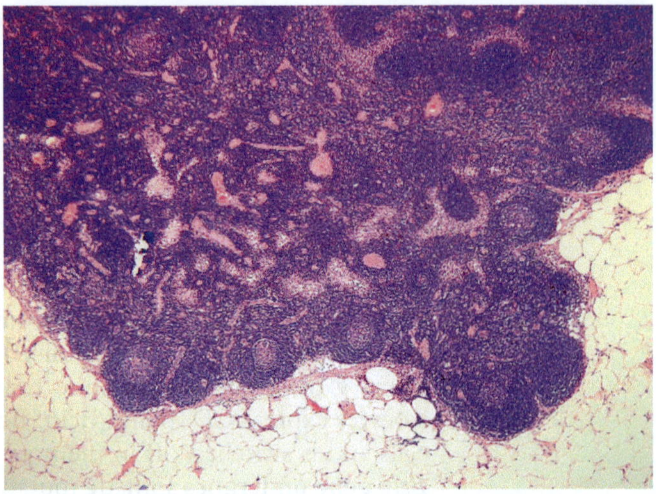

Fig. 4.2. A mildly hyperplastic lymph node showing primary and secondary follicles with prominent sinuses.

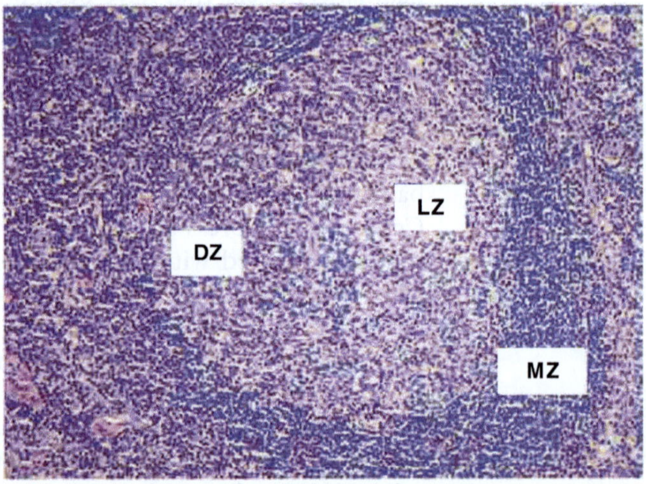

Fig. 4.3. Distinct polarization is seen in the germinal center with a basal dark zone (DZ) and an overlying light zone (LZ) surrounded by the mantle zone of small lymphocytes (MZ).

have indented nuclei with moderately condensed chromatin and moderate quantities of pale cytoplasm.

Post-germinal center memory B cells circulate in the peripheral blood and make up some of the cells in the follicular marginal zones of the lymph node, spleen, and mucosa-associated lymphoid tissue. Marginal zone B cells with clear cytoplasm are seen outside the mantle zone and are most conspicuous in mesenteric nodes, but may not be seen at other sites. The cells in this compartment express Pan-B cell antigens, sIgM and low levels of sIgD and MUM1/IRF4. They do not express CD5, CD10, or Bcl6.

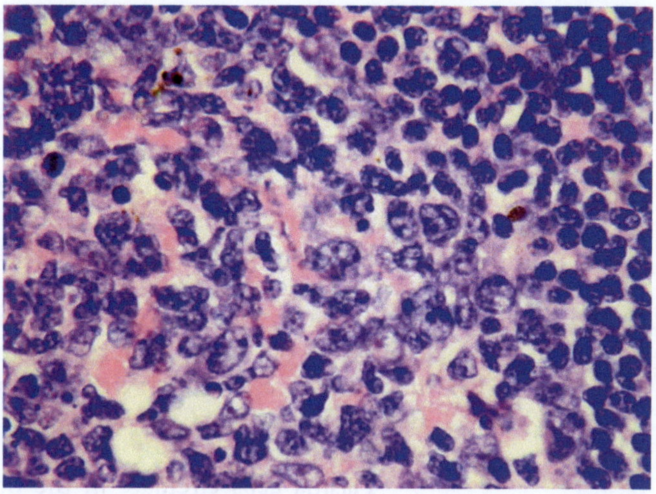

Fig. 4.4. Cells in the dark zone are mostly centroblasts that are more closely packed and have vesicular nuclei with nucleoli. Also present are follicular dendritic cells which have irregular nuclei, violaceous nuclear membrane, solitary nucleolus, and scant pale cytoplasm.

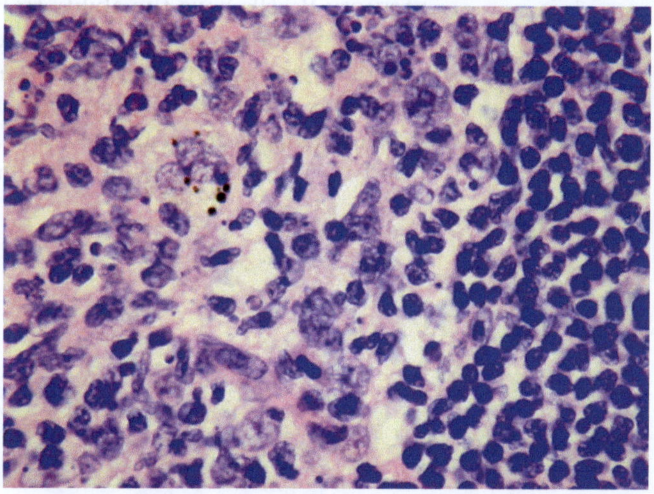

Fig. 4.5. The light zone is composed of centrocytes with scanty cytoplasm and irregular nuclei that do not show visible nucleoli. Apoptotic bodies are prominent.

A number of other cells may be found in lymphoid follicles including FDC, small follicular helper T lymphocytes and macrophages. FDC form a meshwork which capture and retain immune complexes on their surface for presentation to B cells. The nuclei of FDC are distinctive, often with folded violaceous nuclear membranes, occasionally binucleated, a solitary small nucleolus, and scant pale blue cytoplasm. Their dendritic processes are not identifiable in H & E sections but are highlighted by staining for IgM, which labels immune complexes on these processes. CD21, CD23, D2-40, and CD35 label FDC and their processes. A variable number of small T cells may be present, these staining for CD3, CD4, CD57, and PD-1. Plasma cells are occasionally present in the germinal centers of reactive lymph nodes, and involuting germinal centers often contain interstitial eosinophilic material that represents proteinaceous material from immune complexes.

Polykaryocytes or Warthin–Finkeldey-type giant cells may be seen in some reactive states, occurring in germinal centers and less frequently in the paracortex adjacent to venules. These giant cells contain 4–60 nuclei that are clustered like grapes. The individual nuclei are oval with clear chromatin and contain a small but distinct nucleolus. Cytoplasm is scanty (**Figs. 4.6, 4.7, 4.8, 4.9, 4.10**, and **4.11**.)

Plasma cells circulate in the peripheral blood and home to the bone marrow. They express cytoplasmic IgG or IgA, MUM1, CD79a, CD38, and CD138 but lack surface Ig and CD20. They may stain for EMA (epithelial membrane antigen). Both memory B cells and plasma cells show mutation of *IGV* region genes and do not continue to undergo mutation. Post-germinal center memory B cells have the ability to home to sites where they have undergone antigen stimulation. As such, B cells that arise in mucosa-associated lymphoid tissues (MALT) tend to return to such sites and those that arise in lymph nodes tend to home to nodal sites and bone marrow. The plasma cell myeloma corresponds to a bone marrow homing plasma cell (**Fig. 4.12**).

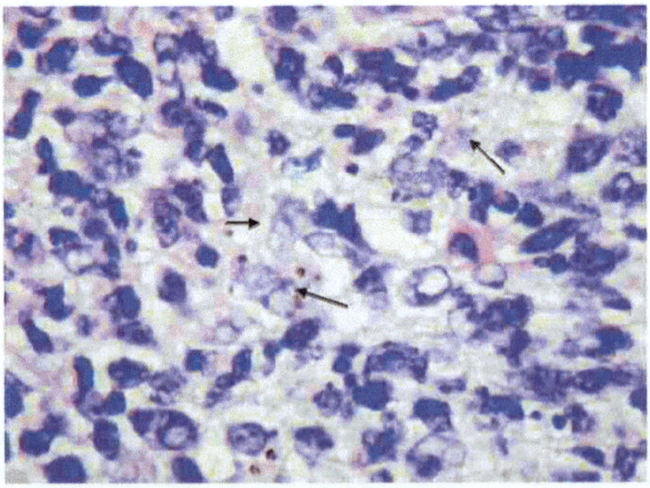

Fig. 4.6. FDC, densest in the dark zone, show abundant poorly defined pale cytoplasm and irregular nuclei with small nucleoli (arrows). Also present are tingible body macrophages with phagocytosed nuclear debris.

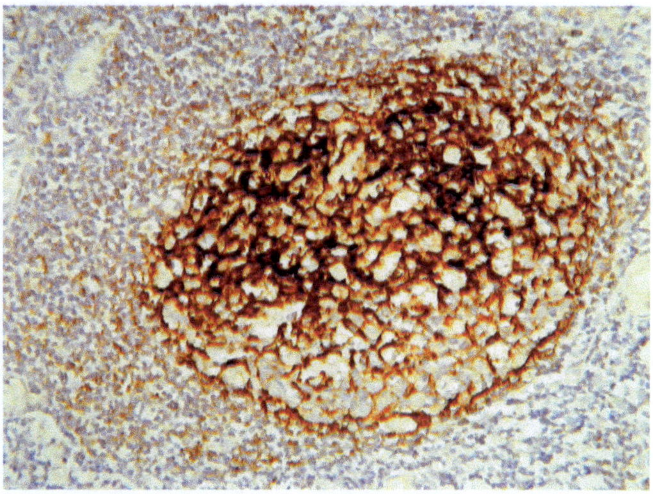

Fig. 4.7. CD21 reveals a meshwork of FDC in the germinal center with fine extensions into the mantle zone. The meshwork is densest in the basal dark zone.

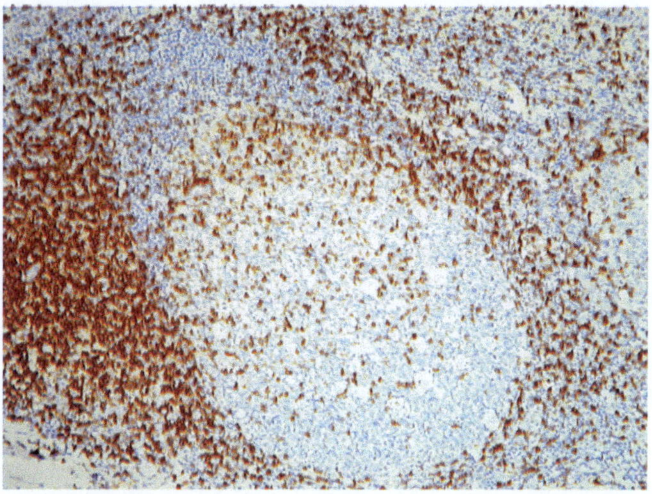

Fig. 4.8. Follicular helper CD4+ T lymphocytes are seen within the germinal center, densest in the light zone.

T Cell Differentiation

In contrast to the B cell lymphomas where there is a relatively well-defined normal counterpart for most subtypes, and for which some key molecular alterations and chromosomal translocations have been described, the pathobiology of peripheral T cell lymphomas is less well understood so that the classification of such lymphomas is less satisfactory.

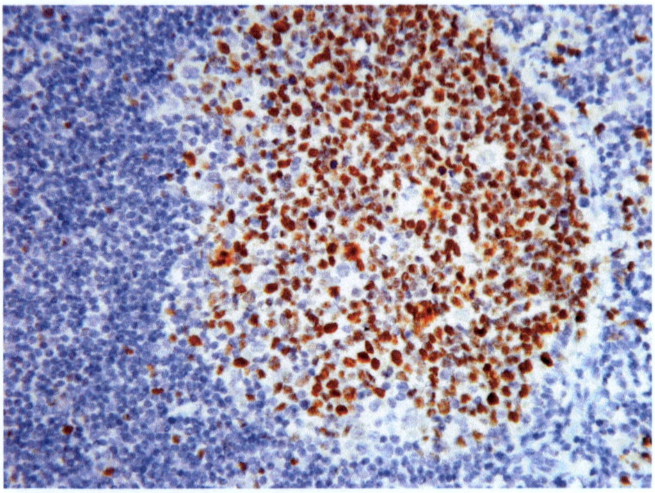

Fig. 4.9. Germinal center cells express Bcl6 which is not seen in the mantle zone.

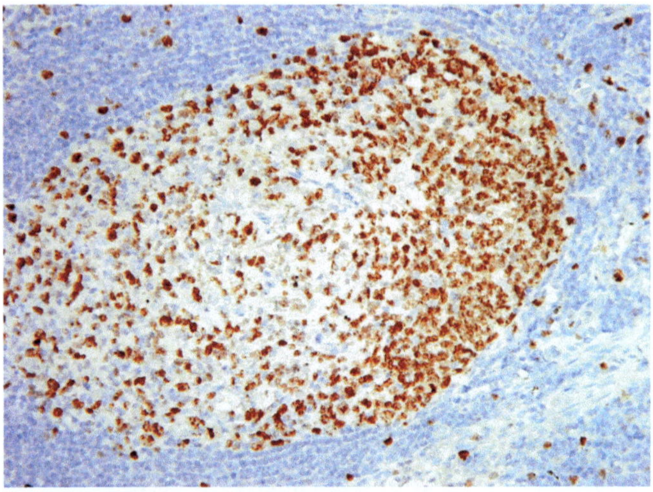

Fig. 4.10. Proliferative activity shown with Ki67 and mitosis is greatest in the dark zone of the reactive germinal center.

Most of the stages of T cell differentiation occur extranodally. T lymphocytes arise from a precursor in the bone marrow that undergoes maturation and acquisition of function in the thymus. Antigen-specific T cells mature in the thymic cortex where those cells that recognize self-peptides are eliminated by apoptosis, mediated by cortical epithelial cells and thymic nurse cells. Cortical thymocytes express terminal deoxynucleotidyl transferase (Tdt), CD1a, CD2, CD3, CD5, and CD7. CD3 is first expressed in the cytoplasm and, following complete T cell gene rearrangement, is exported to the cell membrane. Cortical thymocytes are initially negative for both CD4 and CD8, antigens which are co-expressed in maturing thymocytes; later more mature

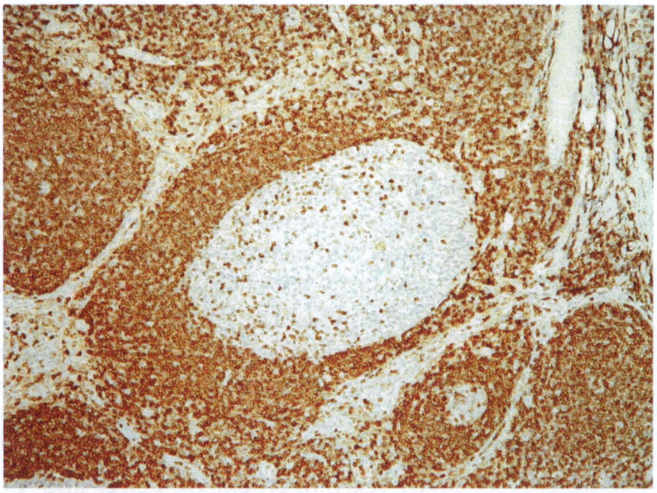

Fig. 4.11. Bcl2 is strongly expressed in the mantle zone and surrounding cortical B cells but not in the germinal center.

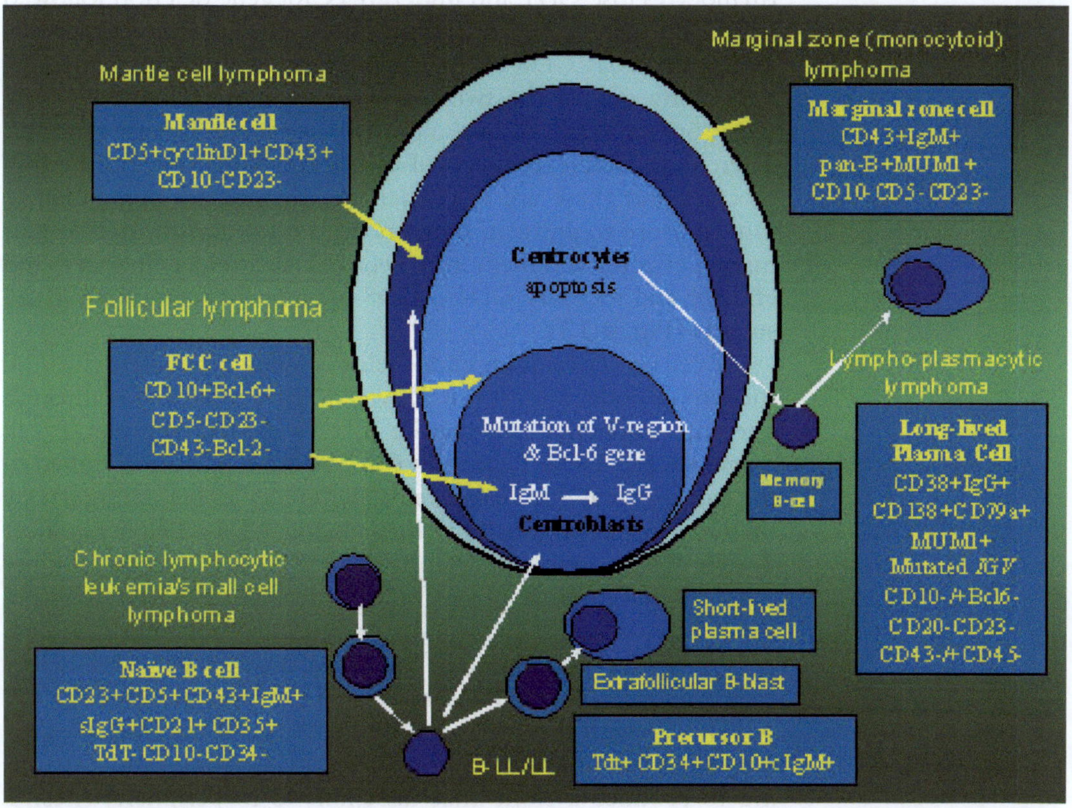

Fig. 4.12. B cell differentiation, associated markers, and neoplasms.

T cells express only CD4 or CD8. These stages of T cell maturation are reflected in T-lymphoblastic leukemia/lymphoma (T-ALL/LBL).

Medullary thymocytes are phenotypically similar to mature T cells in peripheral lymphoid organs. There are two classes of T cell: αβ T cells and γδ T cells, the distinction being based on the structure of the T cell receptor. The αβ and γδ chains are each composed of a variable (V) and constant (C) portion and are both associated with the CD3 complex, which has γ, δ, and ε chains. In the thymus, associated with the distinct and sequential patterns of surface antigen expression and loss during T cell development, there is progressive and orderly rearrangement of the genes encoding the T cell receptor (TCR). Pro-thymocytes undergo rearrangement of the TCRδ gene, immediately followed by rearrangement of TCRγ and TCRβ genes, to become immature thymocyte population. Common thymocytes retain cCD3, CD7, CD2, and CD5, and acquire CD1 as well as co-express CD4 and CD8. The pro-thymocytes, immature thymocytes, and common thymocytes reside within the thymic cortex. Common thymocytes lose CD1 and undergo TCRδ gene deletion followed by TCRα gene rearrangement. They acquire the completely assembled TCR-CD3 surface membrane complex and differentiate along one of the two pathways retaining CD4 and losing CD8, or vice versa, to become mature or medullary thymocytes. There is variable expression of cCD3 and Tdt in medullary thymocytes and these are lost when the thymocytes peripheralize. On exposure to antigen, they undergo blast transformation into mature effector and memory CD4+/CD8– (helper/inducer) and effector and memory CD4–/CD8+ (supressor/cytotoxic) T cell subsets (**Fig. 4.13**).

T cells enter via high-endothelial venules to circulate through the lymph node, and, if not activated, leave after 6–8 h through efferent lymphatics. All mature T cells express the pan-T cell markers CD2, CD3, CD5, and CD7. Most T cells are confined to the paracortex and are largely small lymphocytes belonging to one of three major populations, these being CD4+ helper/inducer T cells, CD8+ supressor/cytotoxic T cells, or NK+ natural killer cells. A small number of small CD4+ T cells are scattered within the follicles where they promote and modulate the reaction of B cells through the secretion of cytokines. These follicular T-helper cells produce a chemokine that causes induction and proliferation of FDC. As with B cells, T cells in the node can become activated to form T immunoblasts, enlarging, proliferating, and expanding to produce a clone that disseminates to peripheral sites. T immunoblasts morphologically resemble their B cell counterpart, having moderate quantities of basophilic cytoplasm and large, round nuclei with one central nucleolus or an irregularly shaped nucleus with two marginal nucleoli. Most mature T cells bear αβ chains of TCR, and a small number express γδ chains of TCR.

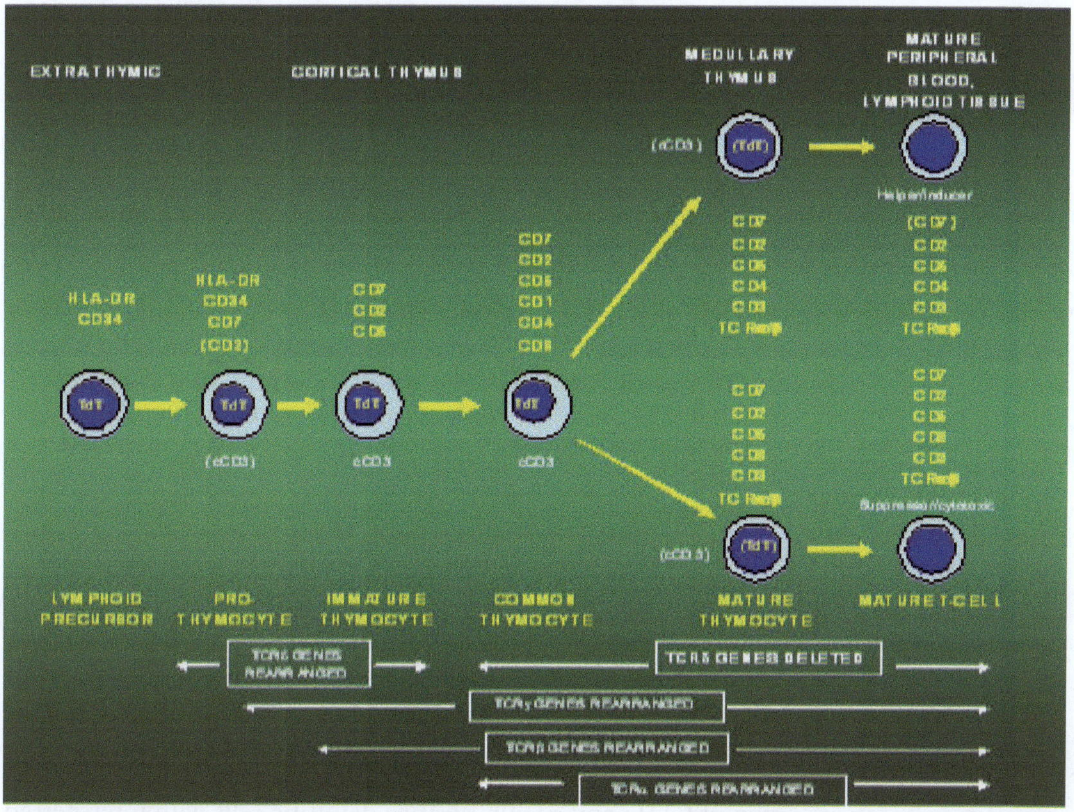

Fig. 4.13. Schematic representation of T cell ontogeny. Key: Markers in parentheses indicate that only a subpopulation of the cells expresses the marker.

The precise maturation pathway of natural killer (NK) cells and γδ T cells is not fully understood. NK cells do not have a complete T cell receptor complex and, when activated, express ε and ζ chains of CD3 in the cytoplasm but not in the membrane. They express CD2, CD7, and sometimes CD8 as well as CD16, CD56, and variably CD57. They also contain cytoplasmic cytotoxic granule proteins. NK cells do not rearrange the T cell receptor genes.

A variety of T cell and NK cell lymphomas are recognized, of which several are located in extranodal sites including the spleen, liver, mucosa, skin, and peripheral blood, but discussion in this book will be confined to nodal lymphomas.

The Paracortex

The paracortex of the lymph node lies between and deep into the follicles. It is composed largely of T cells intermixed with scattered B cells. The state of activation of the node determines the number of T cell and B cell blasts present. High-endothelial vessels are present in the paracortex. The T cell population in the paracortex occurs as nodules with variable appearances ranging from clearly defined nodules to ill-defined aggregates. The nodules are based on a framework of interdigitating dendritic cells (IDC) with distinct vesicular, deeply clefted nuclei, and small nucleoli. Their abundant pale cytoplasm interdigitates between adjacent lymphocytes. IDC stain for S100β and HLA-DR, and some IDC express CD1a on their membranes indentifying them as Langerhans cells. In this lacework of dendritic cells are embedded numerous CD4+ T cells and lesser numbers of CD8+ T cells. These T nodules frequently occur in strict association with a peripheral B follicle in the overlying cortex, together forming a composite nodule. These composite nodules represent a dynamic micro-anatomical structure that continuously changes and remodels in response to the antigen stimulation and in the course of the immune response. In well delineated or primary T nodules, a peripheral rim of concentrically arranged IDC surround a core of almost exclusively small CD4+ T cells. High-endothelial venules border primary T nodules. Secondary T nodules are less well demarcated and show a starry sky appearance because of the larger numbers of IDC interspersed among large numbers of CD4+ T cells admixed with some CD8+ T cells. High-endothelial venules are scattered throughout the secondary T nodule. These nodules represent the site of T cell interaction with antigen presented by IDC, resulting in activation and proliferation of antigen-specific T cells. A third pattern of the paracortical T nodule or the tertiary nodule is represented by the paracortical changes in dermatopathic lymphadenitis, where adjacent T nodules coalesce and the paracortex is almost completely replaced by a semicircular proliferation of CD1a and S100β-positive dendritic cells with interspersed CD4+ and CD8+ T cells associated with several B cell follicles (**Figs. 4.14**, **4.15**, **4.16**, **4.17**, **4.18**, **4.19**, **4.20**, and **4.21**).

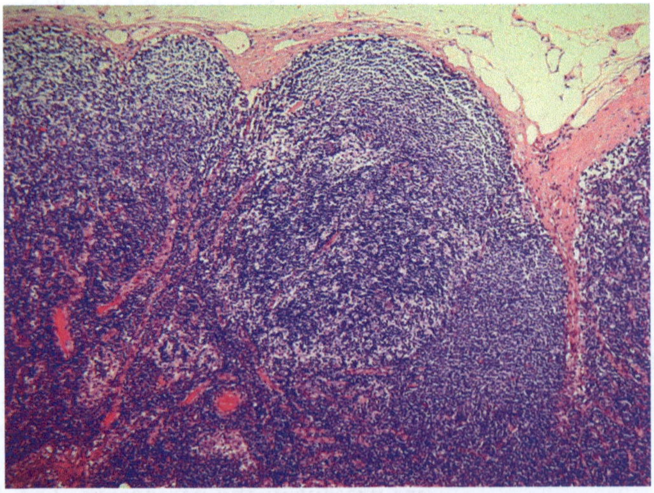

Fig. 4.14. A primary T nodule in the paracortex comprising a rim of IDC (large pale cells) and small lymphocytes. Lymphoid follicles in the overlying cortex make up a composite nodule. High-endothelial venules circumscribe the T nodule.

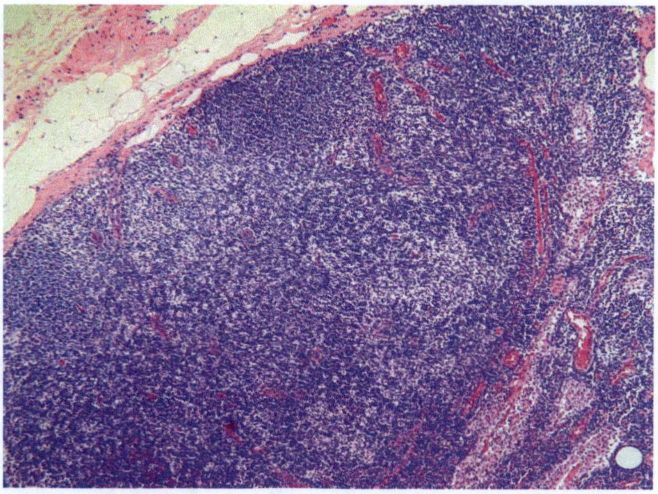

Fig. 4.15. Secondary T nodules are less well demarcated, and abundant IDC scattered throughout the nodule produce a starry sky appearance.

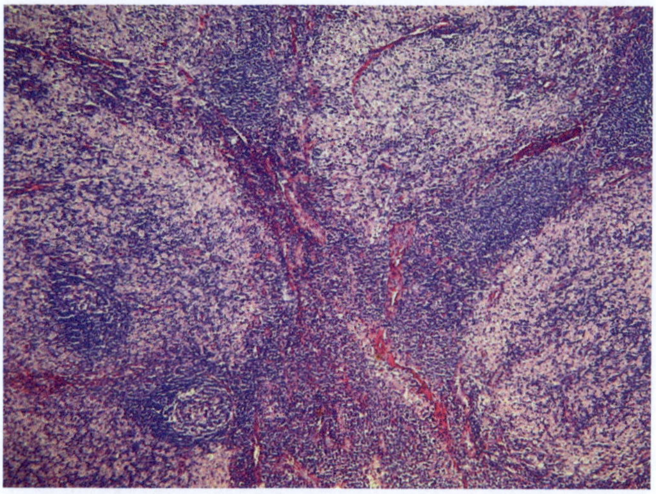

Fig. 4.16. Large tertiary T nodules composed mostly of IDC are characteristic of dermatopathic lymphadenopathy.

The so-called plasmacytoid T cells have undergone numerous nomenclature changes. They are now called plasmacytoid dendritic cells (PDC) and are derived from circulating blood mononuclear cells that are the principal source of interferon-α. PDC may occur in groups and nodules in the paracortex associated with high-endothelial venules; the nodules mimicking germinal centers. They are less readily recognizable when they occur as single cells or in loose aggregates. These cells are medium sized with a faintly stained nucleus and inconspicuous nucleolus. Similar to plasma cells, the nucleus is located eccentrically within moderate quantities of intensely basophilic cytoplasm filled

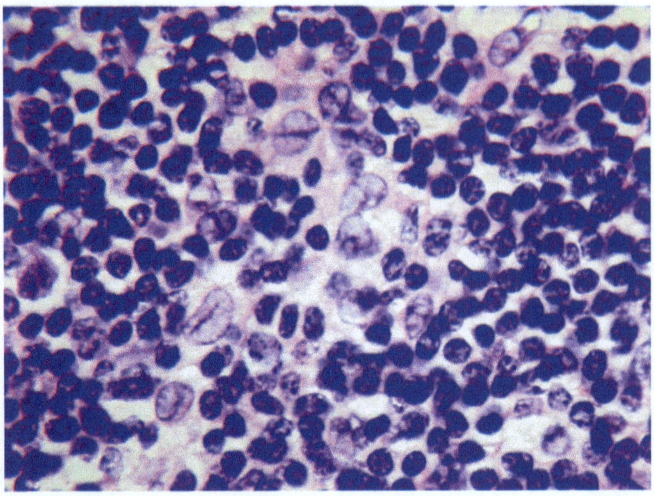

Fig. 4.17. IDC have irregular multilobated nuclei with small nucleoli and large quantities of pale ill-defined cytoplasm.

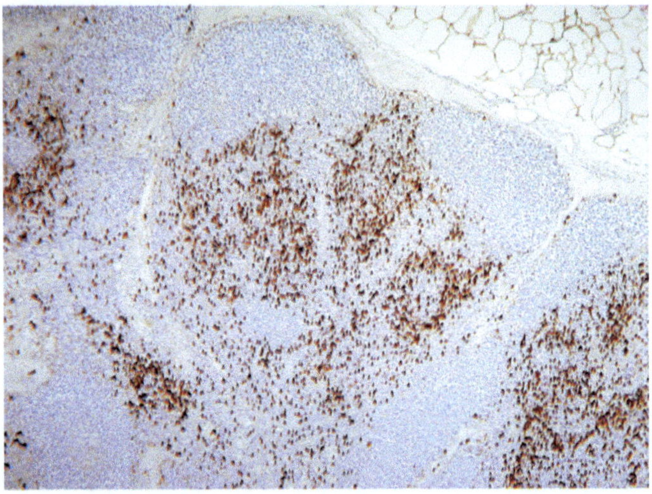

Fig. 4.18. Composite nodule of two follicles associated with underlying T nodules delineated by IDC (anti-S100).

with abundant rough endoplasmic reticulum. They were initially thought to be T cells because they express CD4, a marker now recognized also to be expressed by cells of the monocyte lineage. In addition, they express a number of myelomonocytic specific markers as well as CD123 (receptor interferon-α), CD68, HLA-DR, and CD45RA, the latter confirming their hematopoietic origin. They do not bear lineage specific markers of B and T cells, NK cells, and myeloid cells.

The preferential localization of PDC adjacent to high-endothelial venules and also within their lumen supports the contention that these interferon-producing cells represent a stage in

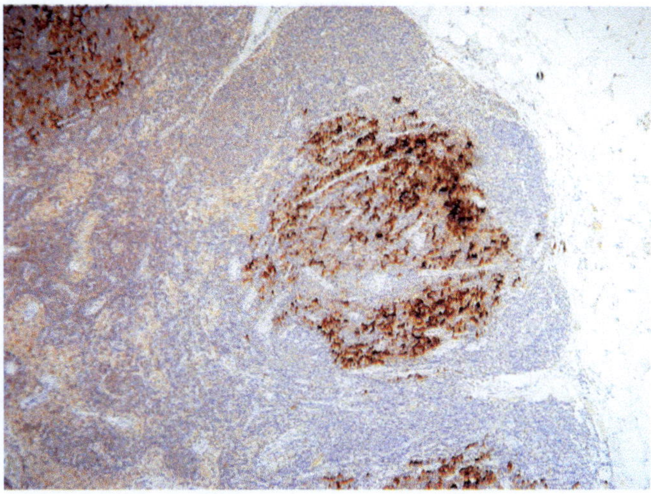

Fig. 4.19. CD1a staining of Langerhans cells in a T nodule.

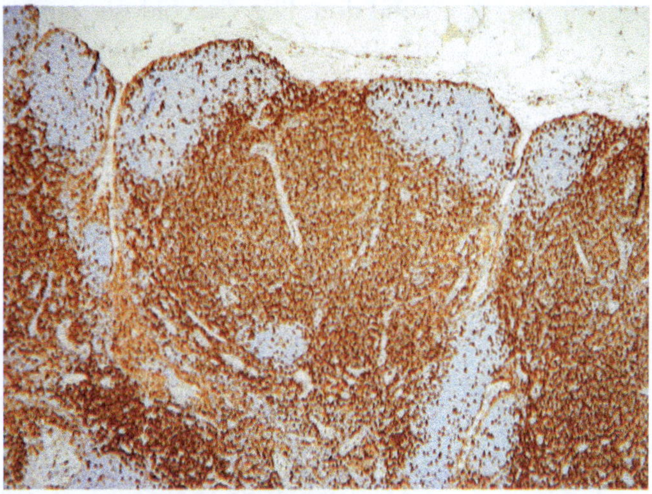

Fig. 4.20. CD4+ cells within a T cell nodule.

the development of circulating dendritic cells. Subsequent confirmatory studies indicate that these cells can differentiate into dendritic cells under the influence of appropriate stimuli, such as viruses, IL-3, CD40L, and non-bacterial DNA, with a potential role in antigen presentation. Plasmacytoid monocytes or plasmacytoid dendritic cells are present in most reactive lymph nodes and are typically seen in Kikuchi disease as the crescentic monocytes that rim areas of extensive apoptosis. A marked increase in plasmacytoid monocytes is seen in hyaline–vascular Castleman disease and classical Hodgkin lymphoma as well as in a range of inflammatory lymphadenopathies, including reactions to infections like tuberculosis and toxoplasmosis, non-infectious

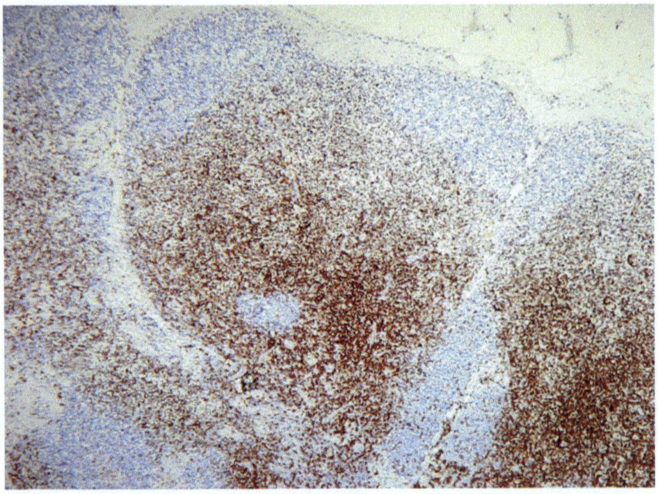

Fig. 4.21. CD8+ cells make up a smaller component of the T nodule.

conditions like sarcoidosis and in association to epithelial neoplasms, and lymphoproliferative and myeloproliferative processes.

A rare blastic plasmacytoid dendritic cell neoplasm that tends to involve multiple sites has been described. It shows a predilection for skin (100% of cases), followed by bone marrow and peripheral blood (60–90%), and lymph nodes (40–50%). Up to 20% are associated with or develop into a myelomonocytic leukemia or acute myeloid leukemia (**Figs. 4.22** and **4.23**).

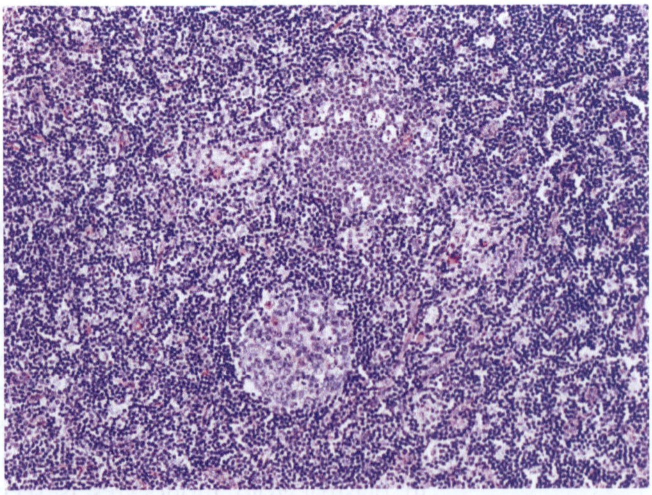

Fig. 4.22. Reactive lymph node showing a cluster of PDC above a germinal center (*arrows*). By comparison, the PDC form less-defined homogenous aggregate devoid of a mantle rim of small lymphoid cells.

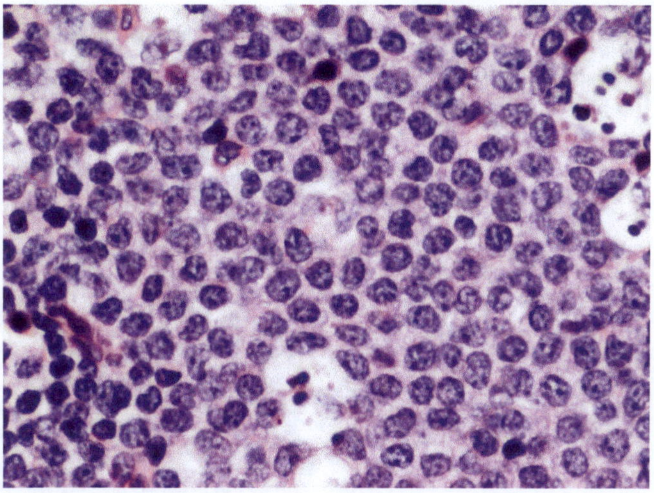

Fig. 4.23. PDC have intermediate-sized oval nuclei, dispersed chromatin, and inconspicuous nucleoli. They have moderate quantities of pale eosinophilic cytoplasm. Numerous tingle body macrophages are present.

High-Endothelial Venules

The high-endothelial venules found in the paracortex are readily recognized by their plump, cuboidal to cylindrical lining endothelial cells which typically have large round vesicular nuclei and abundant cytoplasm. The luminal surface of these post-capillary venules has a cobblestone appearance because of lymphocytes inserting in the crevices between adjacent endothelial cells. The uneven surface is thought to result in turbulence in blood flow enhancing lymphocyte margination and adhesion. Migration of lymphocytes into the lymph node parenchyma occurs generally by diapedesis or by emperipolesis. This transendothelial lymphocyte trafficking is mediated by specific adhesion molecules expressed by the lymphocytes, the selectins, which interact with ligands present on the endothelial cell lining, the vascular addressins. Integrins present on the lymphocyte surface that interact with adhesion molecules belonging to the immunoglobulin gene superfamily also contribute to the penetration of the post-capillary venule wall.

Medullary Area

The medulla is composed of cords of cells that include lymphocytes, plasmacytoid lymphocytes, plasmablasts, and mature plasma cells, in varying proportions. It is the primary site of plasma cell proliferation, differentiation, and the production of antibodies. Under intense antigenic stimulation, the medullary cords may extend into the cortex. Medullary cords are separated by wide medullary sinuses which contain percolating lymph, numerous monocytes, plasma cells, and mast cells (**Fig. 4.24**).

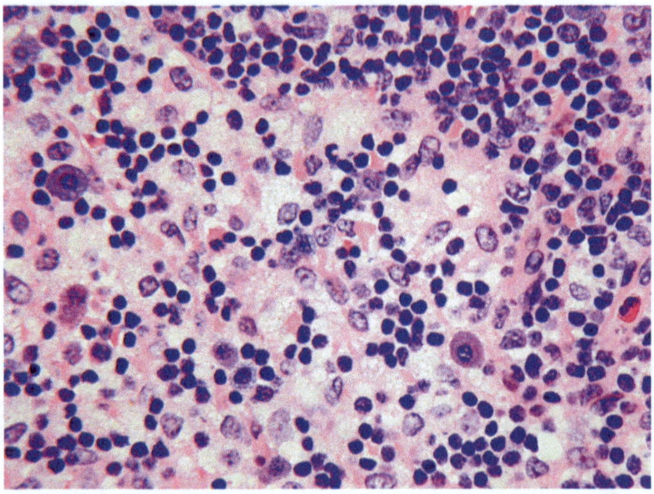

Fig. 4.24. Medullary sinuses contain plasma cells, small lymphocytes, macrophages, and the occasional mast cells (*arrow*).

Connective Tissue Framework

The lymph node is invested in a thin fibrous capsule which is in continuity with fibrous trabeculae that penetrate the parenchyma of the node. Both capsule and fibrous trabeculae may become prominent with lymphadenitis.

Section II

Chapter 5

Nodular Lymphoid Infiltrates

Key words: Follicular lymphoma, mantle cell lymphoma, marginal zone lymphoma, growth centers, Hodgkin lymphoma, post-transplantation lymphoproliferative disorders, germinal center colonization, reactive follicles, progressive transformation of germinal centers, rheumatoid lymphadenitis, dermatopathic lymphadenitis, drug-induced.

Cellular proliferations that result in a pattern of nodules or spheres are very distinctive. This is the most frequent benign and neoplastic growth pattern encountered in lymph nodes. The rounded nodules or spheres are the result of localized aggregates of cells that are different to the mixed background of lymphoid cells that normally make up the lymph node.

A distinction needs to be made between a true follicular growth pattern and nodular proliferations. A true follicular growth pattern reflects a proliferation of cells intrinsic to the lymphoid follicle and can be benign or neoplastic in nature. The follicular pattern of growth is imparted because of retention or preservation, and often expansion of the follicular dendritic cell (FDC) meshwork which can be readily demonstrated with a number of antibodies in routinely fixed, paraffin-embedded sections as previously discussed. By convention, the term "follicular lymphoma" is used for germinal center cell lymphomas with a follicular pattern of growth, although mantle cell lymphomas and marginal zone lymphomas are also derived from the lymphoid follicle and are associated with expanded meshworks of FDC. While these entities are not termed follicular lymphomas, for convenience, they will also be discussed in this book under the heading "neoplastic follicles."

Compared to the follicular growth pattern, the nodular pattern is less distinct in outline and the nodule of lymphoid cells while rounded is often vague and ill-defined. The nodular pattern is largely imparted because the accumulated cells produce

A.S.-Y. Leong, *A Pattern Approach to Lymph Node Diagnosis*,
DOI 10.1007/978-1-4419-7176-0_5, © Springer Science+Business Media, LLC 2011

a localized distension of a normal anatomical compartment of the node, especially, the lymph node sinuses. Pseudo-follicles or growth centers seen in chronic lymphocytic leukemia/small lymphocytic lymphoma also produce a nodular pattern as a result of localized collections of blastic cells. By definition, other localized accumulations of cells that are non-lymphoid, with different and distinct tinctorial properties or appearance to the background lymphocytes, are not included among the nodular infiltrates. These are often sharply demarcated and, more often than not, are of variable shape and size, e.g., metastatic tumor.

A nodular growth pattern is also a characteristic of Hodgkin lymphoma, occurring in most of the subtypes of classical Hodgkin lymphoma and nodular lymphocyte-predominant Hodgkin lymphoma.

A vaguely nodular pattern can also be imparted by proliferations in the paracortex as the T cells are also arranged into nodules that form a functional relationship between the antigen-presenting interdigitating dendritic reticulum cells and the T cell subsets. This is seen in dermatopathic lymphadenitis and drug-induced lymphadenopathy.

A number of other neoplastic and non-neoplastic lesions can produce rounded accumulations of cells that are localized or scattered throughout the node. Only those lesions that present primarily with a follicular or nodular pattern will be discussed in detail in this chapter. Other entities in **Table 5.1** identified in italics are discussed elsewhere in this book.

Follicular Pattern

The most important pattern of growth that requires recognition is the follicular pattern. Follicles may be benign or neoplastic. The distinction of neoplastic follicles from benign follicles is one of the most common diagnostic problems encountered in consultation practice. A benign follicle, described in detail in a previous section, is composed of a germinal center surrounded by a rim of dark-staining mantle cells. The germinal center shows polarization and displays a basal dark zone composed mostly of centroblasts and a light zone (orientated closer to the capsule) composed mostly of centrocytes. In contrast, neoplastic follicles are generally devoid of the mantle rim or, if present, are thin and incomplete, and they do not display polarization. Recognition of true neoplastic follicles has histogenetic as well as prognostic relevance as a follicular lymphoma (FL) is a proliferation of B cells and generally implies an indolent disease that, in the far majority of cases, is not curable.

Table 5.1
Follicular and nodular patterns.

Neoplastic "follicles"
Follicular lymphoma
Mantle cell lymphoma
Marginal zone lymphoma
Neoplastic nodules
Growth centers in CLL/SLL
Hodgkin lymphomas – NLPHL, NSCHL, LRCHL, MCCHL, LDCHL
Post-transplant lymphoproliferative disorders
Colonization of germinal centers
Others – lymphoplasmacytoid lymphoma, lymphoblastic lymphoma, prolymphocytic leukemia
Reactive follicles
Progressive transformation of germinal centers
Rheumatoid
Toxoplasmosis
HIV
Kimura disease
Castleman disease
Syphilis
Kikuchi disease
Systemic lupus erythematosus
Infectious mononucleosis
Other viral lymphadenitis
Paracortical nodules
Dermatopathic lymphadenitis
Drug-induced lymphadenopathy

Neoplastic Follicles

Follicular Lymphoma (FL)

Clinical

Follicular lymphomas (FL) are neoplasms of follicular-center B cells, typically of both centrocytes and centroblasts that partially or completely replace the lymph node with a follicular growth pattern. It is the most common form of low-grade non-Hodgkin lymphoma in the West but is of lower prevalence in Asia, Eastern Europe, and Africa. Individuals below the age of 20 years are rarely affected and pediatric patients are predominantly males.

The disease is mostly widespread at presentation, principally involving lymph nodes, and often also the spleen and bone marrow. Bone marrow involvement may be associated with spillage into the peripheral blood, and with widespread nodal disease there may be a spread into the gastrointestinal tract or soft tissue. Primary involvement of the skin, breast, ocular adnexa, testis, and gastrointestinal tract is less common and clinically different from nodal FL.

Despite widespread disease, patients are usually asymptomatic. FL is generally indolent but runs a progressive course. Without treatment it may undergo spontaneous remission for varying periods. While chemotherapy is effective in controlling the disease, it is rarely curative except for the infrequent localized case. In 25–35% of patients with FL, transformation to a high-grade lymphoma occurs, usually diffuse large B cell lymphoma (DLBCL) or sometimes resembling Burkitt lymphoma. This transformation is usually associated with a non-responsive, rapidly progressive clinical course and death (**Table 5.2**).

Table 5.2
Follicular lymphoma (FL) – clinical

- Most common NHL in the Western world, less common in Asia, Africa, and Eastern Europe
- Median age in sixth decade, uncommon below 20 years of age
- Pediatric patients are predominantly males
- Usually present as stage III or IV disease
- Involves lymph nodes, bone marrow, peripheral blood, spleen, Waldeyer ring
- Primary extranodal FL of skin, GI tract, breast, testis, and ocular adnexa are clinically different from nodal FL
- Indolent course, long survival but rarely curable except in the infrequent localised disease
- 25–30% transform to DLBCL with a non-responsive, rapidly progressive course

Morphology

The neoplastic follicles are generally closely packed, have uniform rounded shapes which may be ill-defined with absent or attenuated mantle zones, and are dispersed throughout the node. Preexisting nodal architecture is destroyed with loss of the sinus structure and the neoplastic follicles can replace the hilar fat and extend into perinodal tissue. Besides the mixture of centrocytes and centroblasts that form the neoplastic population of follicular-center B cells, there are also follicular dendritic cells (FDC) and reactive T cells in the follicles. The neoplastic cells, most commonly centrocytes, recognized by their morphology and immunohistochemical characteristics, can also be found in between follicles.

The phenomenon of "colonization" of non-neoplastic follicles by FL cells may be infrequently observed in lymph nodes otherwise involved by typical FL. Such changes may also be seen in lymph nodes adjacent to those containing FL.

When the interfollicular area is populated by large centroblasts, a separate primary diagnosis of DLBCL should be made, irrespective of the grade of the follicular component. Staining for FDC with CD21, CD35, or D2-40 is required in this regard as the WHO classification defines a diffuse area as "an area of the tissue completely lacking follicles defined by CD21+/CD23+ FDC." An estimate of the proportion of each component should be made (>75% follicular; 25–75% follicular; <25% follicular). In about 10% of FL, a marginal zone pattern is produced around a few neoplastic follicles as a result of marginal zone differentiation (**Figs. 5.1**, **5.2**, **5.3**, **5.4**, **5.5**, and **5.6**).

Grading

The grading of FL is controversial. Grading is done by counting or estimating the number of centroblasts in 10 representative neoplastic follicles, expressed per 40× objective high-power microscopic field (hpf). Grade 1 = 0–5 centroblasts/hpf; grade 2 = 6–15 centroblasts/hpf, and grade 3 = >15 centroblasts/hpf. Over the years since its introduction, this method of grading has not shown significant clinical differences between grades 1 and 2 and it is recommended that these two grades be combined. If distinct areas of grade 3 FL are present in an otherwise grade 1–2 FL, it is recommended that a separate diagnosis of grade 3 FL be made. Grade 3 FL is further subdivided into grades 3A when centrocytes are still present and 3B when the follicles are composed entirely of

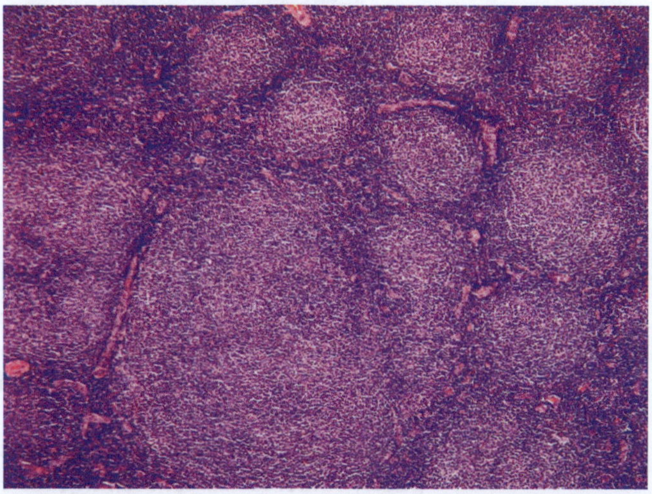

Fig. 5.1. FL. Rounded follicles replace the node. A distinct mantle is absent and the largest follicle displays a floret pattern resulting from the confluence of several follicles. There is no polarization in the neoplastic follicles.

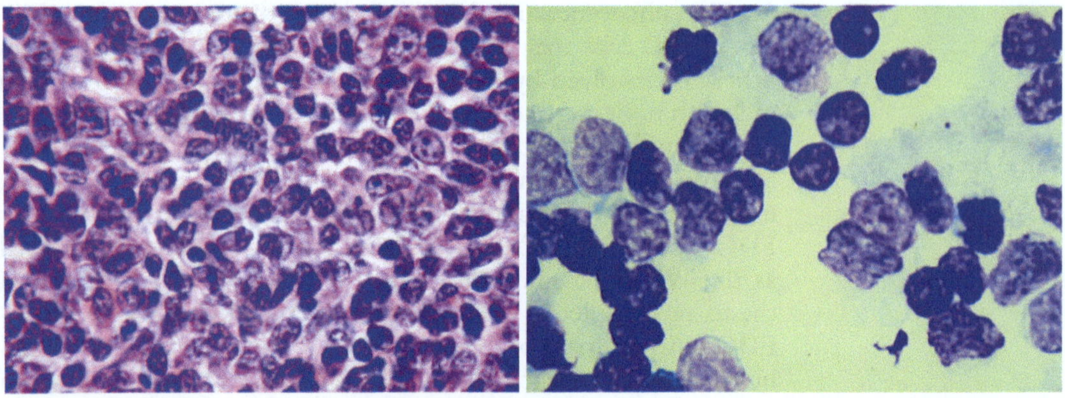

Fig. 5.2. The neoplastic follicles are composed of mostly centrocytes and a smaller component of centroblasts (grade 1). FDC cells are also present. Inset shows imprint of centrocytes.

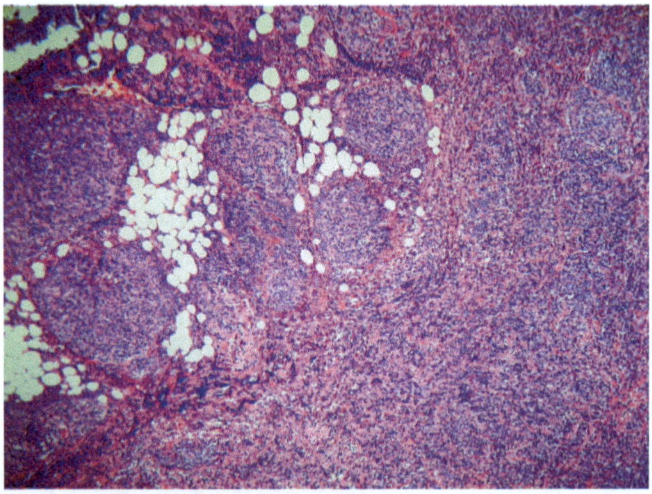

Fig. 5.3. FL with extension into perinodal fat.

centroblasts or immunoblasts. The vast majority of FLs are grade 1–2, whereas pediatric cases are more likely to be grade 3.

While the 2008 WHO Classification recommends that any area of DLBCL in a FL be reported as a separate primary diagnosis, with an estimate of the proportion of the two components, prognosis is not significantly altered even when very large diffuse areas occur in grade 1–2 FL. In most studies reported, however, grade 3 FL with >25% diffuse areas have a worse prognosis than purely follicular cases. Staining for FDC is essential to distinguish large confluent follicles or interfollicular involvement from areas of DLBCL, the latter lacking FDC (**Figs. 5.7**, **5.8**, **5.9**, **5.10**, **5.11**, **5.12**, **5.13**, and **5.14**; **Table 5.3**).

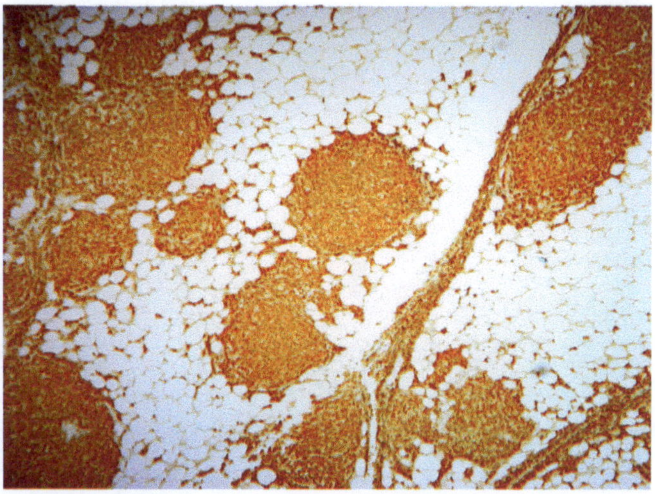

Fig. 5.4. Neoplastic follicles in the perinodal fat stain for Bcl2.

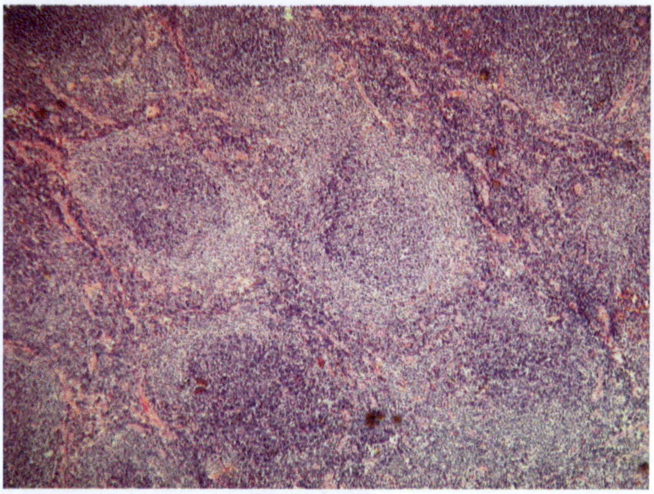

Fig. 5.5. Marginal zone differentiation in FL. A pale marginal zone encircles the neoplastic follicles.

Immunohistology

The neoplastic cells usually express surface, and less frequently, cytoplasmic immunoglobulin (IgM+/IgD+, IgG+, or rarely IgA+) with light-chain restriction, express B cell-associated antigens (CD20, CD79a) and are Bcl2+/Bcl6+/CD10+. They are negative for CD5, CD23, and CD43. Markers of follicular dendritic cells, namely CD21, CD23, CD35, and D2-40 are useful in demonstrating the follicular nature of the disease. They show a meshwork of dendritic cells in the neoplastic follicles. The neoplastic follicles may contain numerous other non-neoplastic cells including T cells and histiocytes.

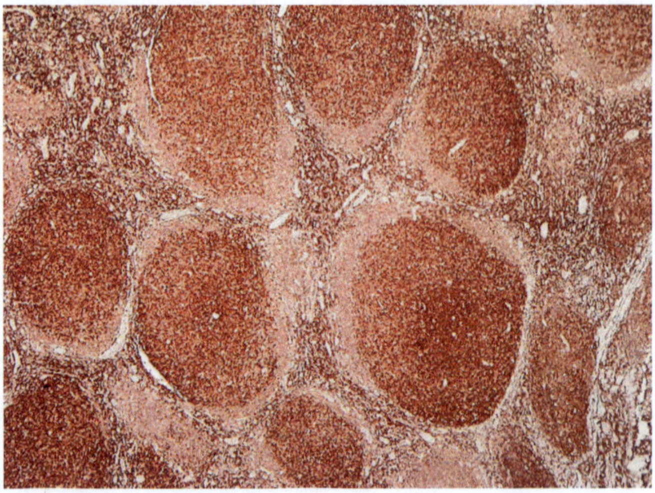

Fig. 5.6. Bcl2 stains neoplastic cells in the follicles and interfollicular areas. In contrast, the marginal zones are pale.

Genetics

FL is characterized by the translocation t(14;18)(q32;q21) involving the *IgH* chain gene on chromosome 14 and the *Bcl-2* gene on chromosome 18, and *bcl2* gene rearrangements. Up to 90% of grade 1–2 FL show t(14;18) but this varies with the technique employed, FISH being the most sensitive. *Bcl2* rearrangements are much less frequent in grade 3B FL.

Immunoglobulin heavy and light chain are rearranged with variable regions (**Table 5.4**) showing extensive and ongoing somatic hypermutations but detection is dependant on the primers used and 10–40% of cases may not yield monoclonal products (**Figs. 5.15**, **5.16**, **5.17**, and **5.18**).

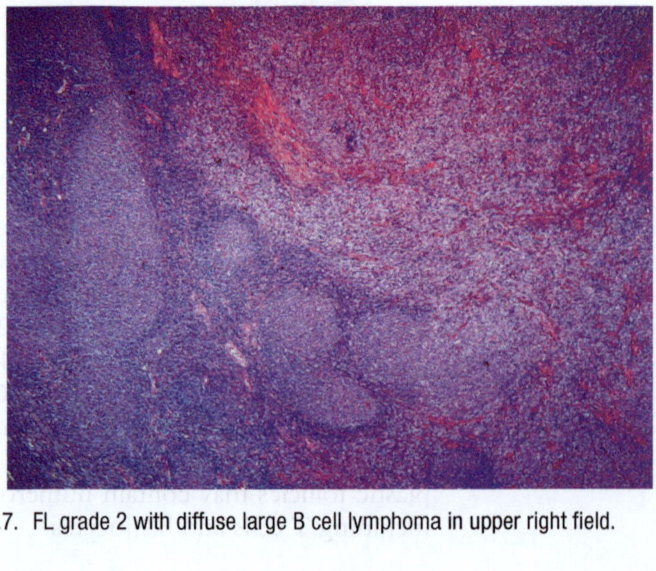

Fig. 5.7. FL grade 2 with diffuse large B cell lymphoma in upper right field.

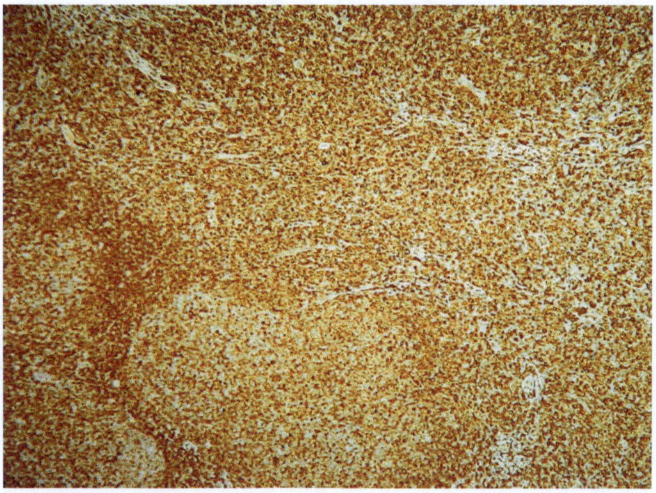

Fig. 5.8. Both the FL and diffuse large cell lymphoma stain for CD20. FDC were present only in the follicular areas (not shown).

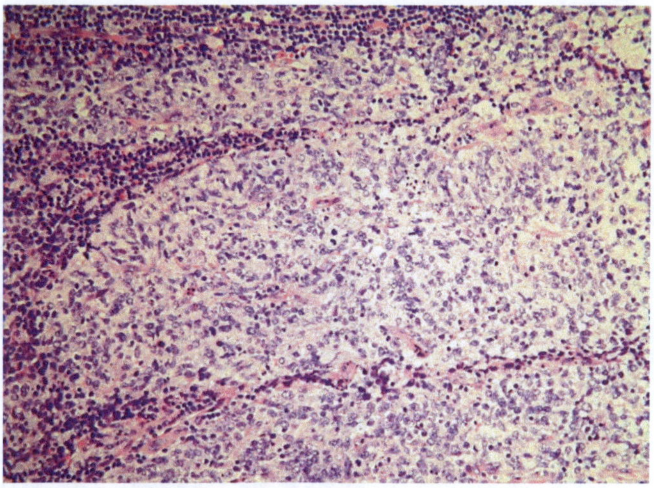

Fig. 5.9. A large cell lymphoma infiltrating in an apparently diffuse pattern.

Follicular Hyperplasia Versus Follicular Lymphoma

The distinction of follicular hyperplasia from FL is a common problem encountered even by experienced pathologists. One important characteristic of benign follicles is the presence of polarity. Often the three zones of the follicle are identifiable, namely an outermost mantle zone with a light and dark basal zone within the germinal center. The latter comprises centroblasts/non-cleaved cells, which, because of their heavy chromatin and basophilic cytoplasm (RNA-rich) impart darker appearance. Centroblasts have

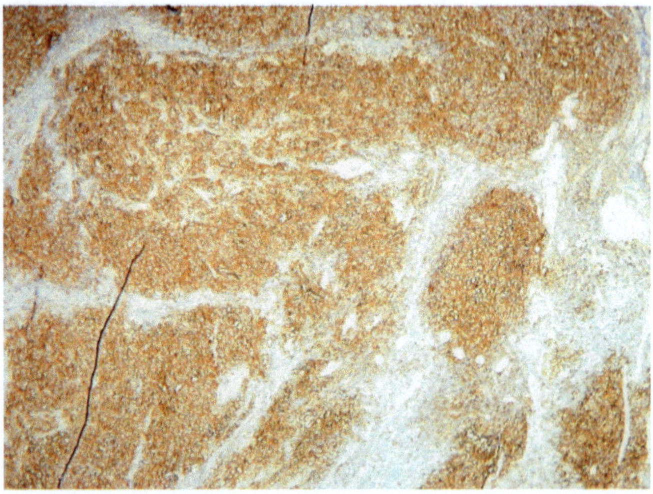

Fig. 5.10. CD21 reveals FDC and a distinct follicular pattern. The apparently diffuse areas are the result of confluence of follicles.

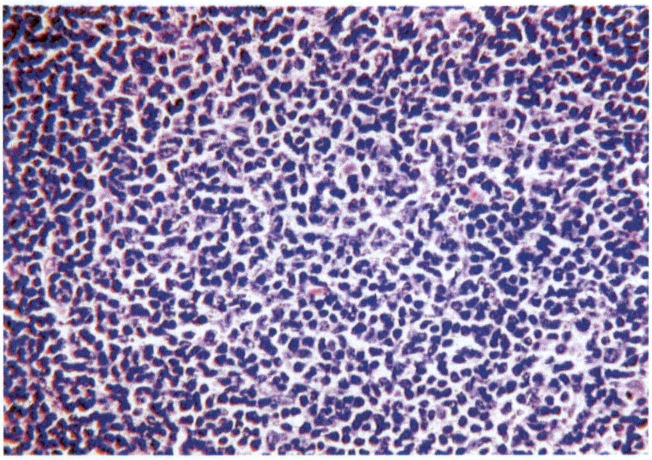

Fig. 5.11. FL grade 1–2 composed almost entirely of small- to intermediate-sized cells with irregular nuclei (centrocytes).

rounded vesicular nuclei with several small basophilic nucleoli and scant cytoplasm. The light zone comprises mostly centrocytes/cleaved cells mixed with dendritic reticulum cells so that there is less increased internuclear space, which, together with the less-dense chromatin of the cells impart the lighter appearance. Centrocytes are recognized by their scanty cytoplasm and their twisted, angulated, or folded nuclei that do not show distinct nucleoli. The mantle zone, which comprises small lymphocytes with coarse chromatin, is a distinct dark rim around the germinal center. It is eccentric and thickest towards the subcapsular sinus or the mucosal surface in the case of the tonsil. The light

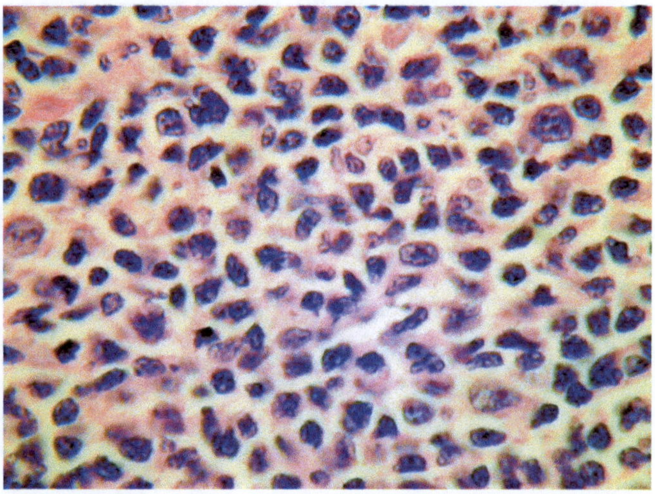

Fig. 5.12. FL grade 1–2, scattered larger centroblasts with distinct nucleoli are present among the centrocytes.

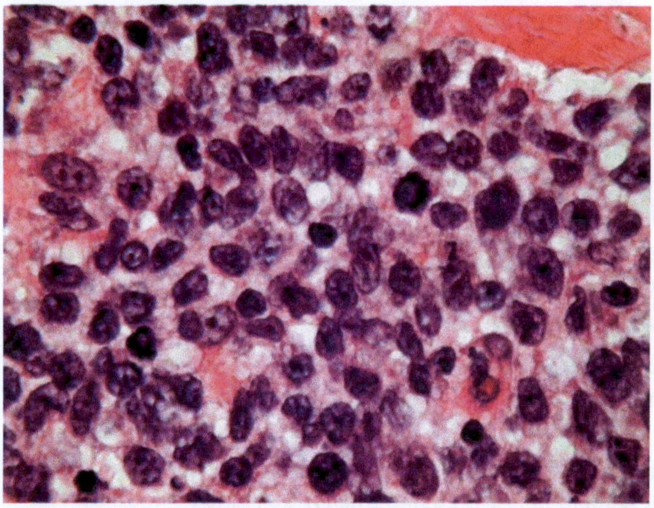

Fig. 5.13. FL grade 3A, there are more than 15 centroblasts present per high power field and centrocytes are present.

zone of the germinal center is similarly oriented peripheral to the dark zone. The polarization into light and dark zones may be difficult to discern in large hyperplastic follicles but the mantle rim is preserved.

Neoplastic follicles do not demonstrate the polarization/zonification characteristic of benign follicles, and neoplastic follicles are usually less well defined. They are usually not surrounded by the mantle cell rim. If mantle zones are present, they are invariably thin and incomplete. Besides being tightly packed, neoplastic follicles are generally uniform in shape and size and do

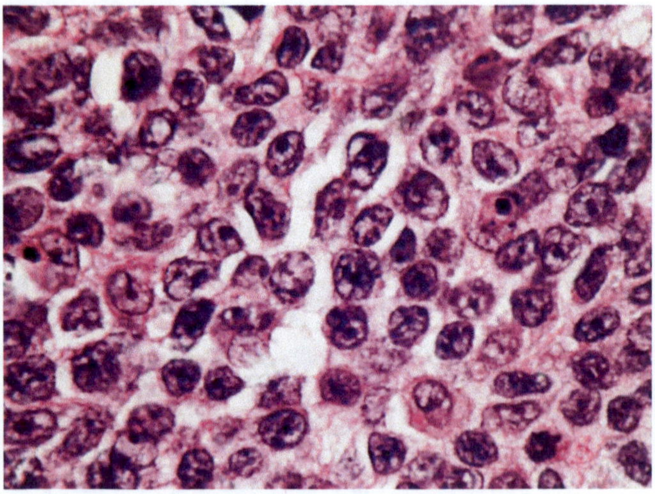

Fig. 5.14. FL grade 3B, composed almost entirely of centroblasts.

Table 5.3
Follicular lymphoma – morphology

- Lymph node enlarged by numerous crowded, uniform-appearing follicles
- Mantle zone attenuated or lost
- Absence of polarization in follicles
- Follicles composed of a mixture of centrocytes and centroblasts
- Absence of tingible-body macrophages
- Follicles present throughout node; may spill into perinodal tissue and hilar fat
- Nodal architecture lost, sinus pattern not discernable
- Grading: Grade 1–2 = 1–15 blasts/hpf; grade 3 = >15 blasts/hpf grade 3A = centrocytes present; grade 3B = only centroblasts present
- Prognosis worse in grade 3 FL with >25% DLBCL transformation
- Additional diagnosis of DLBCL is made when interfollicular areas are populated only by centroblasts, FDC should not be present in the DLBCL areas
- Marginal zone differentiation around neoplastic follicles occurs in 10% of cases

not display the variation that is generally characteristic of reactive follicles. Furthermore, they do not show the degree of mitotic or apoptotic activity so prominent in reactive follicles. Neoplastic follicles may display a marked preponderance of centrocytes, and tingible-body macrophages are not present. Interfollicular areas may contain neoplastic cells, whereas hyperplastic nodes contain a polymorphous population of small lymphocytes, immunoblasts, and plasma cells. Extranodal extension is frequently seen in lymphomas. Benign follicles tend to be of variable sizes and are located in the cortex of the node, whereas neoplastic follicles

Table 5.4
Follicular lymphoma – immunohistology and genetics

- Membranous/cytoplasmic IgM+/IgD+/≥ IgG > IgA
- B cell markers – CD20, CD79a
- Neoplastic follicles Bcl2+, Bcl6+, CD10+, CD45RA+ (MT2)
- CD21, CD35, CD23, D2-40 show expanded meshwork of FDC
- t(14;18)(q32;q21) involving *Bcl2* and *IgH* genes; *Bcl2* rearrangements
- *IgH* and *IgL* rearranged; extensive and ongoing somatic hypermutations in variable regions

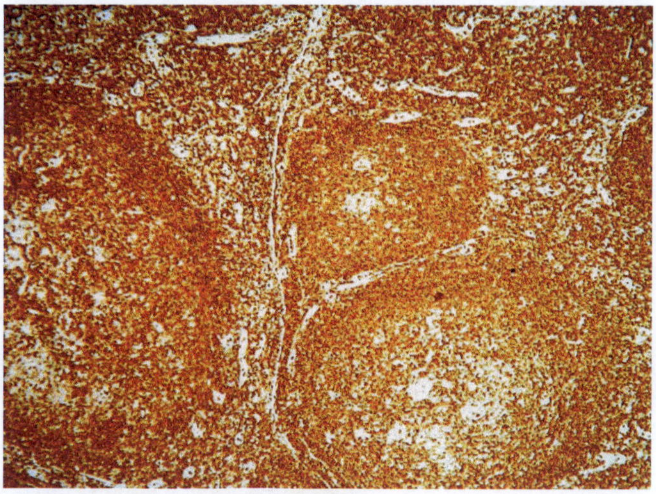

Fig. 5.15. FL. Neoplastic follicles stain for CD20.

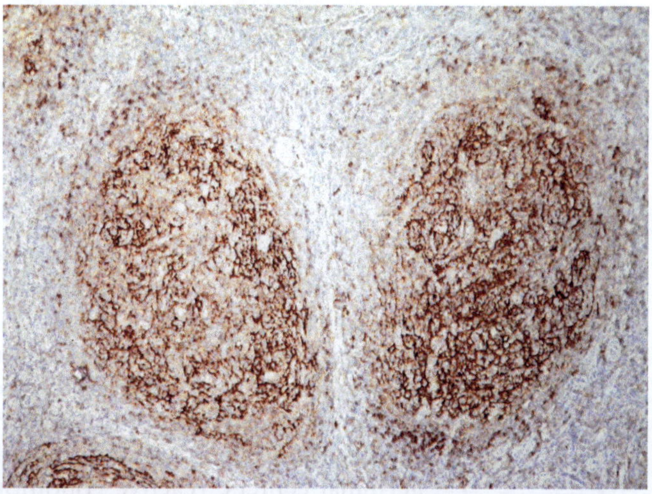

Fig. 5.16. Expanded meshwork of CD21+ FDC in the neoplastic follicles. Finer extensions of FDC in the attenuated mantle zone are also visible.

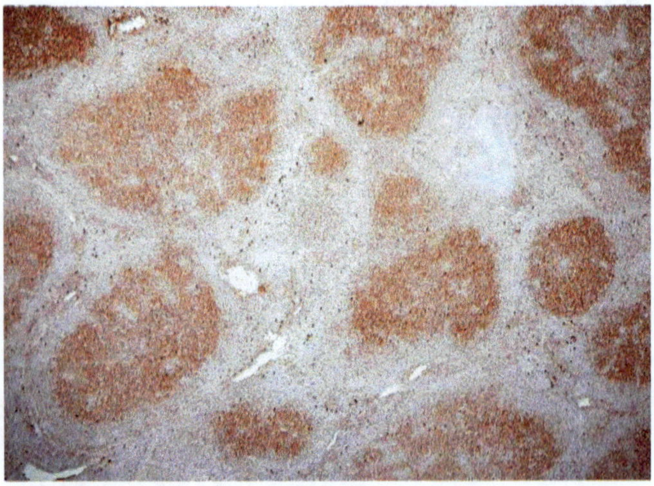

Fig. 5.17. Igκ light-chain restriction in the neoplastic follicles.

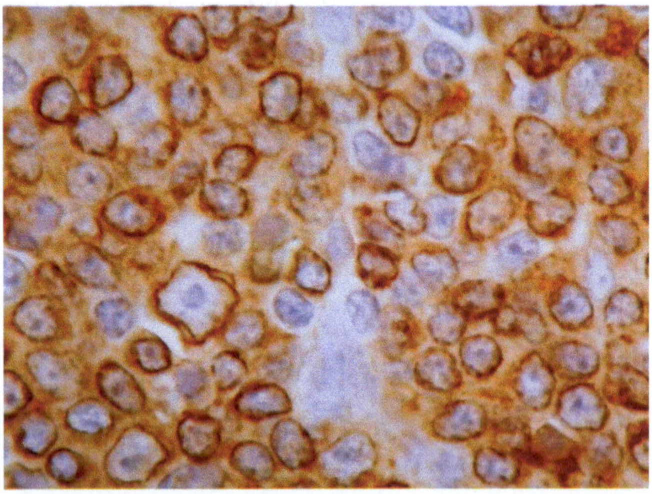

Fig. 5.18. Igκ light-chain restriction in both centroblasts and centrocytes. Distinct staining present in the perinuclear endoplasmic reticulum, cytoplasm, and occasional cell membrane.

tend to be dispersed throughout the node, involving both cortex and medulla, and extend into perinodal tissues and hilar fat. They are of uniform size and appearance, and are closely packed, often lying back-to-back. The normal sinus structure of the lymph node is usually identifiable in reactive hyperplasia but this is not the case in FL. Demonstration of this feature is enhanced with a reticulin stain. Besides hyperplasia of lymphoid follicles and enlargement of germinal centers, reactive conditions often also produce expansion of all other anatomical compartments of the lymph node which can be a helpful pointer to its benign nature.

Follicular hyperplasia is seen in reactive conditions particularly in the early phases of HIV infection, rheumatoid arthritis, toxoplasmosis, syphilis, post-transplantation lymphoproliferative disorders, and giant lymph node hyperplasia of the plasma cell type (Castleman disease).

Immunostaining for Bcl2 antigen shows immunoexpression within neoplastic follicles, but this is absent in reactive follicles with only the mantle cells staining positive to produce a marked contrasting rim around the negative germinal centers. In addition, CD45RA (MT2) is immunoexpressed in almost 60% of neoplastic follicles and has been exploited for diagnostic purposes as only weak or no scattered positivity is seen in reactive germinal center cells. This differential staining with MT2 has been postulated to be due to differences in the sialation of the CD45 protein present on the neoplastic B lymphocytes.

The staining pattern of FDC within neoplastic follicles can a useful identifier of FL. FDC can be labeled with CD21, CD35, CD23, or D2-40. Hyperplastic follicles reveal a dense FDC meshwork conforming to the polarization of the germinal centers. There is densely meshed FDC staining of the light zone and a loosely arranged, much less compact staining of the dark zone, with an accompanying delicate FDC meshwork in the mantle zone. This is different to the staining pattern in neoplastic follicles, which shows less dense, sharply defined, and expanded, often thicker dendritic processes and sometimes merging FDC meshwork. There are variable numbers of benign CD3+/CD4+ T lymphocytes within the reactive follicle and these are distributed in the light zone and at the junction of the light and mantle zones. The reticulin stain can be employed to show compression of reticulin surrounding the expanding neoplastic follicles compared to reactive ones but is often difficult to interpret and has lost popularity as a diagnostic discriminator (**Table 5.5**; **Figs. 5.19**, **5.20**, **5.21**, and **5.22**).

Other Follicular Patterns

Two other lymphomas proliferate in a follicular pattern; however, as they do not originate from cells of the germinal center, the pattern of growth is different. It is therefore important to determine whether the spherical structure or nodule is composed of one layer or two or three layers of cells. If there is more than one layer, then it is important to identify whether the structure has a normal arrangement of colors at low magnification, or an inverse arrangement, or intermingling of colors. When more than one layer of cells form a nodule, it is likely that the structure

Table 5.5
Distinction between follicular hyperplasia and follicular lymphoma

Feature	Reactive follicle	Neoplastic follicle
Polarization	Present	Absent, predominance of one cell type
Mantle zone	Present	Absent or thin and incomplete
Size and shape	Variable, not back-to-back	Uniform and rounded, crowded
Mitosis	Frequent	Not as frequent
Apoptosis	Frequent	Not as frequent
Tingle-body macrophages	Frequent	Absent
Interfollicular cells	Polymorphous	Extension of neoplastic cells
Sinus structure	Identifiable	Often not discernable
Other anatomical compartments	Often expanded	Seldom expanded
Extracapsular invasion	None	Very often present
Bcl2 staining	None	Positive
MT2 (CD45RA) staining	Mostly negative	Often positive
CD21, CD23, CD35, or D2-40	Dense DRC meshwork with polarization	Expanded DRC meshwork
CD3 and CD4	Distinctive distribution	Diffuse distribution
Reticulin stain	No compression	Compression of surrounding reticulin

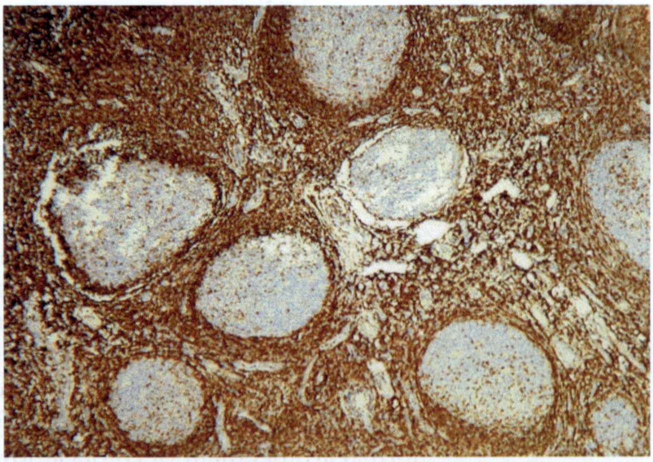

Fig. 5.19. Reactive node. Hyperplastic follicles are distributed mainly in the cortex and germinal centers are negative for Bcl2.

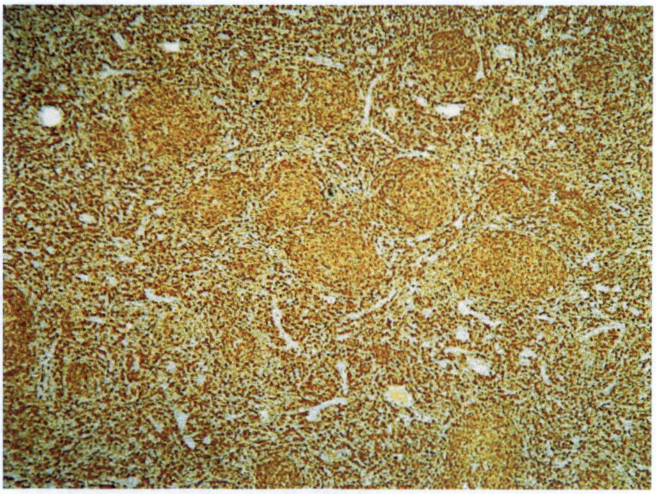

Fig. 5.20. FL. Neoplastic follicles are crowded, often back-to-back or confluent, dispersed throughout the lymph node, and stain for Bcl2.

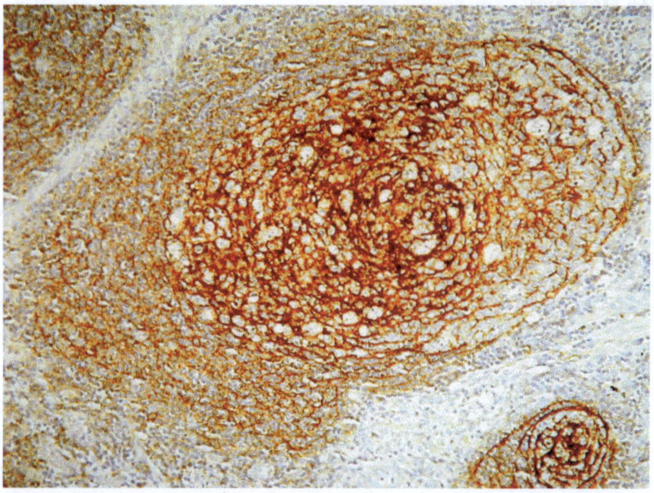

Fig. 5.21. Reactive node. Hyperplastic follicles show polarization. CD21+ FDC are denser in the light zone compared to the dark zone. The same cells are present in the eccentric mantle zone.

represents a proliferation of cells that are derived from the follicular compartment, and hence, may represent either a proliferation of marginal zone cells, mantle cells, or follicular-center cells. Thus, aside from follicular-center cell lymphoma, mantle cell lymphoma and marginal zone lymphoma also produce distinctive patterns, reflecting the expansion of the follicular compartments that they arise in.

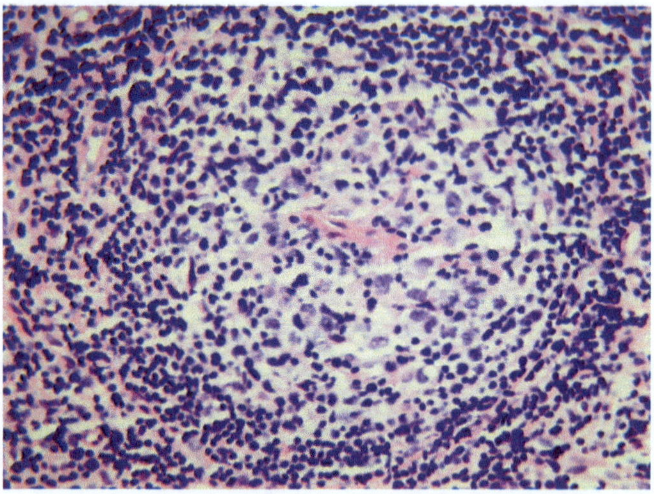

Fig. 5.22. FL. There is no polarization in the neoplastic follicle which contains a mixture of centrocytes and centroblasts and a surrounding attenuated rim of mantle cells.

Mantle Pattern

In mantle cell lymphoma and in rare mantle cell hyperplasia, variable numbers of follicles may show an exuberant proliferation of mantle cells resulting in broad and expansile mantle zones. Because of the massive expansion, adjacent mantle zones may fuse, and neoplastic mantle cells may replace or constrict the germinal centers that become inconspicuous so that the lymph node appears to be replaced by nodules of small dark lymphocytes. The lymphocytes in the mantle zones display nuclear irregularities unlike those of the regular round contours of small lymphocytes.

Benign mantle zone hyperplasia may be seen in giant lymph node hyperplasia of the hyaline vascular type (Castleman disease), mantle zone hyperplasia, and lymphocyte-rich classic Hodgkin lymphoma. In the unstimulated lymph node, germinal centers may be small and the mantle zones very thick as in primary lymphoid follicles.

Mantle Cell Lymphoma

Clinical

Mantle cell lymphoma (MCL) comprises up to 10% of non-Hodgkin lymphomas. The median age of presentation is 60 years and there is a male predominance of 2:1. While peripheral lymphadenopathy is the commonest presentation, MCL frequently involves extranodal tissues including the oropharynx and gastrointestinal tract. In the latter site, it can present as multiple lymphomatous polyposis. The spleen and bone marrow are other important sites of this disease. Most patients present with high-stage disease and peripheral blood involvement is common; the occurrence of marked lymphocytosis may mimic prolymphocytic leukemia. The median survival is 3–5 years and cure is uncommon.

The postulated normal counterpart is the peripheral B cell of the inner mantle zone, mostly naïve pre-germinal center type (**Table 5.6**).

Table 5.6
Mantle cell lymphoma – clinical

- Up to 10% of all NHL
- Median age 60 years
- Male predominance (2:1 male: female ratio)
- Peripheral lymphadenopathy, +/−splenomegaly, and bone marrow involvement
- May present in the oropharynx or as multiple lymphomatous polyposis in the GI tract
- Spleen and bone marrow may be involved with peripheral lymphocytosis
- High stage at presentation
- 3–5 years median survival; cure uncommon
- Normal counterpart – peripheral B cell of inner mantle zone, naïve pre-germinal center cells

Morphology

The propensity to grow around germinal centers produces a mantle growth pattern. When the germinal centers are completely replaced, the pattern is nodular, and less commonly a diffuse pattern may occur when the nodules become confluent. The neoplastic cells are a monotonous population of small- or intermediate-sized lymphoid cells with oval or angulated and clefted nuclei. Chromatin is granular and nucleoli inconspicuous. Centroblastic and plasma cell differentiation is not a feature of MCL and a blastoid variant occurs only uncommonly (**Figs. 5.23**, **5.24**, **5.25**, and **5.26**; **Table 5.7**).

Immunohistology

The tumor cells are positive for B cell-associated antigens CD20 and CD79a and co-express CD43 and CD5. All cases express Bcl2 and cyclin D1 but are usually CD10 and Bcl6 negative. The staining of the nodular infiltrates for Bcl2 should not be mistaken for that of follicular lymphoma. Residual germinal centers, when present, are negative for Bcl2. There is intense expression of surface IgM/IgD. CD21, CD35, and D2-40 display a proliferation of FDC in a pattern which can be distinctive and often contribute to diagnosis. The staining of FDC is especially useful when the pattern of growth is confluent and may be mistaken for a diffuse pattern of infiltration. Ki67 has been used as a prognostic marker (**Figs. 5.27**, **5.28**, **5.29**, **5.30**, **5.31**, and **5.32**).

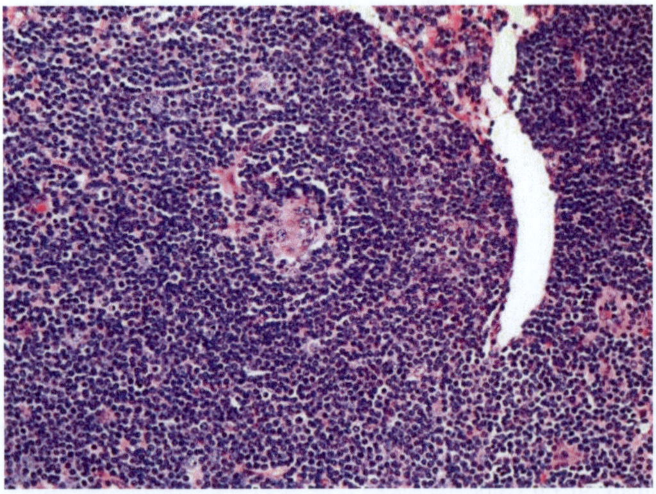

Fig. 5.23. MCL. A mantle cell pattern is imparted by the proliferation of mantle cells around a small germinal center.

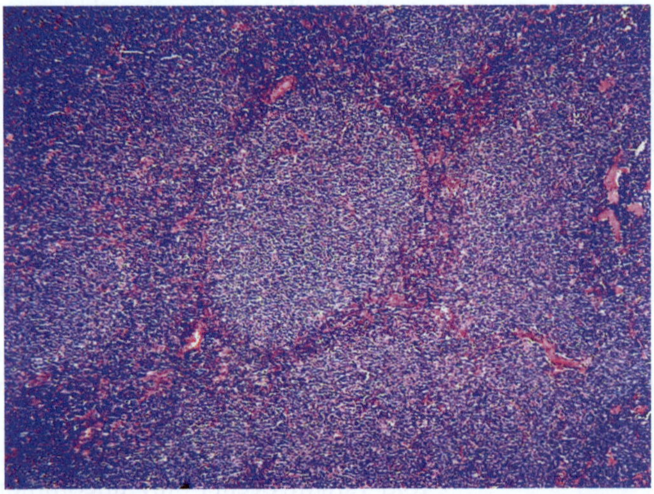

Fig. 5.24. In this case of MCL, germinal centers are not present and the pattern of growth is nodular.

Genetics

MCL shows rearranged immunoglobulin genes, *IG* genes show somatic hypermutations, but variable region genes are unmutated in the majority of cases. MCL is characterized by t(11;14)(q13;q32) with juxtaposition of the *cyclin D1* gene on chromosome 11 to the *IgH* gene on chromosome 14. The deregulated expression of *cyclin D1* is thought to overcome the supressor effects of RB1 and p27kip1, leading to the development of MCL. MCL also carries a high number of chromosomal imbalances, some such as t(8;14)(q24;q32) with *MYC* translocation being associated with an aggressive clinical course. Very

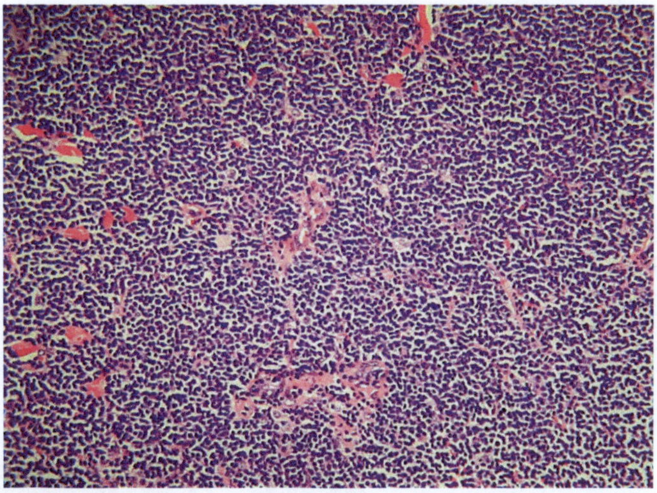

Fig. 5.25. MCL. Confluence of nodules can be mistaken for a diffuse growth pattern but stains for FDC will frequently disclose the nodular confluence.

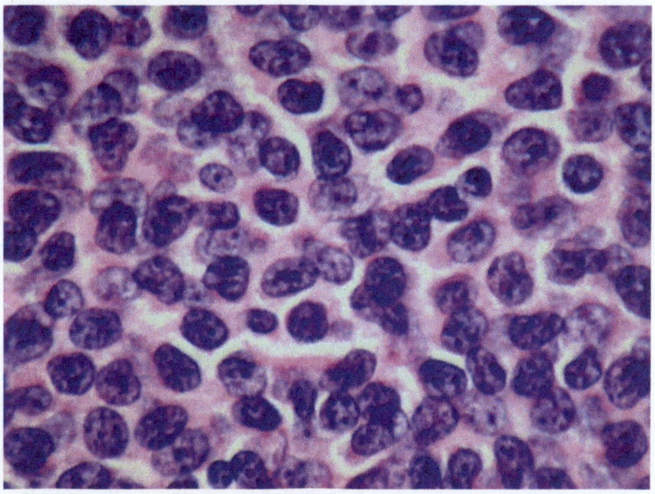

Fig. 5.26. MCL composed of small- to medium-sized neoplastic cells with scanty cytoplasm, angular nuclei, coarse chromatin, and indistinct nucleoli. Blastic and plasmacytoid differentiation is not a feature.

rarely MCL may be negative for cyclin D1 and t(11;14) but are otherwise indistinguishable from conventional MCL. Such cases show high expression of cyclin D2 or cyclin D3 and carry a t(2;12)(p12;p13) translocation, fusing *cyclin D2* to the *kappa light-chain* gene locus (**Table 5.8**).

Table 5.7
Mantle cell lymphoma – morphology

- Small- to medium-sized cells
- Angular nuclei, granular chromatin, inconspicuous nucleoli
- Patterns – Mantle growth pattern
  - Nodular pattern: replaces germinal centers
  - Diffuse pattern: nodules become confluent
- Centroblastic and plasma cell differentiation not seen
- Blastoid variant uncommon

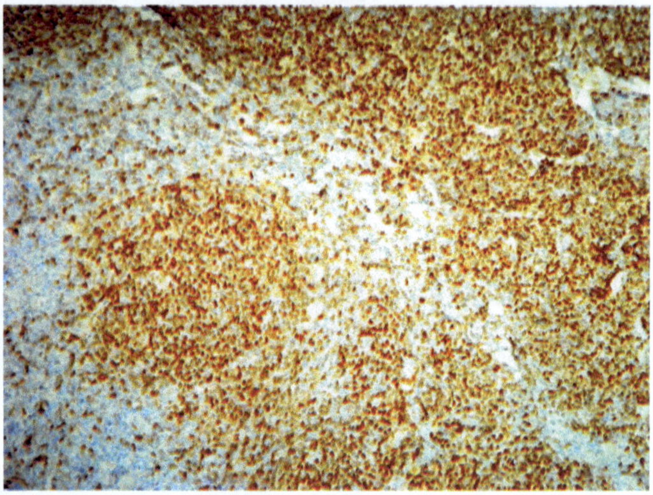

Fig. 5.27. MCL. There is strong nuclear staining for cyclin D1 in the neoplastic nodules.

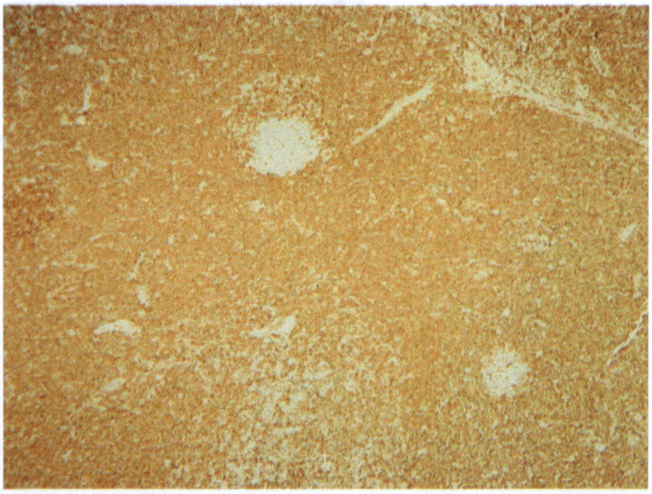

Fig. 5.28. The nodules of MCL stain for Bcl2. Two residual germinal centers in the field do not stain for the antigen.

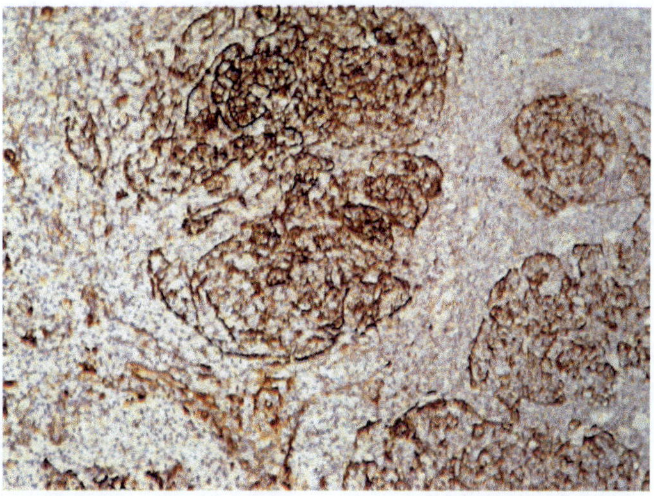

Fig. 5.29. The FDC meshwork of MCL nodules is revealed by CD21. Unlike FL, the dendritic processes are not fragmented and are thicker and appear more distinct.

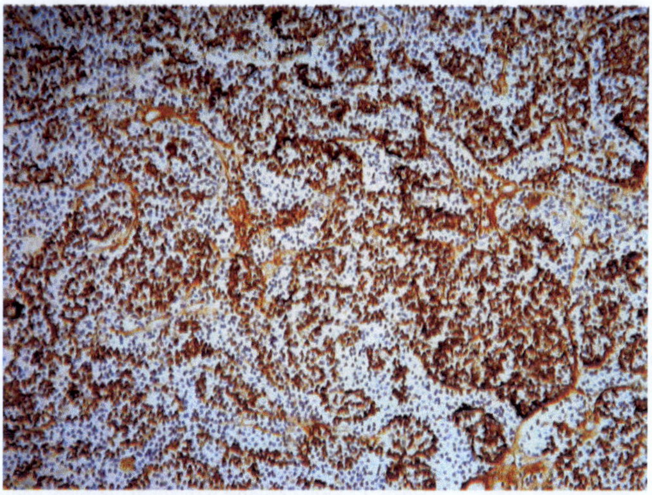

Fig. 5.30. Apparently diffuse growth pattern of MCL due to confluent proliferation of FDC as revealed by CD21 and CD35.

Marginal Zone Pattern

The marginal zone pattern is represented by spherical structures or nodules with three layers. The outermost layer is composed of monocytoid B cells that have abundant pale-staining cytoplasm and rather uniform-appearing oval nuclei. This pale marginal zone is contrasted against the inner dark rim of mantle cells, with the paler germinal center forming the third and innermost layer in the marginal zone pattern. Sometimes adjacent expanded marginal

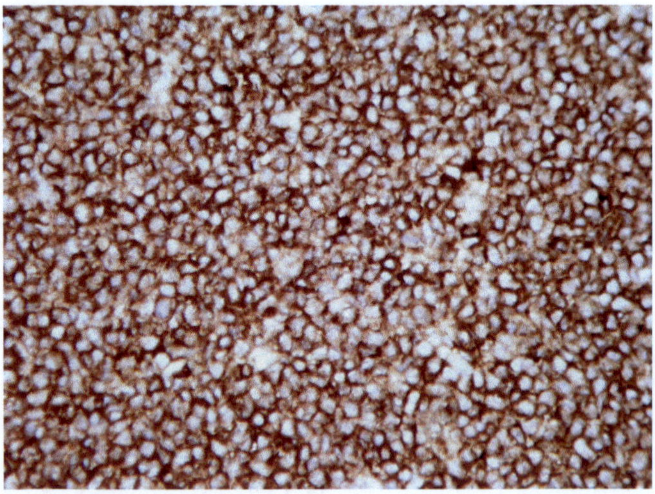

Fig. 5.31. MCL stained for CD5.

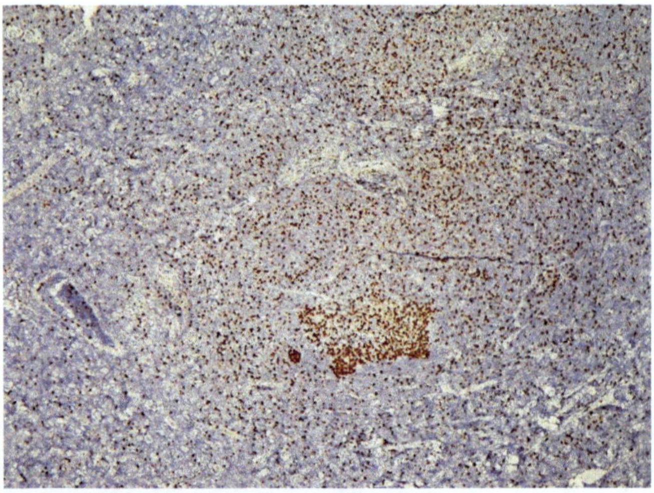

Fig. 5.32. Ki67 reveals a residual germinal center just below the center of the field. This is surrounded by MCL with a proliferative index of 43%.

zones may become confluent to produce a pale infiltrate throughout the node with scattered residual-constricted germinal centers. In approximately 30% of cases of nodal or extranodal marginal zone B cell lymphoma, the malignant cells completely surround one or more reactive follicles producing this distinct third layer or ring. Rarely the neoplastic monocytoid B cells can invade or colonize the follicle center either partially or completely with a pattern that may be indistinguishable from a true follicular pattern. However, unlike follicle-center cells, monocytoid B cells are negative for CD10, Bcl6, and MUM1. They are IgM and IgG positive but CD43 and CD5 negative.

Table 5.8
Mantle cell lymphoma – immunohistology and genetics

- B cell-associated antigens CD20+, CD79a+
- Intense IgM+/IgD+
- Bcl2+, CD43+, CD5+
- Cyclin D1+
- Bcl6–, CD10–
- Ki67 prognostic marker (>40% proliferative index poor prognosis)
- CD21, CD35, and D2-40 show expanded FDC meshwork
- t(11;14)(q13;q32) between *cyclin D1* and *IgH* genes
- *IG* rearranged, variable region genes not mutated, *IG* show somatic hypermutation

In about 10% of FL, malignant monocytoid B cells surround several malignant follicles in a marginal zone pattern. The monocytoid cells in such cases often form sheets, islands, and clusters in the interfollicular areas to result in an interfollicular growth pattern. Similar cells are also often seen in the sinuses.

In the early stages of CLL/SLL, growth centers or pseudofollicles may completely surround one or more reactive follicles and simulate a marginal zone pattern. This layer is composed of cells that are identical to those seen within the growth centers of later stages of this disease, i.e., prolymphocytes.

Lastly, several other situations may also produce a marginal zone pattern. Rare cases of peripheral T cell lymphoma, especially so called T-zone lymphomas may show scattered reactive follicles with sheets of interfollicular malignant T cells which sometimes surround one or more benign follicles to produce a marginal zone pattern. Benign diseases such as the early phase of HIV and toxoplasmosis may show monocytoid B cells in the sinuses and adjacent to follicles, rarely surrounding the reactive follicles to form a third layer. Other cells such as benign plasma cells, lymphoplasmacytoid cells, and mast cells may also surround benign follicles to simulate a marginal zone pattern.

Nodal Marginal Zone Lymphoma (Monocytoid B Cell Lymphoma)

Clinical

Nodal marginal zone lymphoma (MZL) is morphologically and immunophenotypically similar to extranodal marginal zone (MALT) lymphoma but without evidence of extranodal or splenic involvement. It makes up less than 2% of all lymphoid neoplasms, most cases occurring in adults with a median age of about

60 years, and with an equal distribution between males and females. Its occurrence in children is reported to be associated with hepatitis C virus infection. Presentation is mostly asymptomatic except for localized or generalized peripheral lymphadenopathy with occasional bone marrow and peripheral blood involvement. The presence of extranodal marginal zone lymphoma should be excluded especially as about one-third of the latter present with nodal involvement.

Prognosis is good with 60–80% of patients surviving longer than 5 years. Transformation to a large B cell lymphoma may occur and diagnosis requires the presence of sheets of large cells.

The postulated normal counterpart is the post-germinal center marginal-zone B cell (**Table 5.9**).

Table 5.9
Nodal marginal zone lymphoma (monocytoid B cell lymphoma) – clinical

- Less than 2% of all lymphoid neoplasms
- Mostly adults, median age 60 years; equal male: female distribution
- Pediatric patients uncommon; associated with hepatitis C virus infection
- Asymptomatic
- Localized or generalized peripheral nodal involvement
- Bone marrow and peripheral blood may be involved
- 30% of extranodal MZL show nodal involvement and require exclusion
- Prognosis good, 60–80% survive beyond 5 years
- Transformation to DLBCL may occur
- Postulated normal counterpart is the post-germinal center marginal-zone B cell

Morphology

The monocytoid tumor cells have medium-sized nuclei that are indented or irregular with moderate quantities of pale cytoplasm. They surround reactive follicles to produce the distinctive inverted follicular pattern, i.e., pale cells surrounding central dark cells instead of the usual dark mantle cells surrounding a paler germinal center. The reactive follicles may display features of progressive transformation of germinal centers. The expanded marginal zone is made up of variable numbers of monocytoid B cell, plasma cells, and scattered transformed B cells. When large numbers of plasma cells are present, distinction from lymphoplasmacytic lymphoma becomes difficult and the presence of a FDC meshwork suggestive of colonization of follicles favors the diagnosis of marginal zone lymphoma. Scattered clusters of

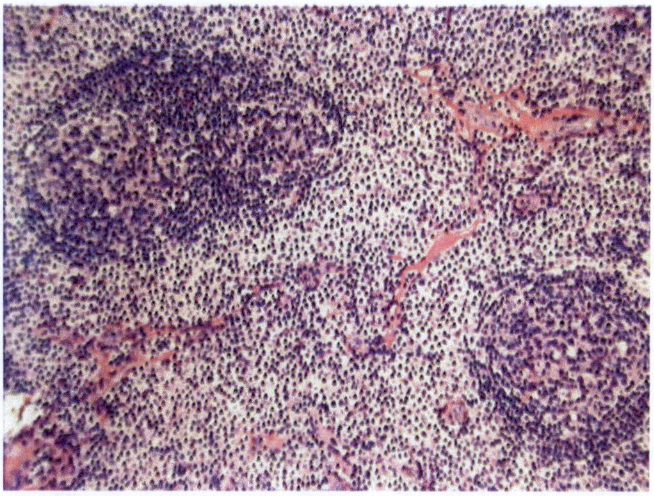

Fig. 5.33. MZL with characteristic marginal zone or inverted follicular pattern. The encircled germinal centers show progressive transformation.

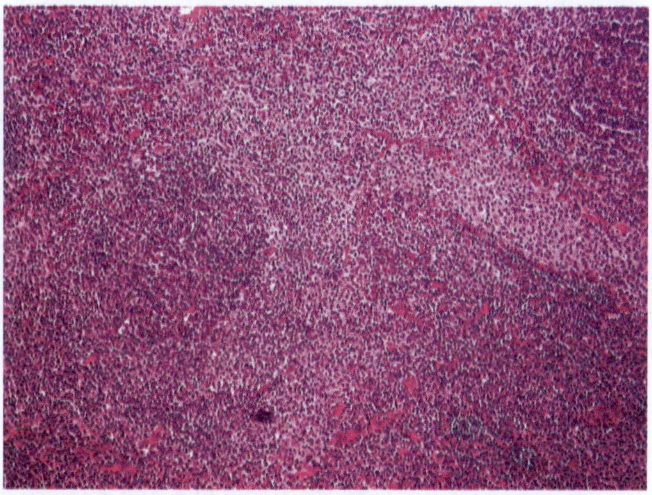

Fig. 5.34. The pale cells of MZL surround a reactive follicle and extend into an adjacent lymph node sinus (S).

epithelioid histiocytes may be present, often surrounding small groups of monocytoid cells (**Figs. 5.33**, **5.34**, **5.35**, and **5.36**; **Table 5.10**).

Immunohistology

The monocytoid cells do not express a distinctive immunophenotypic profile. They express the B cell-associated antigens CD20 and CD79a, with CD43 co-expressed in about half of the cases. Bcl-2 is positive in most cases. CD5, CD10, CD23, Bcl-6, MUM1, and cyclin D1 are negative. Surface/cytoplasmic

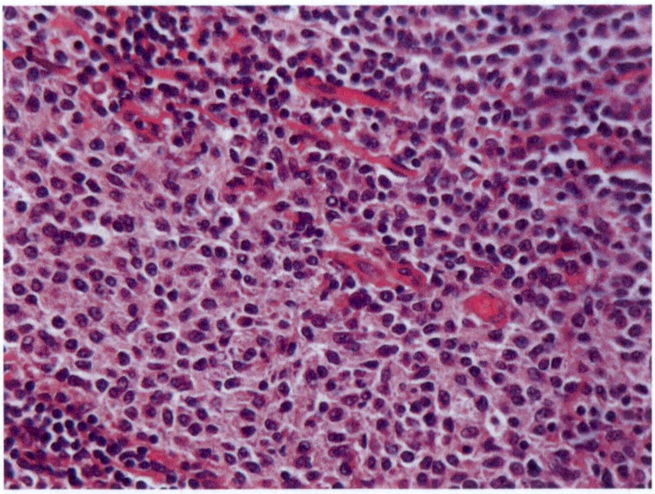

Fig. 5.35. MZL cells have irregular-shaped nuclei and moderate amounts of pale eosinophilic cytoplasm.

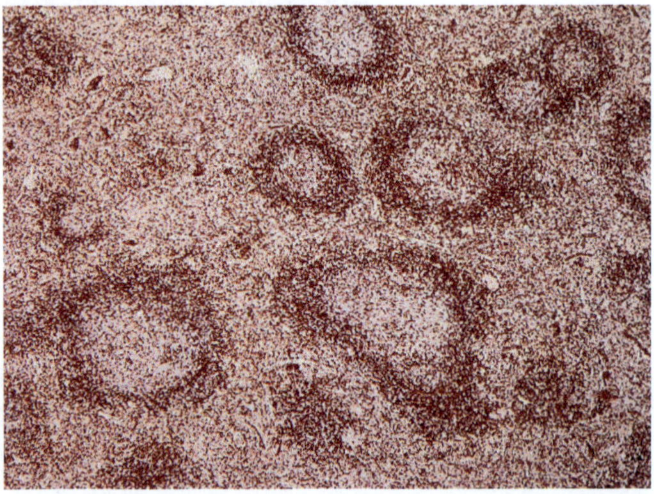

Fig. 5.36. CD5 stains the mantle cells and follicular and interfollicular T cells but the neoplastic cells of MZL do not express the antigen.

immunoglobulin is expressed, usually IgM, sometimes associated with IgD. Plasma cells show similar monoclonal immunoglobulin.

Genetics

The normal counterpart of the marginal zone lymphoma is thought to be the post-germinal center marginal-zone B cell.

The immunoglobulin genes are clonally rearranged with a predominance of mutated *VH3* and *VH4* families. The translocations associated with extranodal marginal zone lymphoma have not been detected (**Tables 5.6** and **5.11**).

Table 5.10
Nodal marginal zone lymphoma – morphology

- Marginal zone or inverted follicular pattern
- Reactive follicles present may display progressive transformation
- May be diffuse
- Colonized follicles revealed by meshwork of FDC
- Moderate quantities of pale cytoplasm, nuclei medium sized, irregular, indented
- Mixed with plasma cells and transformed B cells
- Clusters of epithelioid histiocytes may surround the monocytoid cells

Table 5.11
Nodal marginal zone lymphoma – immunohistology and genetics

- Immunophenotype not specific; CD20+, CD79a+, Bcl2+, CD43+/–
- Surface/cytoplasmic IgM+, IgD+/–, less commonly IgA+ or IgG+
- CD5–, CD10–, CD23–, Bcl6–, MUM1–, cyclin D1–
- Immunoglobulin genes clonally rearranged, predominantly of *VH3* and *VH4* families
- Translocations associated with extranodal marginal zone lymphomas are not detected

Nodular Pattern

Not all spherical structures in the lymph node are follicles. Besides neoplastic and benign follicles, a nodular pattern can be produced by other neoplastic lymphoid proliferations. Such nodules should be distinguished from true follicles. Nodules of neoplastic cells may homogenous or heterogenous in composition. Heterogenous nodules are frequently seen in Hodgkin lymphoma and when lymphoma cells colonized follicles. In contrast, homogenous nodules may be seen when neoplastic cells infiltrate and locally distend lymph node sinuses.

Heterogenous Nodules

Pseudofollicular Pattern

The true follicular pattern should be distinguished from the heterogenous nodular growth centers (also known as proliferation centers or pseudofollicles) that are seen with varying prominence in the majority of chronic lymphocytic leukemia/small lymphocytic lymphoma (CLL/SLL) and in less than 5% of lymphoplasmacytoid lymphomas. Growth centers do not occur in benign disease.

Pseudofollicles are one-layer rounded structures that are often vague and pale staining and are never surrounded by mantle zones. They occur in a dark background of small lymphocytes and may be few or many, far apart, or closely packed. Pseudofollicles are generally of small size and contain small round lymphoid cells mixed with other cells of small, medium, and large size that have features of prolymphocytes and paraimmunoblasts. Prolymphocytes are cells of intermediate size with more dispersed chromatin, small nucleoli, and scant cytoplasm. Paraimmunoblasts are larger cells with oval to round nuclei. Chromatin is dispersed and there is a central eosinophilic nucleolus and small quantities of basophilic cytoplasm. A reticulin stain shows no compression of surrounding reticulin and FDC are not present in the proliferation centers or pseudofollicles.

The presence of proliferation centers per se does not appear to correlate with the clinical course of the disease but the clinical impact of the size and number of such centers requires further studies (**Figs. 5.37**, **5.38**, and **5.39**).

Hodgkin Lymphoma (HL)

Hodgkin lymphoma (HL) is recognized to be a type of B cell lymphoma that is currently classified separately from the B cell lymphomas in the WHO classification. The neoplastic cells of HL

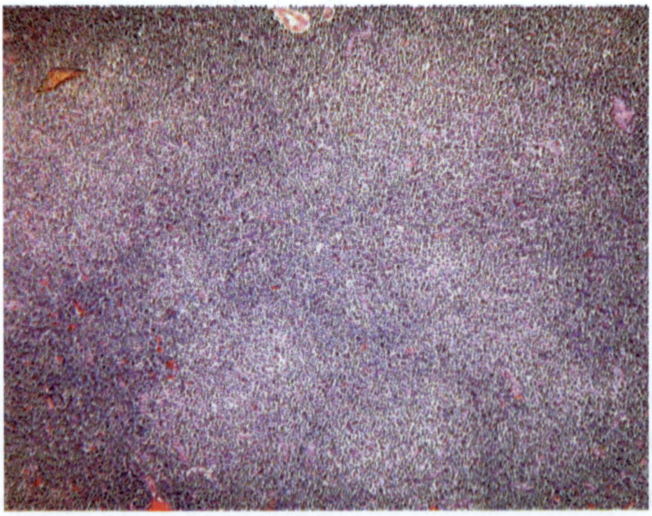

Fig. 5.37. CLL/SLL showing diffuse infiltration with vague nodules of pallor that are growth centers.

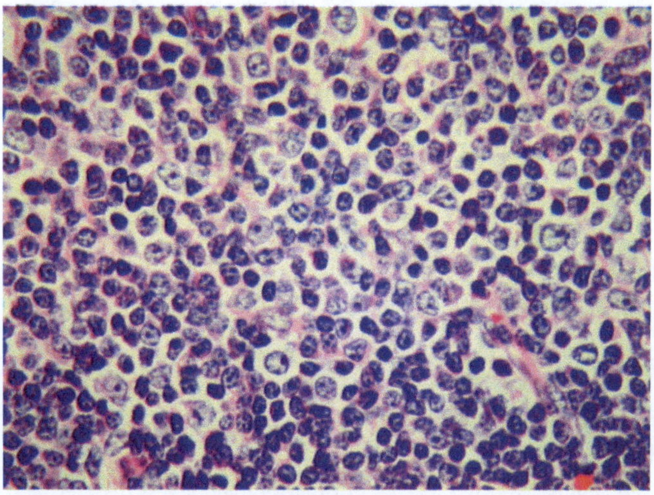

Fig. 5.38. The pallor of the growth center is due to the presence of prolymphocytes and paraimmunoblasts mixed with small lymphocytes.

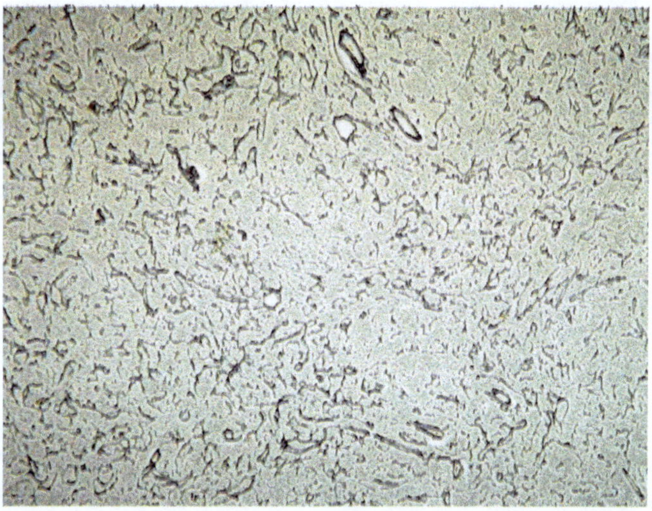

Fig. 5.39. CLL/SLL. Reticulin stain shows no compression of reticulin around the growth centers.

show clonal immunoglobulin gene (*IG)* rearrangements in >98% of cases but have lost much of their B cell specific expression program. Instead they have acquired inappropriate gene products and deregulation transcription factors that promote proliferation and abrogate apoptosis. HL makes up about 12% of all lymphomas. HL is composed of two disease entities, nodular lymphocyte-predominant Hodgkin lymphoma (NLPHL) and classical Hodgkin lymphoma (CHL). The two entities differ in clinical presentation and behavior, as well as pathology. CHL is further divided into four subtypes, namely, nodular sclerosis, mixed cellularity, lymphocyte-rich, and lymphocyte-depleted.

NLPHL, nodular sclerosis, and lymphocyte-rich subtypes present with heterogenous nodular growth patterns. In mixed cellularity CHL, the nodular growth pattern may be less distinct (**Table 5.12**).

Table 5.12
Hodgkin lymphoma

Nodular lymphocyte-predominant Hodgkin lymphoma (NLPHL)
Classical Hodgkin lymphoma (CHL)
• Lymphocyte-rich (LRCHL) – nodular pattern
• Mixed cellularity (MCCHL) – nodularity may be less distinct
• Nodular sclerosis (NSCHL) – nodular pattern
• Lymphocyte depleted (LDCHL) – occurrence infrequent, diffuse pattern

Nodular Lymphocyte-Predominant Hodgkin Lymphoma (NLPHL)

Nodular lymphocyte-predominant Hodgkin lymphoma (NLPHL) is a monoclonal B cell neoplasm characterized by a nodular pattern of proliferation with or without diffuse areas. The nodules are composed of a heterogenous population of large neoplastic cells mixed with a background of small lymphocytes, histiocytes, and epithelioid histiocytes.

This subtype of HL represents 5–6% of all HL, affecting males more frequently than females in a ratio of 3:1. It has a peak incidence of 30–50 years of age. Presentation is often as peripheral lymphadenopathy, frequently asymptomatic and localized to the cervical region. Axillary and inguinal nodes are also commonly involved. B-type symptoms are uncommon, occurring in <10% of cases. Less than 20% of patients present with high-stage disease showing involvement of multiple lymph node groups, bone marrow, liver, spleen, and bones. When this occurs, transformation to large B cell lymphoma should be excluded.

The disease is generally indolent, and in the pediatric age group a "watch and wait" strategy has been adopted. Others are treated with localized radiotherapy without chemotherapy.

Histologically, the typical pattern of NLPHL is one of large, expansile irregular nodules that partially or totally replace the lymph node. Uninvolved nodal tissue is compressed to the periphery. The neoplastic nodules are of variable size, mostly larger than reactive follicles and typically closely packed. They are composed of numerous small lymphocytes mixed with epithelioid histiocytes, FDC, and lymphocyte-predominant (LP) cells. The latter, commonly known as popcorn cells, have large nuclei with prominent nuclear folds or multilobation, and nucleoli are usually multiple, basophilic, and small. Multinucleation is less common. LP cells have moderate quantities of pale cytoplasm. The LP cells appear to be at a plane of focus different than that of surrounding small lymphocytes and are often "hidden" or partly obscured by these cells. This phenomenon is most likely the result of lymphocyte rosetting that occurs around the LP cells. Occasional cells may resemble classical Reed–Sternberg cells and internodular spread of similar cells may be present.

LP cells express the pan-B cell markers CD20, CD79a, and CD75. They are CD45+/Bcl6+/OCT-2+/BOB.1+/EMA+/– and CD15– and CD30–. This phenotypic profile allows distinction from CHL. In keeping with their B cell lineage, they also express J chain and have been described to express IgG and Igκ. Small T cells form spontaneous rosettes around the LP cells. These cells are CD3+/CD4+/CD57+/Bcl6+ and are thought to be intrafollicular T-helper cells, as they stain for PD-1. Unlike in CHL, NLPHL is negative for Epstein–Barr virus. FDC are found within the nodules of NLPHL and are useful to highlight focal areas of nodularity in a pattern that otherwise may appear diffuse. The nodules of NLPHL may be associated with progressive transformed germinal centers (PTGC) and require distinction (*see* below). A diffuse pattern has rarely been ascribed to NLPHL and most such cases have been reclassified as T cell/histiocyte-rich B cell lymphoma, NLPHL with large areas of a diffuse pattern, or CHL. Only very rare cases of NLPHL with an entirely diffuse pattern exist (**Figs. 5.40**, **5.41**, **5.42**, **5.43**, **5.44**, **5.45**, **5.46**, **5.47**, **5.48**, and **5.49**; **Table 5.13**).

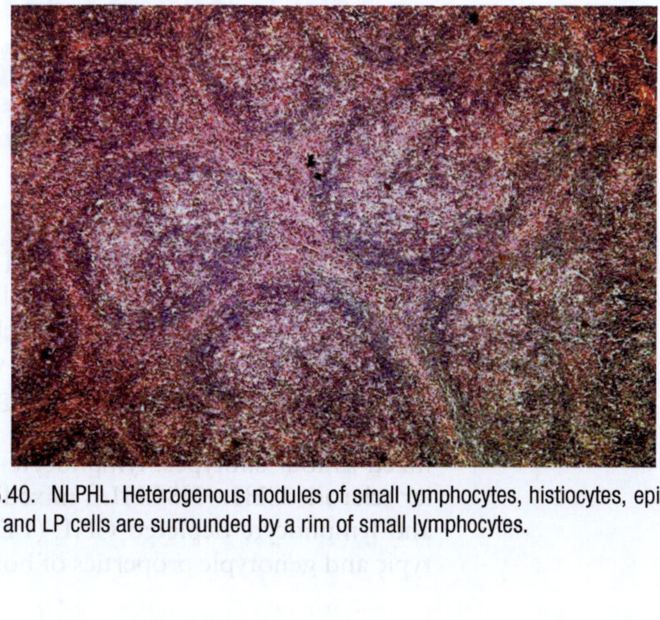

Fig. 5.40. NLPHL. Heterogenous nodules of small lymphocytes, histiocytes, epithelioid cells, and LP cells are surrounded by a rim of small lymphocytes.

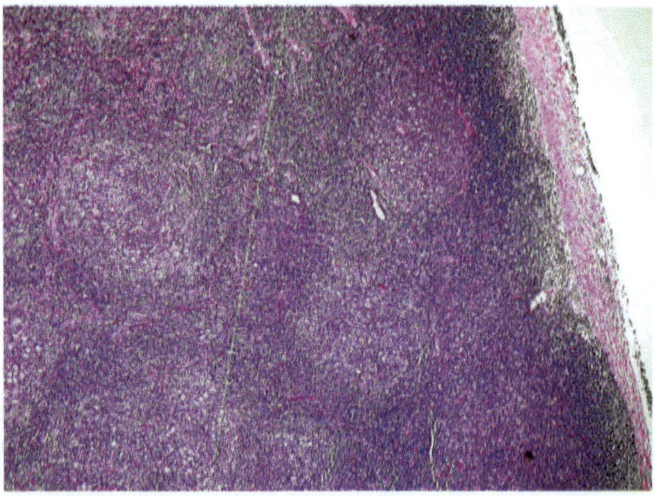

Fig. 5.41. Another example of NLPHL in which the nodules are less-well defined as the rim of surrounding small lymphocytes is not present.

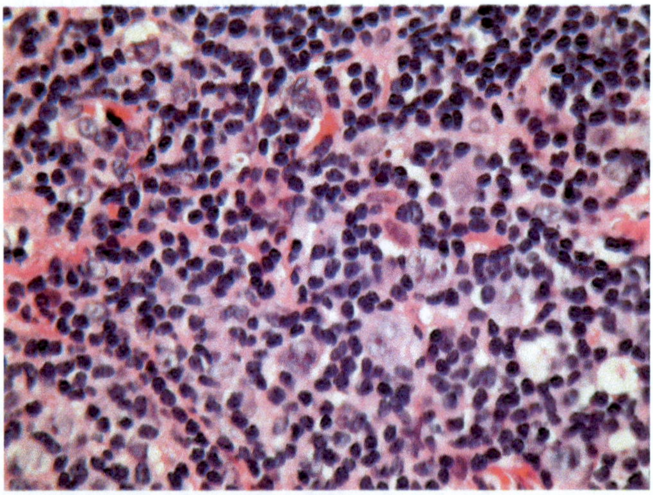

Fig. 5.42. NLPHL. The nodules comprise mostly small lymphocytes and prominent multilobated LP cells.

Classical Hodgkin Lymphoma (CHL)

Classical Hodgkin lymphoma (CHL) is a monoclonal neoplasm, in most cases derived from B cells. This lymphoma is composed of mononuclear Hodgkin cells (HC) and multinucleated Reed–Sternberg cells (RSC) in a variable background of heterogenous reactive cells comprising small lymphocytes, epithelioid histiocytes, plasma cells, and eosinophils. CHL is recognized as four subtypes: lymphocyte-rich CHL (LRCHL), nodular sclerosis CHL (NSCHL), mixed cellularity CHL (MCCHL), and lymphocyte-depleted CHL (LDCHL). The immunophenotypic and genotypic properties of both HC and RSC in these four

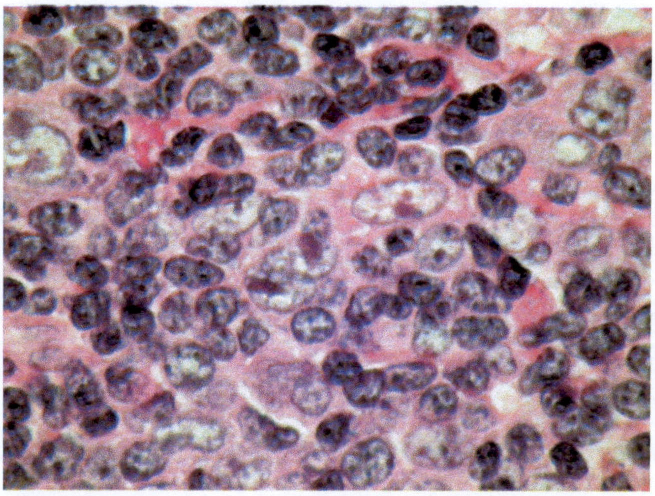

Fig. 5.43. NLPHL. Several LP or popcorn cells are present in the background of small lymphocytes. The LP cells are often partly obscured by small lymphocytes.

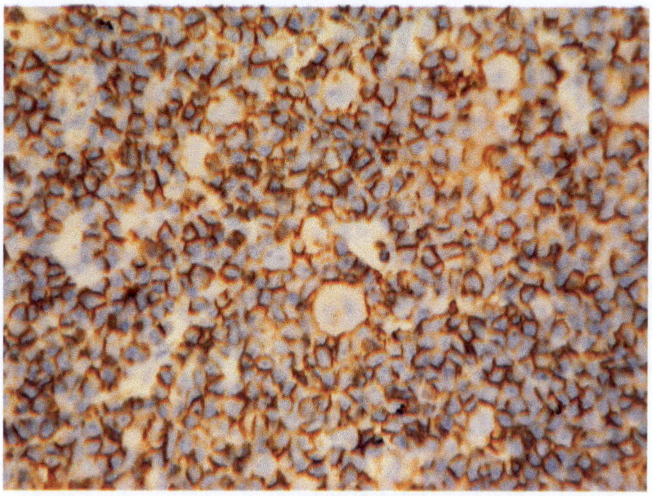

Fig. 5.44. NLPHL. Unlike RSC, LP cells typically stain for CD45.

subtypes are identical but they show differences in clinical presentation and their association with Epstein–Barr virus.

Nodular Sclerosis Classical Hodgkin Lymphoma (NSCHL)

Nodular sclerosing classical Hodgkin lymphoma (NSCHL) is a subtype of CHL with a distinctly nodular pattern of growth. This lymphoma is made up of heterogenous nodules of small lymphocytes and other inflammatory cells with variable numbers of intermingled RSC that are circumscribed by bands of collagen. At least one nodule must be surrounded by the fibrous bands. Formalin fixation may produce a retraction artifact around the HC and RSC to produce a lacuna cell appearance.

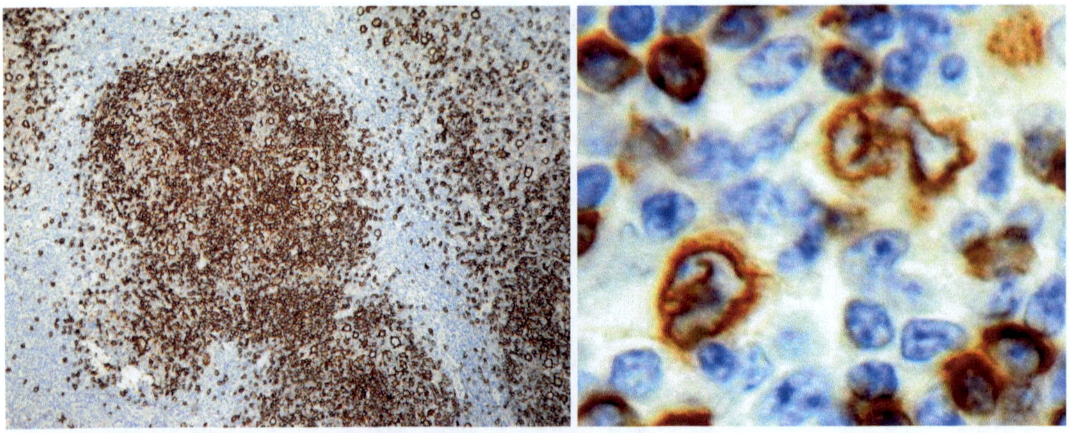

Fig. 5.45. The nodules of NLPHL comprise predominantly of CD20+ cells. LP cells are also CD20+/CD79a+. *Inset:* CD79a staining of LP cells.

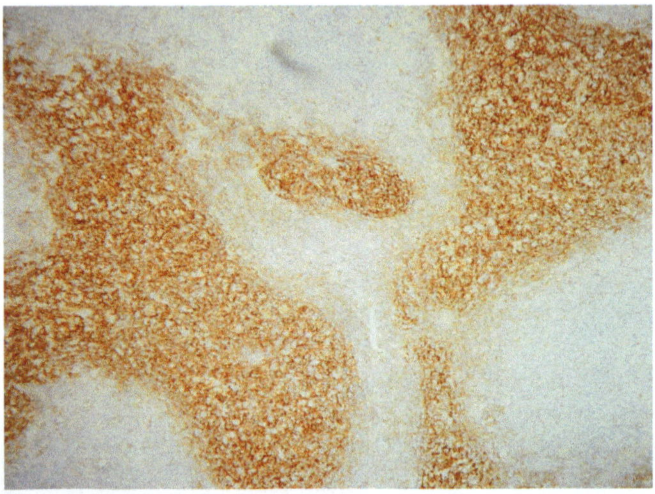

Fig. 5.46. NLPHL. CD23 reveals a proliferation of FDC in the nodules with confluence of adjacent nodules.

This subtype forms about 70% of all CHL with a peak incidence at 15–34 years of age and equal male to female ratio. Mediastinal involvement is very common, and bulky disease is seen in about half the cases and presentation is often with B symptoms and with stage-II disease (**Figs. 5.50**, **5.51**, **5.52**, **5.53**, and **5.54**; **Table 5.14**).

Mixed Cellularity Classical Hodgkin Lymphoma (MCCHL)

Mixed cellularity CHL (MCCHL) comprises about 20–25% of CHL. MCCHL may show a vaguely nodular pattern of growth with classical RSC among a mixed inflammatory background but without nodular sclerosing fibrosis. Peripheral nodes are commonly involved, and the spleen is involved in 30%, bone marrow

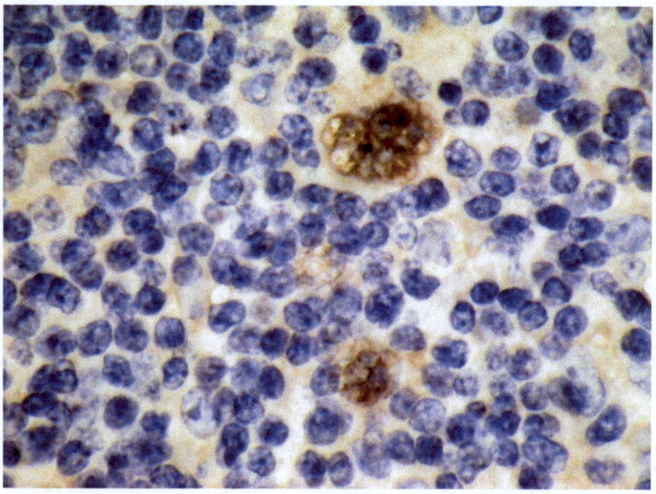

Fig. 5.47. NLPHL. LP cells stain for OCT-2.

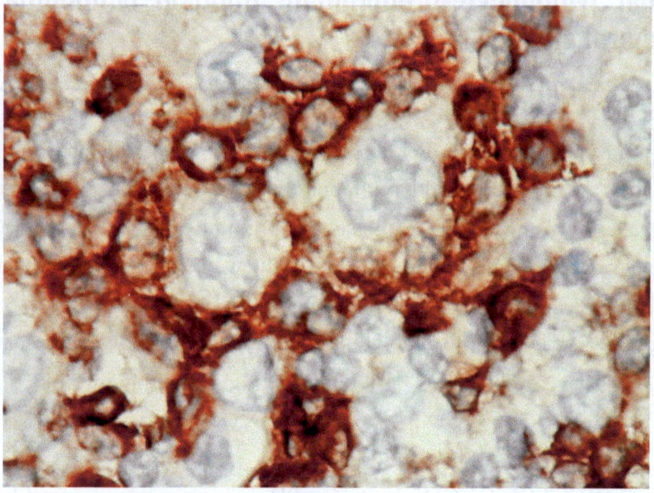

Fig. 5.48. NLPHL. CD3 staining reveals small T cells rosetting around the LP cells.

in 10%, and the liver and other organs in <3% of cases. B symptoms are frequent.

The lymph node architecture is effaced, although an interfollicular pattern may be seen. Sclerosis may be present but not in the form of the circumscribing broad bands of fibrous tissue that identifies NSCHL. Background reactive cells are a mixture of small lymphocytes, eosinophils, plasma cells, and epithelioid histiocytes. RSC are large, have at least two nuclei or lobes, and abundant, slightly basophilic or amphophilic cytoplasm. Nuclear membranes are thick and often irregular; chromatin is pale and there is usually one prominent eosinophilic nucleolus surrounded by a perinucleolar clearing or halo. Diagnostic RSC must have

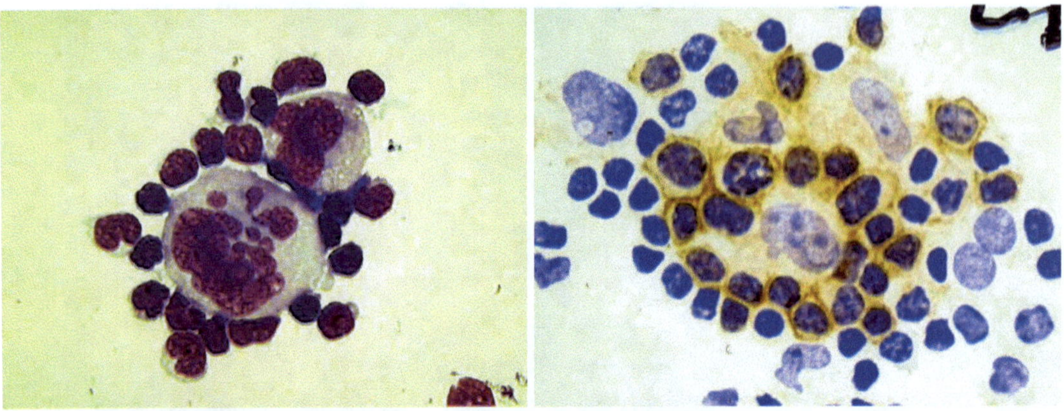

Fig. 5.49. Imprints of LP cells and rosettes. The right panel shows expression of CD4 by the rosetting lymphocytes which also expressed CD57 (not shown).

Table 5.13
Nodular lymphocyte-predominant Hodgkin lymphoma (NLPHL) clinical features and morphology

• About 5% of all HL
• Younger patients (peak incidence 30–50 years), male: female ratio 3:1
• Asymptomatic peripheral lymphadenopathy, often localized to cervical region
• Excellent prognosis but relapses common; may transform to DLBCL
• Total or partial replacement by large cellular nodules with irregular outlines
• May be accompanied by follicular hyperplasia and PTGC
• Nodules composed of small lymphocytes, epithelioid histiocytes, and LP or popcorn cells
• LP cells have marked nuclear lobation, variably prominent nucleoli, and pale cytoplasm
• LP cells are CD45+, CD20+, CD79a+, Oct-2+, Bob.1+, EMA+, CD15–, and CD30–/+
• FDC meshwork within nodules
• Small CD3+, CD4+, CD57+,Bcl6+, PD-1+ cells rosette around LP cells often "hiding" LP cells
• Necrosis and fibrosis absent

at least two nucleoli within two separate nuclear lobes. HC are mononuclear variants of RSC. Necrobiotic or mummified HC and RSC are often seen. While the neoplastic cells form 0.1 to 10% of the cellular infiltrate, they are essential for the diagnosis and need to be with the appropriate background infiltrate. However, diagnostic RSC are not required in a patient with CHL diagnosed at another site. A granulomatous response may be present.

The neoplastic cells of CHL exhibit the phenotype of CHL being CD15+, CD30+, CD20–/+, CD79a–/+, CD45–, Oct-2–, and Bob.1–. CD15 and CD30 are typically expressed in the cell membrane with accentuation in the Golgi. CD15 may be

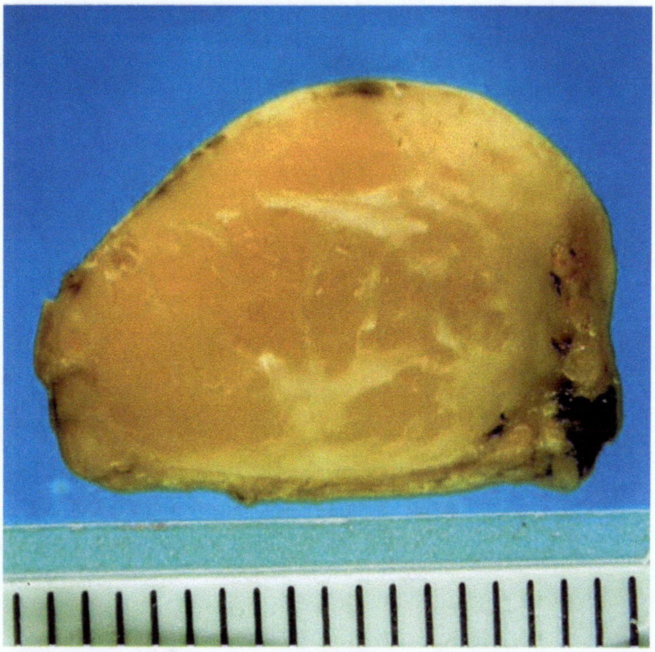

Fig. 5.50. NSCHL in axillary lymph node. Visible bands of fibrous tissue extend from the right half of the node into the remaining nodal tissue.

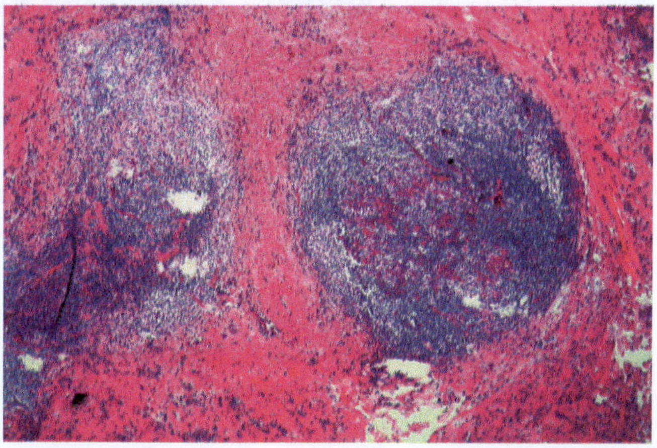

Fig. 5.51. NSCHL. Section from the gross specimen shown in **Fig. 5.46**. Thick bands of collagen encircle heterogenous nodules of lymphoid and inflammatory cells and histiocytes.

only expressed in a minority of the neoplastic cells and may be restricted only to the Golgi. Up to 20% of cases may stain for CD20. The B cell origin of CHL is further supported by expression of B cell-specific activator protein PAX5/BSAP, with weaker staining in RSC than in reactive B cells. IRF4/MUM1 is consistently positive in CHL. EBV-encoded LMP-1 and EBER are expressed much more frequently in MCCHL (about 75%) than in

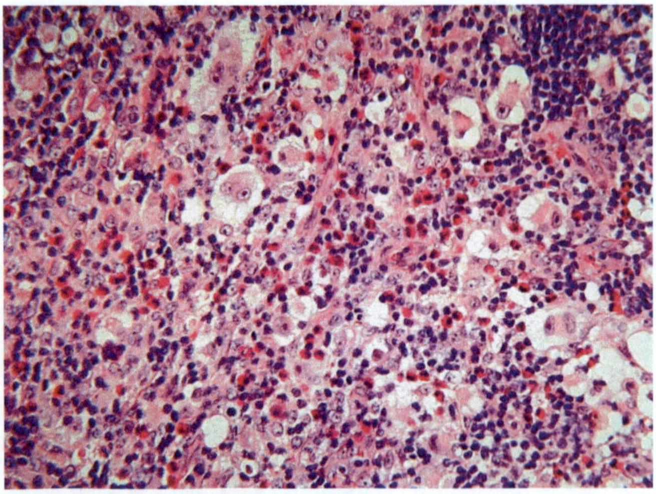

Fig. 5.52. The nodules of NSCHL are composed of small lymphocytes, eosinophils, plasma cells, histiocytes, epithelioid cells, and many lacuna cells with prominent eosinophilic nucleoli.

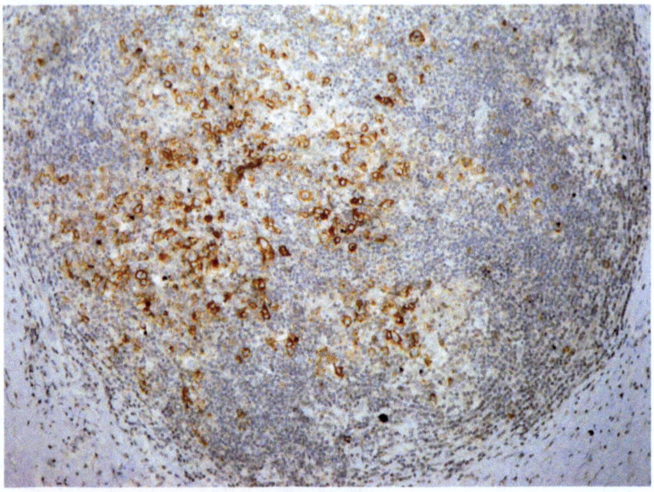

Fig. 5.53. NSCHL. Numerous lacuna cells in the nodule stain for CD15. They were also CD30+.

LRCHL and NSCHL (10–40%) (**Figs. 5.55**, **5.56**, **5.57**, **5.58**, **5.59**, and **5.60**; **Table 5.15**).

Lymphocyte-Rich Classical Hodgkin Lymphoma (LRCHL)

Lymphocyte-rich classical Hodgkin lymphoma has a frequency similar to that of NLPHL, comprising about 5% of all CHL. The median age is similar to that of NLPHL and higher than other subtypes of CHL. Presentation is similar to that of NLPHL with peripheral nodes commonly involved. Mediastinal involvement and bulky disease are uncommon, most patients present with stage I or II disease, and B symptoms being rare.

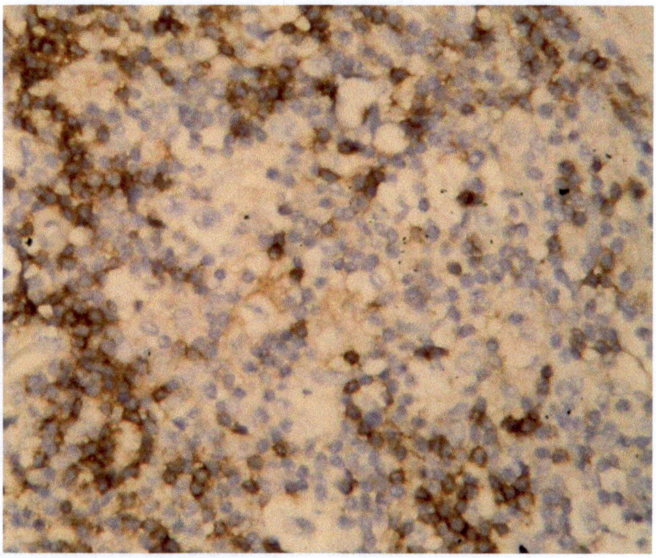

Fig. 5.54. Lacuna cells are CD45– (*arrows*).

Table 5.14
Nodular sclerosis classical Hodgkin lymphoma (NSCHL)

• Makes up 70% of all CHL
• Age peak 15–34 years, male to female ratio equal
• Mediastinal involvement common
• Bulky disease, B symptoms, Stage I or II disease at presentation
• Prominent nodularity
• Nodules of heterogenous lymphoid and inflammatory cells with mixed RSC
• Nodules surrounded by bands of fibrosis – at least one such nodule required for diagnosis
• Retraction artifact around RSC and HC produces lacuna cell appearance
• RSC and HC are CD45–, CD15+, CD30+, CD20–/+, EMA–, Oct-2–, Bob.1–

LRCHL has two growth patterns, commonly a nodular, and rarely a diffuse pattern. The nodules are composed of small lymphocytes with RSC and may harbor small or regressed germinal centers. Neutrophils and eosinophils are generally absent. The RSC may resemble LPs or mononuclear lacunar cells so that the appearances and presentation can be confused with NLPHL, and in the past about one-third of NLPHL have been found to be LRCHL. Distinction of these two entities is based on the demonstration of the typical immunophenotype for RSC, i.e., CD15+/–, CD30+, CD45–, CD75–, and CD20–/+. In contrast, LP cells of NLPHL are CD45+, CD75+, CD20+,

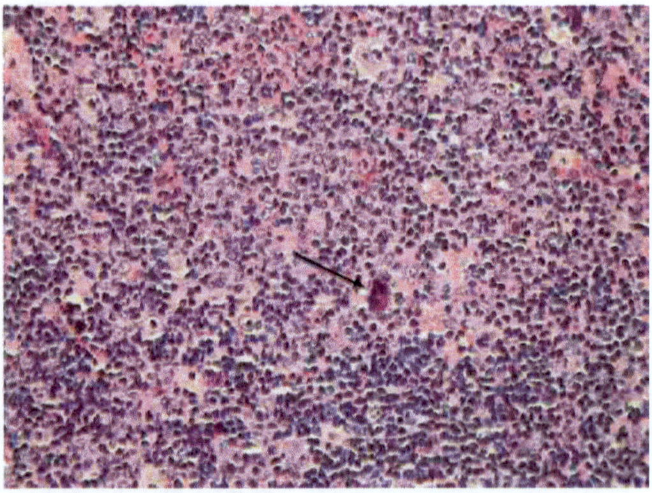

Fig. 5.55. MCCHL comprises epithelioid histiocytes, plasma cells, and occasional eosinophils. Large HC and RSC are present including a large mummified cell (*arrow*).

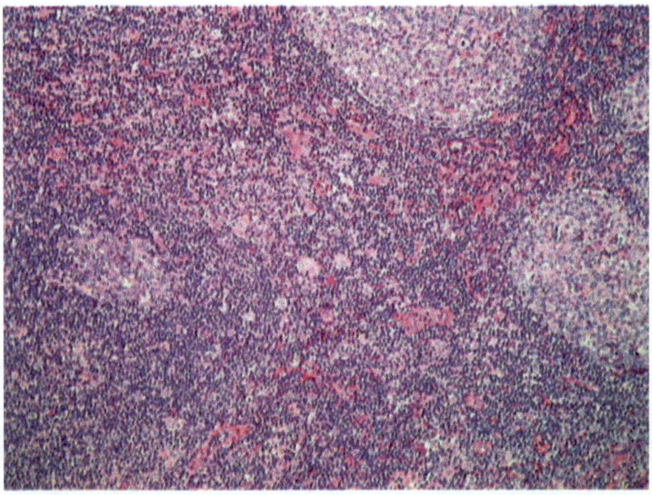

Fig. 5.56. MCCHL. Germinal centers are preserved in this variant which shows interfollicular polymorphous infiltration that includes diagnostic RS cells.

CD79a+, Oct-2+, Bob.1+, and CD15− and CD30−/+. In addition, LP cells show rosetting CD3+ or CD4+, CD57+ T cells, a feature not seen with LRCHL. Rarely, the nodules of LRCHL may be surrounded by fibrous bands with randomly distributed RSC in T cell-rich zones. The WHO classification recommends that such cases are better typed as NSCHL. The diffuse form of LRCHL may show a mixture of histiocytes in the background of small lymphocytes. EBV LMP-1 expression is more frequent in LRCHL than NLPHL but less frequent than in MCCHL.

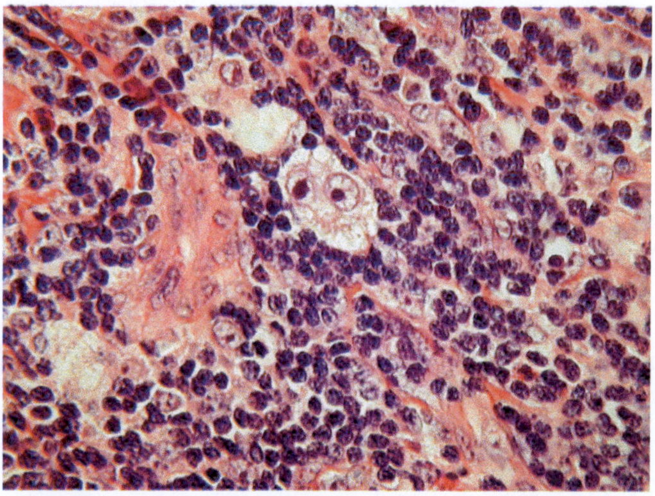

Fig. 5.57. MCCHL. Diagnostic RSC are bilobed with a large eosinophilic nucleolus in each lobe. Nuclei are vesicular and nuclear membranes distinct. Cytoplasm is abundant.

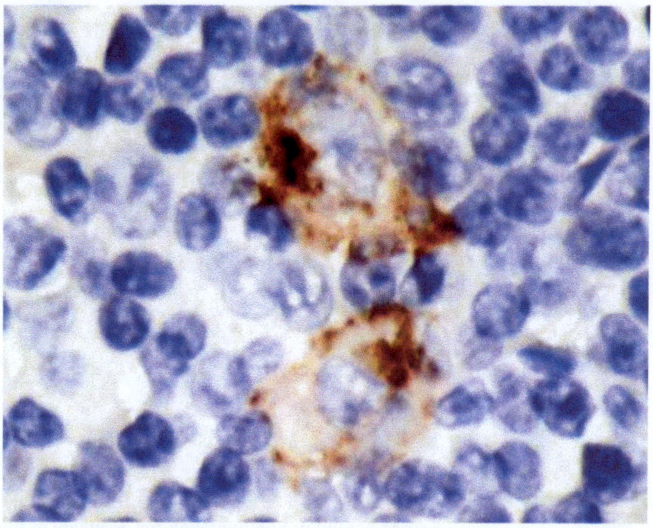

Fig. 5.58. The typical staining pattern of CD15 in HC and RSC is one of cell membrane with dot-like Golgi staining.

Survival and progression-free survival are slightly better than in other subtypes of CHL and similar to that of NLPHL, relapses being more common in the latter (**Figs. 5.61**, **5.62**, **5.63**, **5.64**, **5.65**, and **5.66**; **Table 5.16**).

Lymphocyte-Depleted Classical Hodgkin Lymphoma (LDCHL)

Lymphocyte-depleted classical Hodgkin lymphoma (LDCHL) has a diffuse growth pattern, but for convenience it will be discussed here with other subtypes of CHL. The definition of this subtype has undergone several changes and a proportion of cases

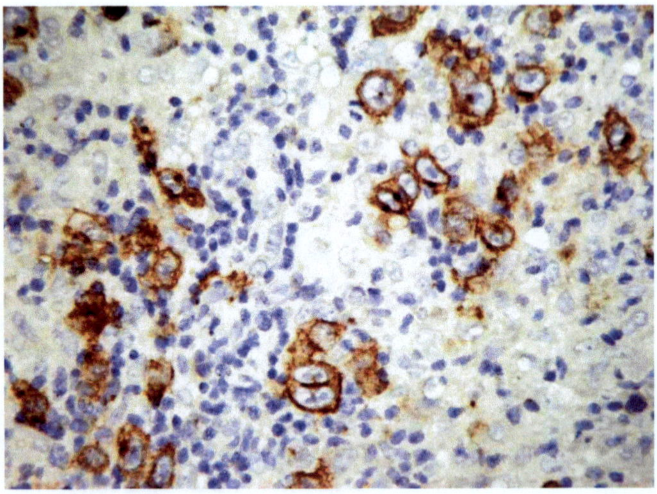

Fig. 5.59. CD30 in MCCHL. The pattern of membrane and Golgi staining is similar to that of CD15, although many more cells stain for CD30.

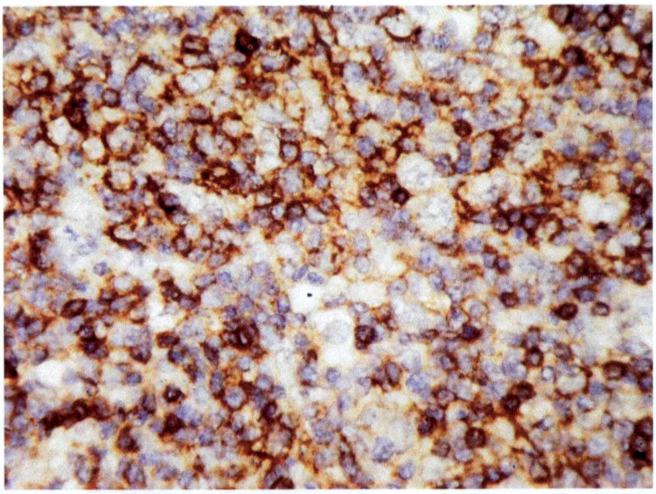

Fig. 5.60. HC and RSC are CD45–. Membrane staining of surrounding small lymphocytes should not be mistaken for positivity in the neoplastic cells.

with this designation has been reclassified as other lymphoma entities, as such, previously described definitions and clinicopathological correlations may not be tenable. It is likely that a *de novo* diagnosis of LDCHL is uncommon.

The morphology of LDCHL is highly variable but shows the unifying features of depletion of non-neoplastic lymphoid cells and an abundance of RSC and HC which can produce a sarcomatous appearance. Differentiation from anaplastic large cell lymphoma may pose a problem but the RSC show the characteristic immunophenotype and express LMP-1 and EBER.

Table 5.15
Mixed cellularity classical Hodgkin lymphoma (MCCHL)

• Peripheral nodes involved, spleen involved in 30%, bone marrow in 10%
• Nodular pattern less pronounced than in other subtypes of CHL
• Interfollicular pattern may occur
• Diagnostic RSC have at least two large eosinophilic nucleoli in two separate nuclear lobes, abundant amphophilic cytoplasm, thick, irregular nuclear membranes, pale chromatin
• Background of small lymphocytes, plasma cells, and eosinophils required for diagnosis
• Mummified (necrobiotic) cells common
• HC are mononuclear forms of RSC
• Sclerosis may be present but does not circumscribe lymphoid nodules as in NSCHL
• Granulomatous reaction common
• LMP-1 and EBER positive in 75% of cases
• Immunophenotype typical of RSC – CD15+, CD30+, CD45–, CD20–/+, Oct-2–, Bob.1–

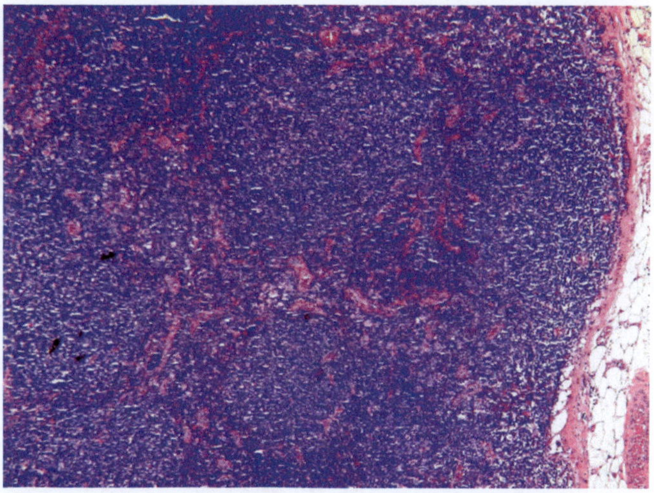

Fig. 5.61. LRCHL. The nodular proliferations are not dissimilar to those of NLPHL except that typical RSC are present. Some nodules contain regressed germinal centers.

Post-transplant Lymphoproliferative Disorders

The post-transplant lymphoproliferative disorders (PTLD) arise as a consequence of immunosuppression in a recipient of a solid organ, bone marrow, or stem cell allograft. The risk varies with the type of allograft and the immunosuppressive regime used. PTLD is a spectrum of lymphoid or plasmacytoid proliferations that range from usually Epstein–Barr virus (EBV)-driven infectious mononucleosis-type polyclonal proliferations to EBV-positive or EBV-negative proliferations that are indistinguishable from a subset of B cell. Less frequently PTLD is similar to T cell lymphomas that occur in the immunocompromised. As with

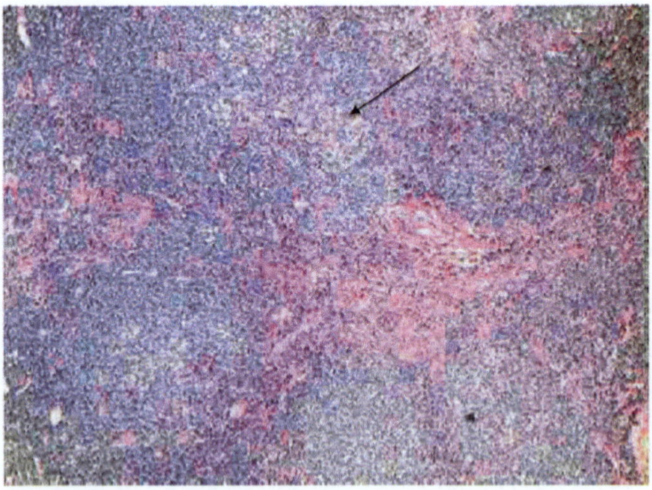

Fig. 5.62. LRCHL with a nodular pattern. The mottled area between the nodules contains RSC and HC (*arrow*).

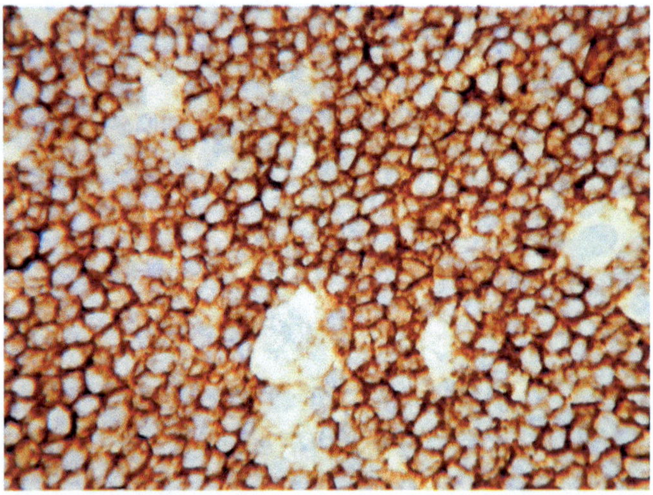

Fig. 5.63. LRCHL. The nodules comprise mostly of small B cells that are CD20+. There is no staining of HC and RSC.

other immunodeficiency-associated lymphoproliferations, PTLD is mainly due to impaired T cell immunity to the EBV. However, approximately 20% of PTLD are EBV negative and may involve other unknown viruses or due to chronic antigenic stimulation by the transplant itself. EBV-negative cases occur after 4–5 years post-transplantation compared to EBV-positive cases that occur earlier to 6–10 months of post-transplantation. Both conditions may regress with reduction of immunosuppression and can be nodal or extranodal, the latter occasionally involving the allograft. Over 90% of PTLD in solid organ recipients are of host

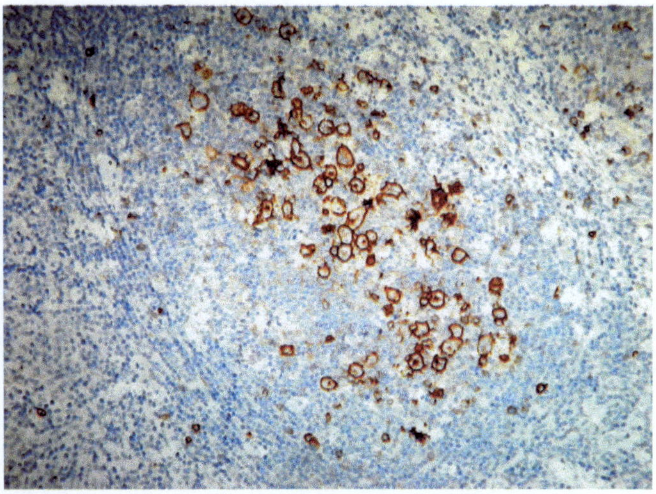

Fig. 5.64. LRCHL, nodular variant with CD30+ RSC within a nodule.

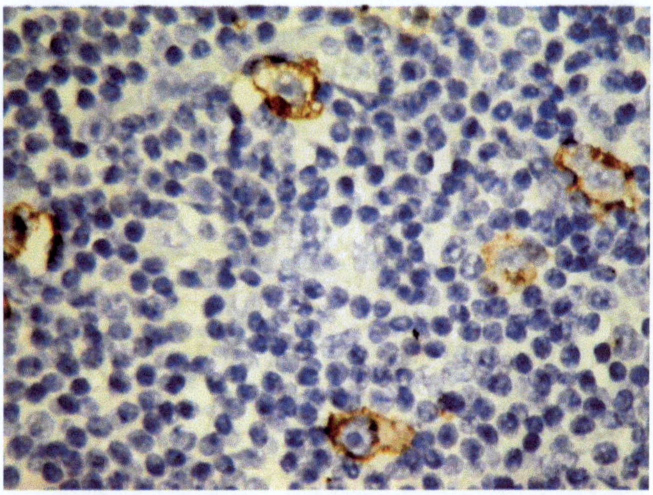

Fig. 5.65. Immunophenotyping of the atypical cells provides the best distinction from NLPHL. The RSC and HC are CD15+. They are also CD30+, OCT-2–, Bob.1–, CD45–, CD75–, CD20–/+, and EMA-.

origin. Donor origin PTLD appears most common in liver and lung allograft recipients and often involves the allograft. Bone marrow allografts are also associated with donor origin PTLD.

Prognosis for "early" lesions, particularly in children, is excellent, PTLD regressing with reduction of immune suppression. Polymorphic and less often monomorphic PTLD may also regress with reduction in immune suppression but rebound and chronic rejection may lead to loss of graft and death.

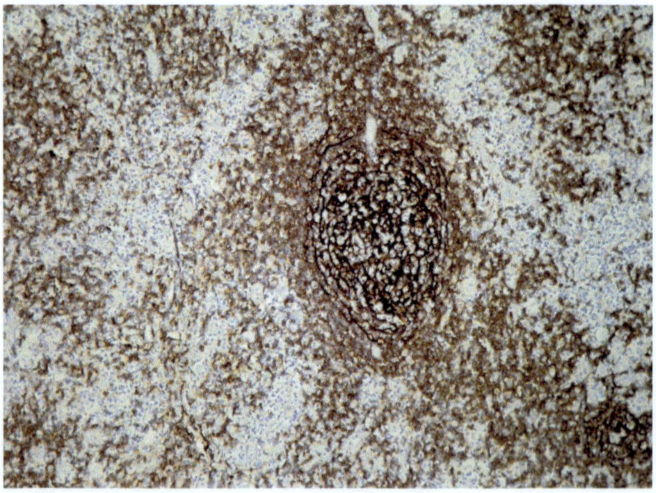

Fig. 5.66. LRCHL. CD23 staining reveals a meshwork of FDC that form the nodule and extend into the internodular areas. The denser area represents a germinal center within the nodule.

Table 5.16
Lymphocyte-Rich classical Hodgkin lymphoma (LRCHL)

- Incidence similar to NLPHL, 5% of all HL
- Presents with stage I or II disease, B symptoms rare
- Nodular pattern prominent, can be confused with NLPHL, diffuse pattern rare
- Nodules may harbor regressed germinal center
- Nodules composed of lymphocytes, plasma cells, eosinophils, and epithelioid cells
- Classic RSC present, occasional cells resemble LP cells of NLPHL
- Distinction from NLPHL based on immunophenotype of RSC, i.e., CD15+, CD30+, CD45−, CD20−/+, Oct-2−, Bob.1−
- Prognosis slightly better than other subtypes of CHL, similar to NLPHL

Plasmacytic Hyperplasia and Infectious Mononucleosis-Like PTLD

The early lesion occurs in young patients who were negative for EBV at the time of transplantation. Nodes and tissues of Waldeyer's ring are typically involved. Architecture is preserved and the plasmacytic hyperplasia shows florid hyperplasia of follicles and paracortex that is expanded by numerous polyclonal plasma cells, small lymphocytes, and generally infrequent immunoblasts. The infectious mononucleosis-like lesion shows expansion of the paracortex by numerous immunoblasts in a background of small lymphocytes. Regression may be spontaneous or occurs following reduction in immune suppression.

Polymorphic PTLD

These polymorphic lesions are composed of immunoblasts, plasma cells, small- and intermediate-sized lymphocytes that efface the nodal architecture or form extranodal tumors. Bizarre cells may be present and there may be areas of necrosis. The proliferation is usually clonal by immunoglobulin gene analysis. These cases may regress following reduction in immunosuppression in a variable number of cases, while others may progress and require treatment for lymphoma.

Monomorphic PTLD

These lesions resemble lymphomas; the majority are of large B cell lymphoma, less commonly Burkitt lymphoma. T cell lymphoma is less common and often extranodal in the skin or liver and spleen. Hodgkin lymphoma has been reported. Response to reduction of immunosuppression may occur (**Figs. 5.67**, **5.68**, **5.69**, and **5.70**; **Table 5.17**).

Colonization of Follicles by Neoplastic Cells

While neoplastic follicles generally show a loss of polarization, some follicles may show only partial replacement by neoplastic cells. While it is not known whether these follicles represent incomplete neoplastic transformation or colonization of benign follicles by neoplastic cells, such changes may result in some degree of heterogeneity of the follicles that may be puzzling. However, the distinct homogenous clustering of atypical cells, especially centroblasts, within the benign germinal center in a background of neoplastic follicles allows a definite diagnosis. This phenomenon may also be seen in lymph nodes adjacent to those involved by FL, and when present in isolation in patients with or without FL elsewhere has been called "in situ" FL (**Figs. 5.71** and **5.72**).

Colonization of follicles by neoplastic cells may also occur in mantle cell lymphoma. Besides growing outwards, the

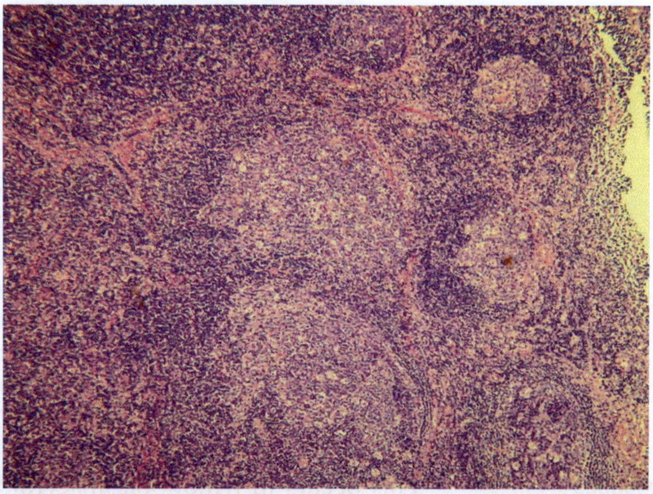

Fig. 5.67. PTLD, plasmacytic hyperplasia. Architecture is preserved and there is follicular hyperplasia and paracortical expansion.

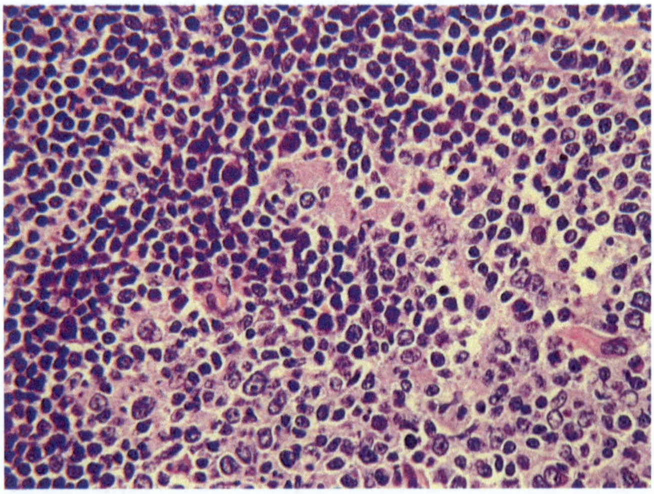

Fig. 5.68. PTLD, plasmacytic hyperplasia. The sinuses and paracortex are engorged with numerous plasma cells and small lymphocytes. The plasma cells stain purple.

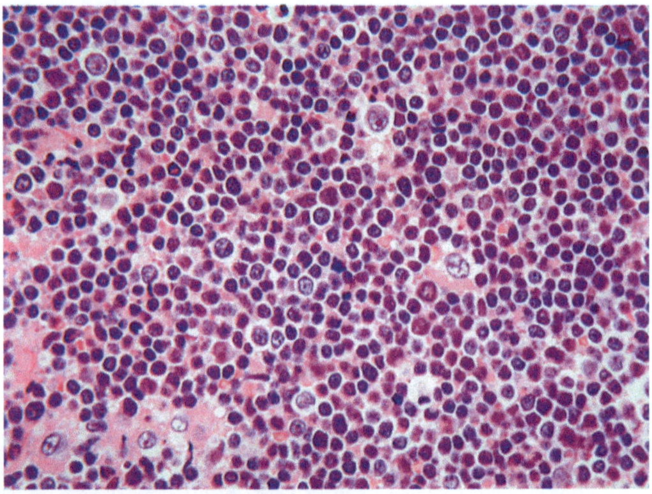

Fig. 5.69. Polymorphic PTLD. Expanded paracortex filled with small lymphocytes, plasma cells, and immunoblasts.

proliferating mantle cells also invade the germinal center. This partial or complete replacement of the germinal center can result in a pattern that can be indistinguishable from a true follicular pattern. However, the massive replacement of the follicle by mantle cells is identifiable because the neoplastic cells have relatively more rounded nuclei with irregular contours unlike the twisted, angulated, or folded nuclei of follicular-center cells. Furthermore, mantle cells are Cyclin D1+ and CD10–.

Homogenous Nodules

This occurs in lymphoplasmacytoid lymphoma when the malignant cells produce focal distension of sinuses. A similar phenomenon may occur in B-prolymphocytic lymphoma but such

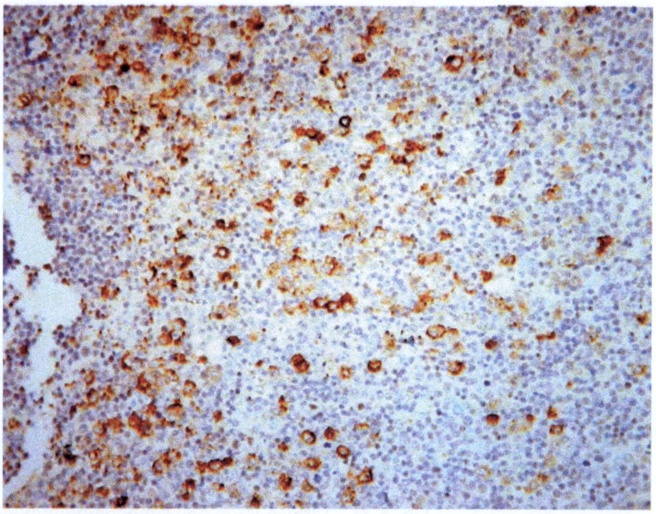

Fig. 5.70. Polymorphic PTLD. Numerous cells in the expanded paracortex stain for LMP-1.

Table 5.17
Post-transplant lymphoproliferative disorders – Clinical and morphology

Clinical

- Following immunosuppression for solid organ, bone marrow, or stem cell allografts
- Due mainly to impaired T cell immunity to EBV
- About 20% EBV–, due to other viruses or chronic antigen stimulation from allograft
- EBV– cases occur 4–5 years compared to 6–10 months post-transplant in EBV+ cases
- Both EBV+ and EBV– cases can respond to reduction of immunosuppression

Morphology

Spectrum of lymphoid and plasmacytoid proliferations:

- Plasmacytic hyperplasia and infectious mononucleosis-like PTLD – architecture partially preserved with proliferation of plasma cells and/or blast cells
- Polymorphic PTLD – proliferation of small angulated lymphocytes, plasma cells, and immunoblasts with loss of normal architecture
- Monomorphic PTLD – resemble lymphomas, mostly large B cell, less commonly Burkitt lymphoma. T cell lymphoma uncommon, extranodal in skin, liver, or spleen

nodular proliferations are usually vague and poorly defined. T-lymphoblastic leukemia/lymphoma may diffusely or partially involve the paracortex, sometimes producing a distinct multinodular pattern or "pseudofollicular" by stretching the fibrous framework.

A nodular pattern may be produced in the paracortical region by nodular T-zone hyperplasia and dermatopathic lymphadenitis. These are subtle nodules of small, medium, or large size that contain mainly small round T lymphocytes and can be identified by

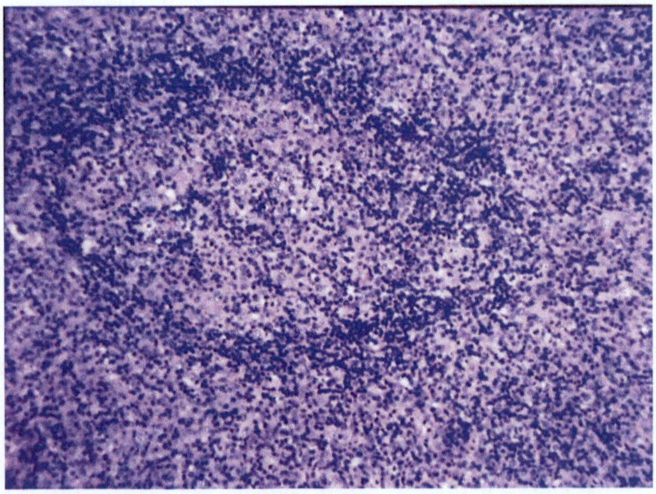

Fig. 5.71. Diffuse large cell lymphoma (immunoblastic sarcoma) showing colonization of a follicle. The follicle retains a mantle rim but contains large blasts in the germinal center.

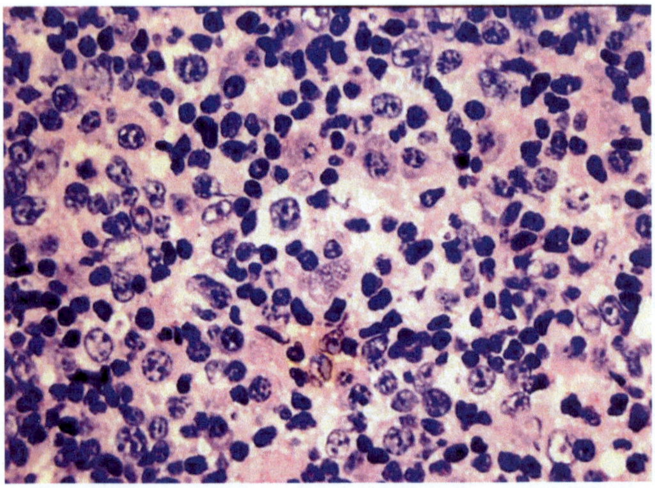

Fig. 5.72. The center of the follicle contains small collections of centroblasts similar to those infiltrating the interfollicular and diffuse areas.

the presence of scattered Langerhans cells or interdigitating dendritic cells and histiocytes, which produce a characteristic mottling appearance (**Figs. 5.73**, **5.74**, **5.75**, and **5.76**).

Reactive Hyperplasia

In non-neoplastic conditions, the pattern of lymph node reaction is often non-specific and is the result of antigenic stimulation of both B and T cells with resulting hyperplasia of follicles

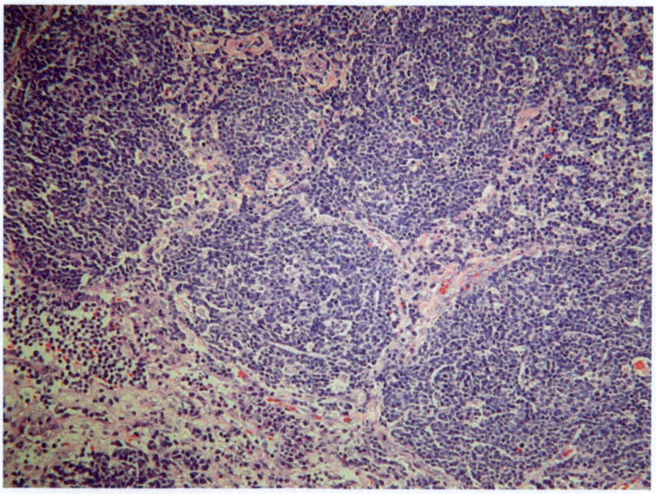

Fig. 5.73. Lymphoplasmacytoid lymphoma with macroglobulinemia showing a nodular pattern of infiltration.

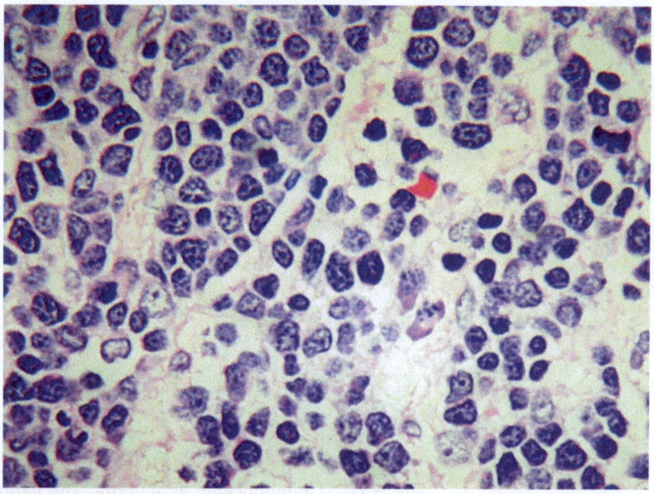

Fig. 5.74. Intermediate-sized plasmacytoid cells with coarse chromatin are mixed with occasional plasma cells.

and paracortex. The extent of hyperplasia in each compartment is influenced by the stage of the disease and the inciting agent. In a few situations, there may be sufficiently distinctive changes to suggest a specific diagnosis that can be confirmed by ancillary investigations, but in many instances, the diagnosis is one of the non-specific lymph node hyperplasias. Often there may be accompanying sinus histiocytosis or a granulomatous reaction and these are discussed separately in another section of this book.

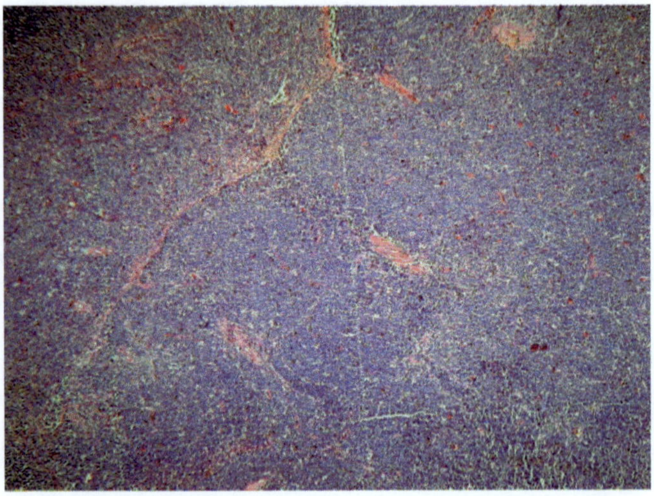

Fig. 5.75. Lymphoblastic lymphoma with a vaguely nodular pattern of growth.

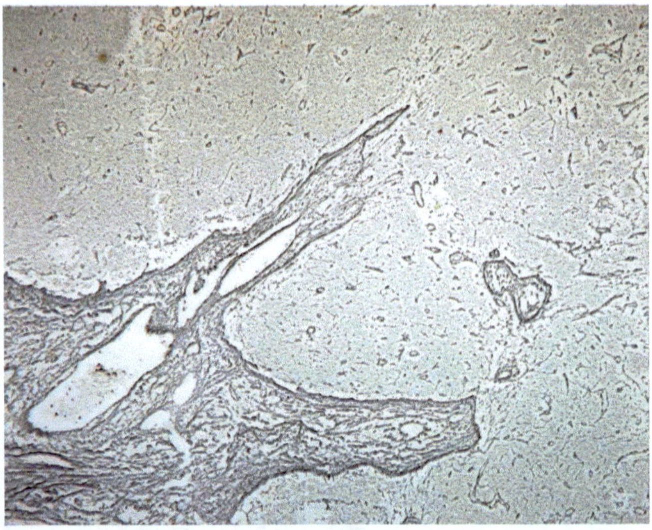

Fig. 5.76. Lymphoblastic lymphoma. The vague nodularity is imparted by tumor cells distending lymph node sinuses shown in the upper field by a reticulin stain.

Follicular and Paracortical Hyperplasia

The diagnosis of persistent lymphadenopathy includes both reactive conditions as well as lymphoma, and a biopsy is required for the distinction. Follicular hyperplasia is the most common pattern of reaction seen in the lymph node and is characterized by enlarged follicles with prominent germinal centers. Follicular hyperplasia is frequently accompanied by some degree of paracortical expansion as the stimulus often activates both B cell and T cells. The assignment of the entities to their most prominent histological feature in **Table 5.18** is largely arbitrary as many have

Table 5.18
Patterns of reactive lymph node hyperplasia

Follicular hyperplasia
• Non-specific follicular hyperplasia
• Progressive transformation of germinal centers
• Rheumatoid lymphadenopathy
• Toxoplasmosis
• Human immunodeficiency virus (HIV) lymphadenitis
• Kimura disease
• Castleman disease
• Syphilis
Paracortical hyperplasia
• Dermatopathic lymphadenopathy
• Kikuchi disease
• Systemic lupus erythematosus
• Viral lymphadenitis, including infectious mononucleosis and measles
• Drug-induced lymphadenopathy

overlapping features. Importantly, the features vary at different stages of the disease.

Non-specific Follicular Hyperplasia

Follicular hyperplasia requires distinction from follicular lymphoma. Follicular hyperplasia is often accompanied by plasma cells in the medullary cords and scattered throughout the interfollicular areas. While it may be possible to identify the inciting etiological agent in some instances with ancillary techniques, in the absence of demonstrable infecting organisms and any specific histological feature, the label of "non-specific hyperplasia" is commonly used. As discussed above, reactive follicles show polarization of centroblasts and centrocytes in the germinal center into dark and light zones, respectively, retain a distinct mantle zone and are generally distributed primarily in the cortex. Reactive follicles are often irregular in size and shape and show tingible-body macrophages and numerous mitotic figures and apoptotic bodies in the germinal centers.

Progressive Transformation of Germinal Centers (PTGC)

Progressive transformation of germinal centers (PTGC) most commonly presents in adolescent and young adult males as solitary painless lymphadenopathy of varying durations. Cervical nodes are most commonly involved, whereas axillary and inguinal nodes less frequently. The disease is benign but may recur and rarely is associated with synchronous or metachronous

Table 5.19
Progressive transformation of germinal centers – clinical

• Adolescent and young adult males
• Solitary painless cervical mass; axillary and inguinal nodes less frequent
• Present for variable periods, sometimes long duration
• Runs a benign course but may recur
• Rarely synchronous or metachronous NLPHL

nodular lymphocyte-predominant Hodgkin lymphoma (NLPHL) (**Table 5.19**).

Morphology

The lymph node shows one or more massively enlarged follicles mixed with a background of reactive follicles. The "transformed" germinal center has a lobated outline and is often four to five times the size of normal germinal centers. The transformed germinal center displays an expanded mantle zone with inward migration of mantle cells into the germinal centers, breaking it up into small clusters of centroblasts. The germinal center becomes smaller with progression of the lesion. PTGC may be seen in NLPHL, non-Hodgkin lymphoma, or reactive lymphadenopathy. Distinction of PTGC should be made from the nodules of NLPHL. In NLPHL, the nodules are closely packed and replace the lymph node. If reactive follicles are present, they are compressed to the periphery of the node. The mantle zone is lost or attenuated and the nodules are composed of a mixture of small lymphocytes, epithelioid histiocytes, and the polylobated LP or popcorn variant of the Reed–Sternberg cell, which are larger cells with pale-staining nuclei and cytoplasm, and prominent eosinophilic nucleoli. The LP cells may also be found among small lymphocytes in the internodular areas. Rarely, fibrocollagenous bands can also produce a distinctive nodular pattern as seen in nodular sclerosing classical Hodgkin lymphoma (**Figs. 5.77, 5.78, 5.79**, and **5.80**; **Table 5.20**).

Rheumatoid Lymphadenopathy

Rheumatoid lymphadenopathy may often be widespread as part of this systemic disease. Hyperplastic follicles are seen in both the cortex and medulla of the lymph node. Follicular enlargement may be striking and is due to expansion of germinal centers with narrowing of the mantle zones. Centroblasts may predominate in the germinal centers and immunoblasts and plasma cells are seen in the medullary cords. Long-term treatment with low-dose methotrexate is associated with an increased risk of lymphoproliferative disorders which may be benign, atypical, or malignant. Lymphomas that develop may be of B cell and less frequently of T cell type. Hodgkin lymphoma can also occur. Some cases are

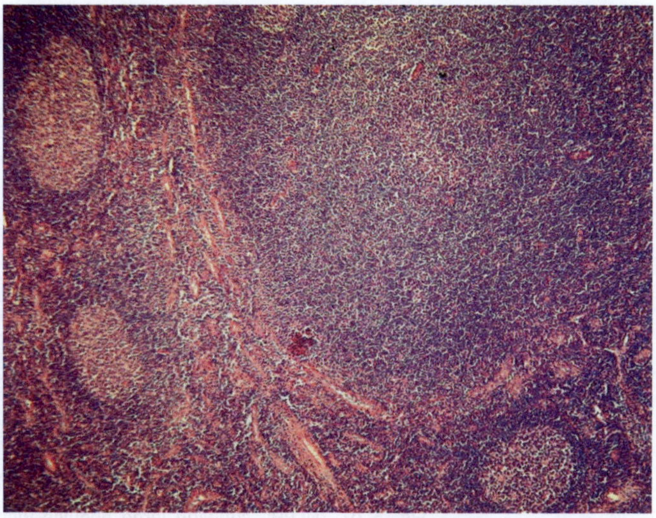

Fig. 5.77. In PTGC, one or more markedly enlarged germinal centers are interspersed between the markedly enlarged follicles. The mantle rim is preserved and small dark mantle cells infiltrate the germinal center breaking it into small collections of centroblasts.

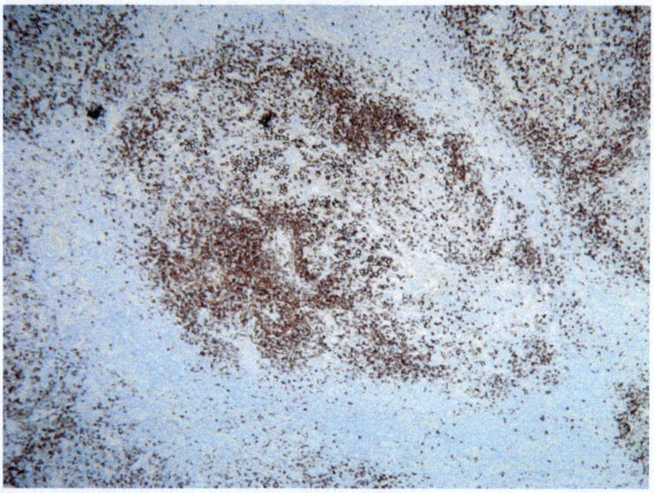

Fig. 5.78. In the "transformed" germinal center, the CD20+ mantle zone is partly preserved and mantle cells infiltrate and break up the germinal center into groups of CD20+ cells.

associated with Epstein–Barr virus (EBV) infection and a proportion of these lymphoproliferative disorders responds to withdrawal of methotrexate, especially those associated with EBV (**Table 5.21**; **Figs. 5.81**, **5.82**, **5.83**, and **5.84**).

Toxoplasma Lymphadenopathy

Toxoplasmic lymphadenopathy or the Piringer–Kuchinka lymphadenitis is the most common manifestation of symptomatic

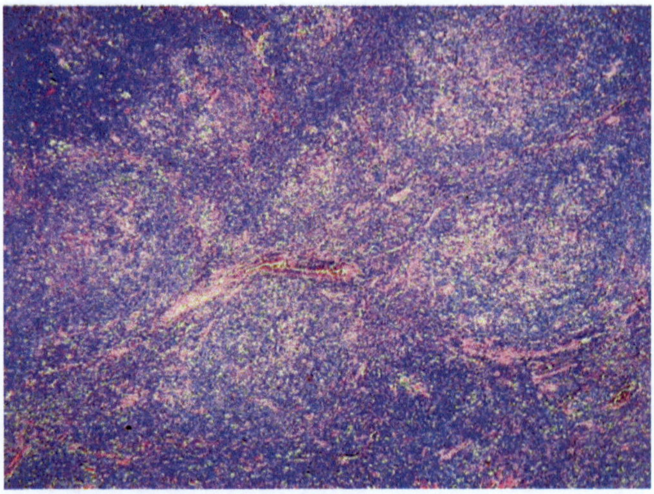

Fig. 5.79. NLPHL showing large nodules with numerous epithelioid histiocytes that result in the eosinophilic pallor within and between nodules.

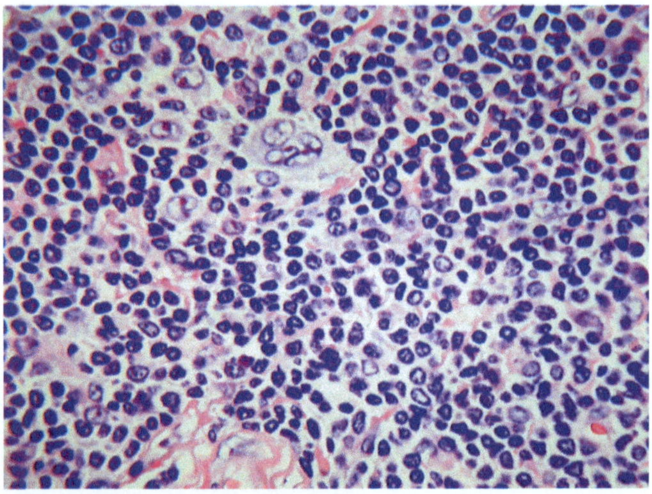

Fig. 5.80. NLPHL. LP cells with pale cytoplasm, large vesicular polylobated nuclei that contain prominent eosinophilic nucleoli are present mixed with small lymphocytes within and between nodules.

infection with *Toxoplasma gondii*. The histologic changes are a mixed pattern of follicular hyperplasia and monocytoid B cell hyperplasia. A prominent finding is the presence of small to large clusters of epithelioid histiocytes scattered throughout the lymph node with encroachment on and involvement of germinal centers. Toxoplasma cysts rarely occur and are best detected with an anti-toxoplasma antibody (**Table 5.22**; **Figs. 5.85** and **5.86**).

Table 5.20
Progressive transformation of germinal centers – morphology

- One or more "transformed" nodules interspersed among hyperplastic follicles
- Nodules very much enlarged, lobulated
- Mantle zone preserved
- Germinal center broken up into small clusters of centroblasts by infiltrating mantle cells
- In contrast, nodules of NLPHL are multiple; hyperplastic follicles compressed to periphery of node; mantle zone lost or attenuated; LP and epithelioid cells present within and between the nodules

Table 5.21
Rheumatoid lymphadenopathy – clinical and morphological

- Systemic rheumatoid disease
- Lymphadenopathy may be widespread
- Follicular hyperplasia marked with striking germinal center enlargement
- Immunoblasts and plasma cells in medullary cords
- Long-term methotrexate treatment associated with lymphoproliferative disorders
- May respond to methotrexate withdrawal especially if EBV-associated

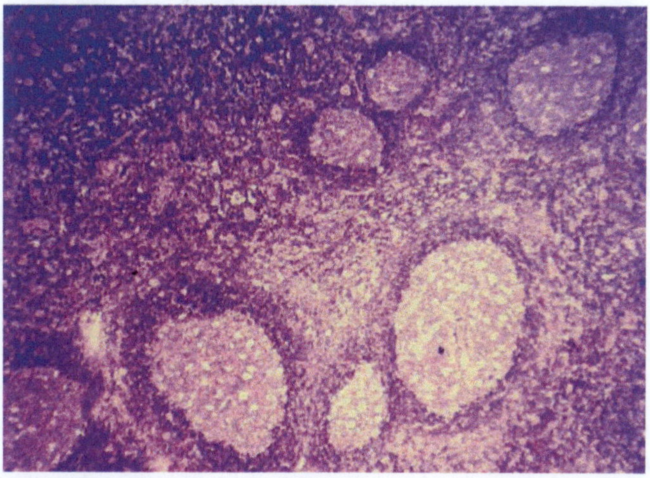

Fig. 5.81. Lymph node from 60-year-old woman with long-standing rheumatoid arthritis. There is marked follicular hyperplasia with enlarged germinal centers that are well demarcated from thin mantle zones.

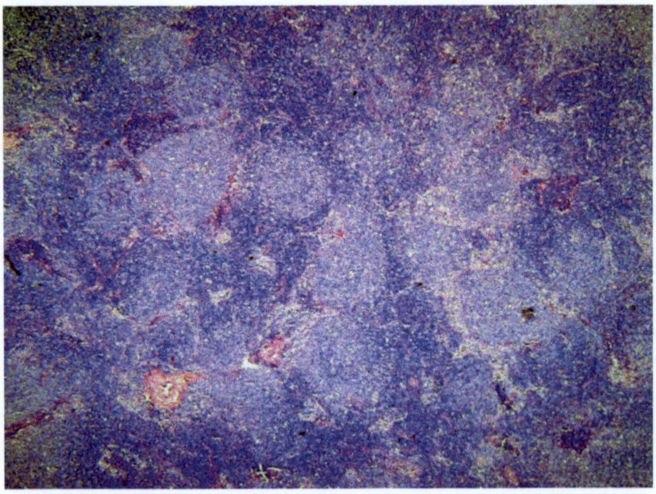

Fig. 5.82. Diffuse immunoblastic lymphoma following 12 years of methotrexate treatment. Germinal centers are without the mantle rim and contain mostly centroblasts and occasional plasma cells. The same cells are present in the interfollicular areas as evident by the purplish infiltrate.

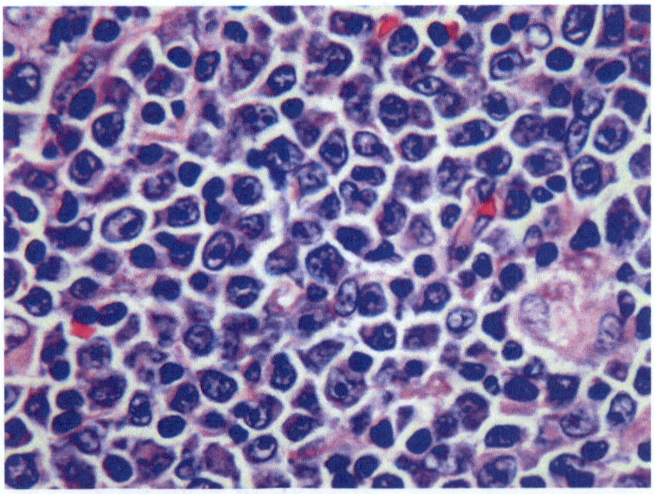

Fig. 5.83. Interfollicular areas are infiltrated by a plasmacytoid immunoblastic infiltrate. The cells showed light-chain restriction for IgMκ and were negative for LMP and EBER (not shown).

Human Immunodeficiency Virus/Acquired Immunodeficiency Disease Syndrome (HIV/AIDS) Lymphadenitis

Lymph node biopsies are now not often performed in HIV+ patients. Persistent lymph adenopathy is a common presentation of AIDS. The enlarged nodes show hyperplastic follicles that may become very large and acquire serrated borders. They may coalesce and form dumbbell and other irregular shapes accounting for the term "geographic follicles." The hyperplastic follicles are present in the cortex and medulla and may extend into the

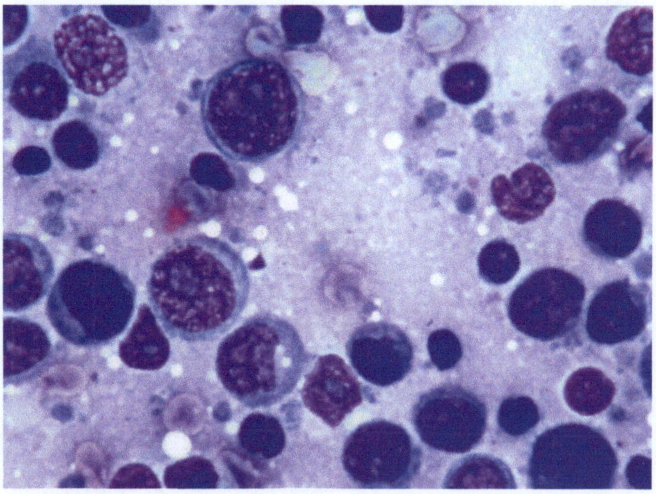

Fig. 5.84. Giemsa-stained imprint showing large cells with coarse chromatin and central nucleoli. Moderate quantities of basophilic cytoplasm are present.

Table 5.22
Toxoplasma lymphadenopathy – morphology

• Follicular hyperplasia
• Paracortical hyperplasia
• Monocytoid B cell hyperplasia
• Small clusters of epithelioid histiocytes throughout node
• Granulomas impinge on and involve germinal centers
• Toxoplasma pseudocysts are very rarely seen

perinodal tissue and mantle zones may be attenuated or disrupted. With continued infection, the lymph node goes through different changes of florid follicular hyperplasia, mixed follicular hyperplasia, and follicular involution; follicular involution and ultimately lymphocyte depletion occurs as a result of cytopathic destruction of CD4+ T cell and follicular dendritic cells. The latter results in involution of follicles so that both T and B cell numbers are reduced. At this stage opportunistic infections may supervene.

Follicular lysis is associated with infiltration of germinal centers by small lymphocytes that result in disruption of the follicles and deposition of PAS-positive material. There is also progressive plasma cell accumulation. The final stage of lymphocyte depletion is the burnt-out stage of AIDS with atrophic follicles, lymphocyte depletion, and extensive diffuse vascular and fibrous proliferation and hyalinization of the node. HIV can be demonstrated by immunostaining various HIV antigens including the core

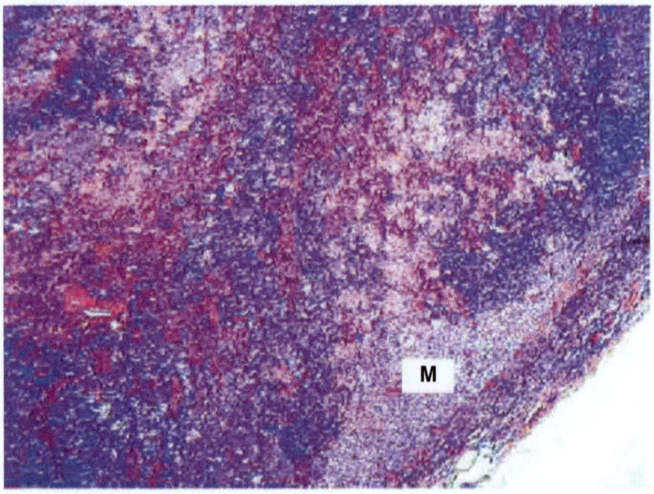

Fig. 5.85. Toxoplasma lymphadenitis showing hyperplasia of follicles and monocytoid B cells (M) and clusters of epithelioid cells.

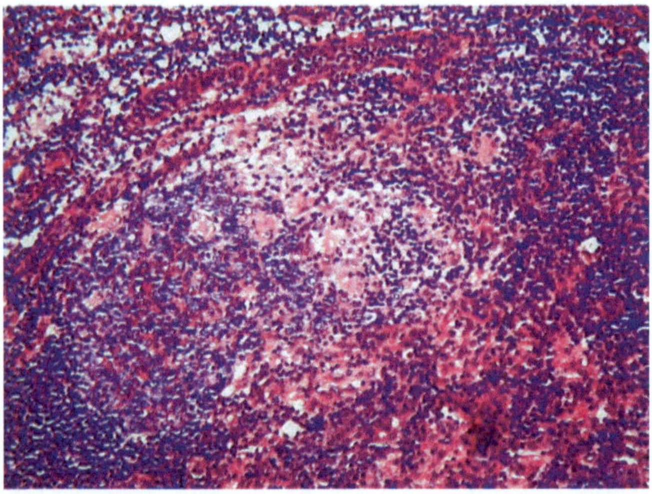

Fig. 5.86. Epithelioid histiocytes encroach on a germinal center and are present within it.

protein p24 that is localized to follicular dendritic cells (**Table 5.23**; **Figs. 5.87** and **5.88**).

Kimura Disease

This is a self-limiting disease that is prevalent but not exclusive to Oriental patients and shows a striking male predominance. It is largely a cutaneus condition but may involve lymph nodes, which may be enlarged, multiple, and matted. If untreated, the condition usually remains static and may regress. There is a mixed hyperplasia involving follicles and paracortex with fibrosis and a marked eosinophilic infiltration. The florid enlargement of ger-

Table 5.23
HIV/AIDS lymphadenopathy – clinical and morphology

Clinical
• At risk population
• Fever, weight loss, diarrhea, hypergammaglobulinemia
• Enlarged nodes at tow or more sites
• Decreased peripheral CD4+ and reversed CD4+/CD8+ T cell ratio
• Positivity for HIV antigen or antibody
Acute stage
• Florid follicular hyperplasia; irregular-shaped follicles
• Mantle zone attenuated or disrupted
• Monocytoid B cell hyperplasia
• Giant cells of Warthin–Finkeldey type
Subacute/chronic stage
• Folliculolysis and follicular effacement
• Involution of germinal centers with hyaline deposition
• Paracortical lymphocyte depletion
• Plasma cells in paracortex
• Paracortical vascular proliferation
Burnout stage
• Atrophic or absent follicles
• Germinal centers hyalinized, with PAS+ deposits and thick vessels
• Paracortical lymphocytes depleted
• Paracortical vascular proliferation and fibrosis
• HIV antigens demonstrated by immunostaining

minal centers shows deposition of a proteinaceous material that is often IgE which is deposited on the meshwork of FDC. The germinal centers may display foci of necrosis or follicular lysis. Eosinophils infiltrate the germinal centers, sinuses, and paracortex and can accumulate as microabscesses. The paracortex also contains plasma cells, small lymphocytes, and mast cells, and there is proliferation of high-endothelial vessel that may be associated with fibrosis. Occasional giant cells of Warthin–Finkeldey type may be present (**Table 5.24**; **Figs. 5.89**, **5.90**, **5.91**, and **5.92**).

Castleman Disease

Castleman disease is a lymphoproliferative disorder that may be divided into following three categories with some degree of overlap: hyaline vascular, localized plasma cell variant, and multicentric Castleman disease.

Hyaline Vascular Variant (HV)

The hyaline vascular variant of Castleman disease (HV) is the most common variant, usually solitary, and involves peripheral

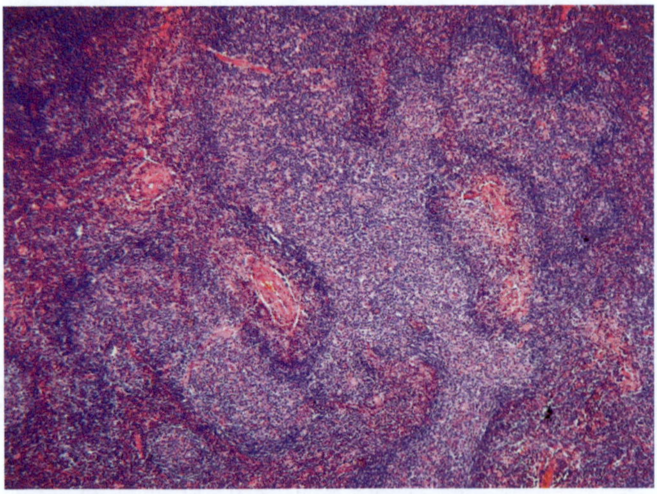

Fig. 5.87. Acute stage showing florid follicular hyperplasia throughout the node. Follicles are of irregular shapes. Mantle zones are thin and disrupted.

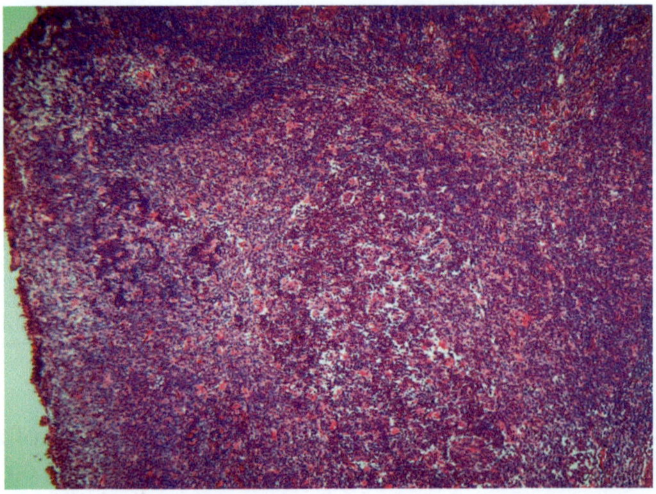

Fig. 5.88. Chronic stage showing large follicle with lysis and infiltration of germinal center by small lymphocytes and plasma cells, and deposition of PAS-positive material.

nodes, mostly mediastinal, or extranodal tissue. It is asymptomatic and occurs most commonly in young adults. The histological features are characteristic and represented by follicles that are mildly enlarged but show a broad mantle of small lymphocytes that assume a concentric onion skin pattern. Often, more than one germinal center may be seen in one follicle, a phenomenon sometimes referred to as "twinning." A single hyalinized vessel penetrates the hypocellular germinal center to produce the appearance of a lollipop. The follicle centers consist mostly of collagenized vessels with plump endothelial cells and prominent

Table 5.24
Kimura disease – clinical and morphology

• Self-limiting disease, common to Orientals
• Striking male predominance
• Involves skin, nodes less often enlarged, multiple and matted
• Mixed hyperplasia of follicles and paracortex
• Enlarged germinal centers contain proteinaceous material, often IgE
• Focal necrosis in germinal centers and eosinophil infiltration
• Eosinophils in paracortex and sinuses, form microabscesses
• Plasma cells, small lymphocytes, mast cells, and vessels in paracortex
• Occasional Warthin–Finkeldey giant cells

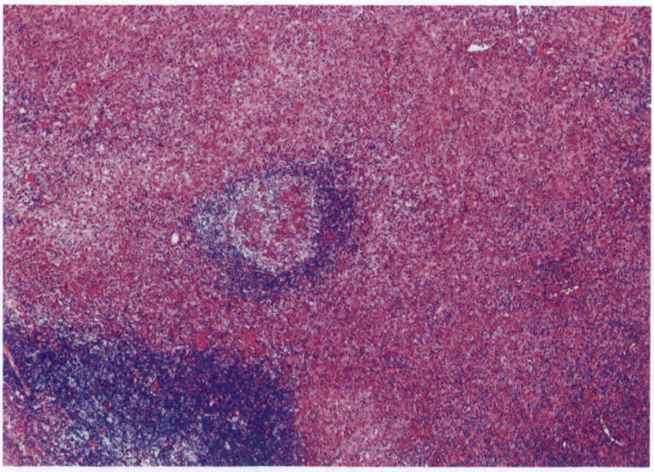

Fig. 5.89. Kimura disease with follicular hyperplasia and fibrosis in the paracortex. The follicle has an enlarged germinal center with eosinophilic precipitate. Eosinophils, plasma cells, and fibrosis account for the purple hue in the paracortex.

follicular dendritic cells (FDC). Interfollicular areas contain a network of collagenized vessels with surrounding fibrosis, scattered small lymphocytes, plasmacytoid, and plasma cells. Collections of plasmacytoid monocytes in the paracortex may be present.

This disease is benign and cured by local excision. A FDC tumor/sarcoma may rarely be associated. Some cases show EBV RNA in the tumor cells (**Figs. 5.93**, **5.94**, **5.95**, **5.96**, **5.97**, **5.98**, **5.99**, **5.100**, **5.101**, **5.102**, **5.103**, and **5.104**).

Plasma Cell Variant (PC)

The plasma cell variant (PC) presents most commonly as abdominal lymphadenopathy with mediastinal and peripheral node less commonly involved. Patients are symptomatic with anemia, elevated polyclonal gamma globulin, and ESR and plasmacytosis in

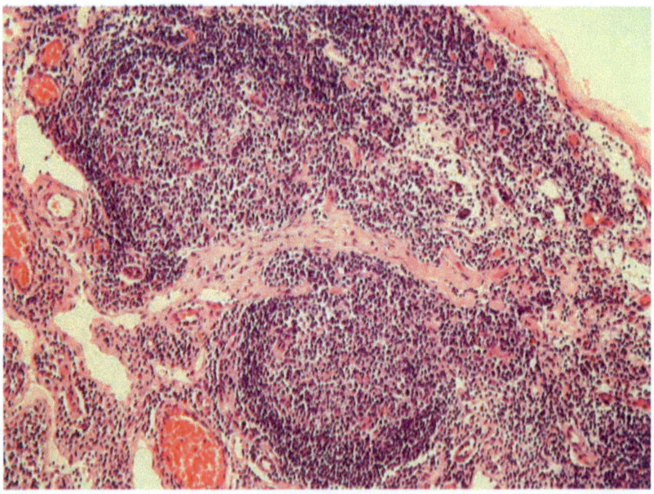

Fig. 5.90. The germinal centers are infiltrated by eosinophils and show foci of necrosis.

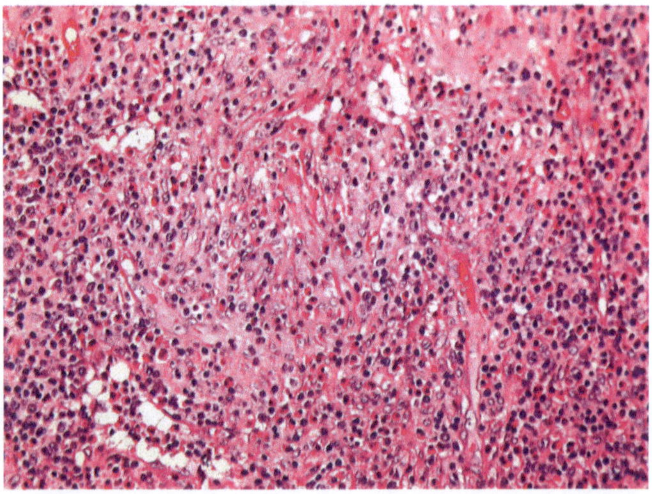

Fig. 5.91. The areas of fibrosis in the paracortex contain high endothelial vessels and an infiltrate of small lymphocytes, eosinophils, plasma cell, and mast cells.

the bone marrow. Both symptoms and abnormal laboratory tests revert to normal after removal of the affected nodes, which is thought to be due to removal of IL-6 secreted by the abnormal nodes and infecting HHV-8 virus that encodes, besides a number of homologues to proteins involved in cell cycle regulation, apoptosis, signal transduction, and immune modulation, the homologue of human interleukin-6 (IL-6) which is thought to be involved in the pathogenesis.

Histologically, in PC, the hyperplastic follicles have a thin rim of mantle cells and are surrounded by sheets of mature plasma

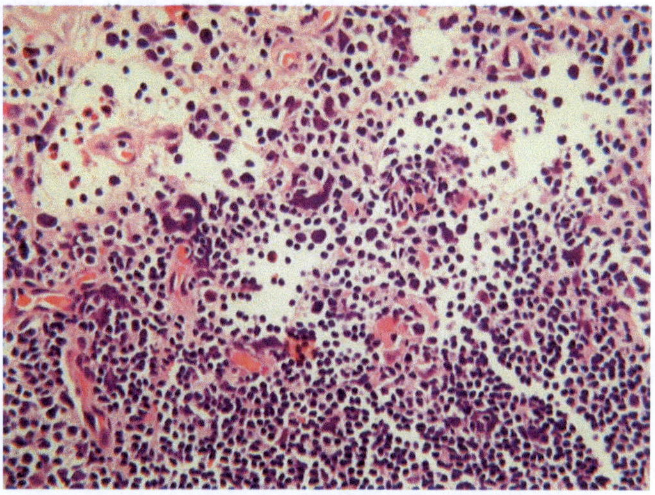

Fig. 5.92. Giant cells are present in an area of necrosis in the paracortex.

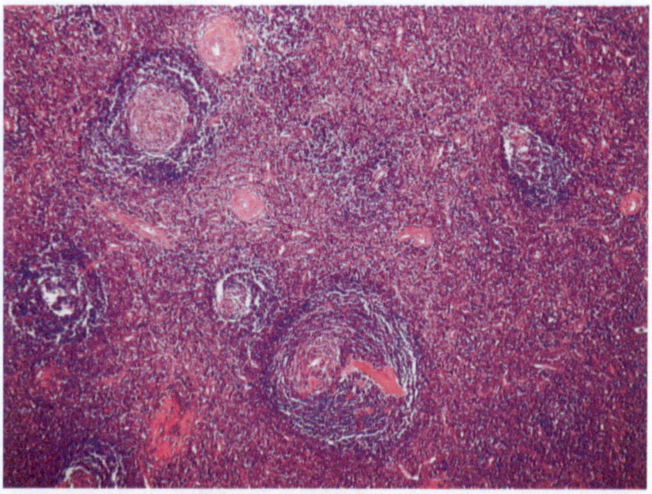

Fig. 5.93. Castleman disease, HV, in a mediastinal node showing variably enlarged follicles with characteristic onion skin arrangement of small lymphocytes around a hypocellular center.

cells that extend into the interfollicular zones. Often some follicles may show penetrating hyalinized vessels with similarities to HC. PC may resemble other lymphadenopathies with severe plasmacytosis such as rheumatoid disease and syphilis except that the plasmacytosis is less severe and the sinus architecture of the node is better preserved in these conditions. In about one-third of cases, the plasma cells show light chain restriction, usually lambda light chain.

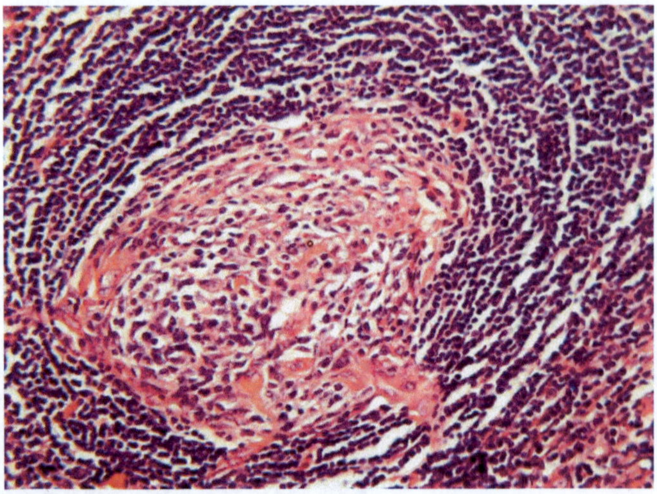

Fig. 5.94. A lollipop appearance is imparted by the hyalinized vessel penetrating the mantle zone into the germinal center which also contains hyalinized vessels and is hypocellular.

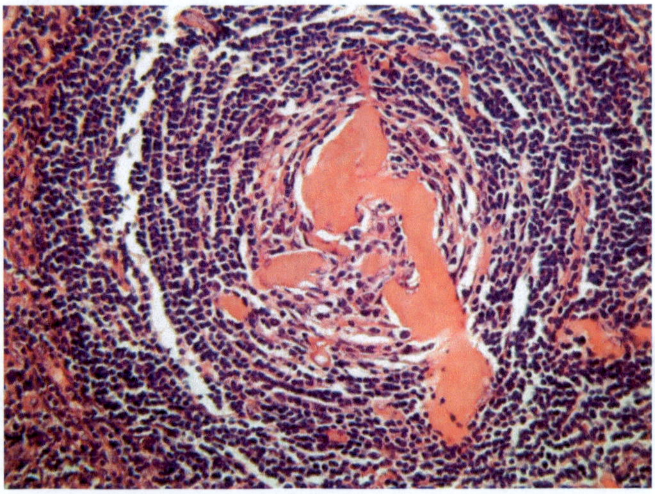

Fig. 5.95. Castleman disease, HV. A penetrating arteriole is completely hyalinized and surrounded by concentric layers of lymphoid cells.

Multicentric Variant (MC)

This variant occurs in an older age group than the other variants and may be primary or associated with HIV infection, Kaposi sarcoma, plasma cell neoplasms, malignant lymphoma, and autoimmune disease. Like PC, it is associated with systemic symptoms and abnormal laboratory findings which is thought to be due to the secretion of IL-6, which can be endogenous or the viral homologue, accounting for the name IL-6 lymphadenopathy that has been suggested for this variant of Castleman disease. POEMS syndrome (polyneuropathy, organomegaly,

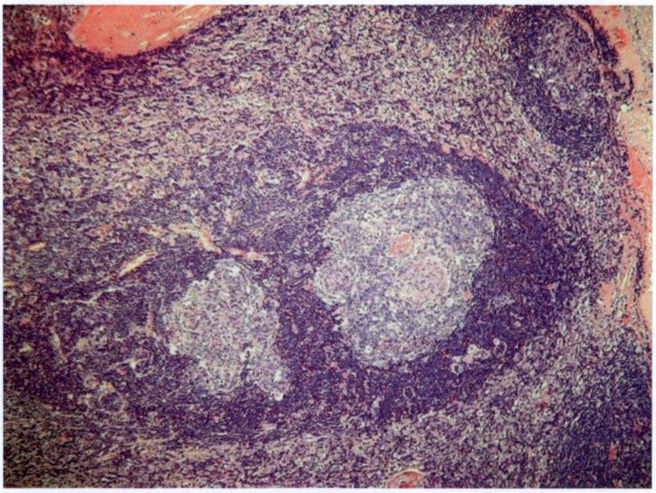

Fig. 5.96. So-called "twining" of germinal centers' seen in Castleman's disease.

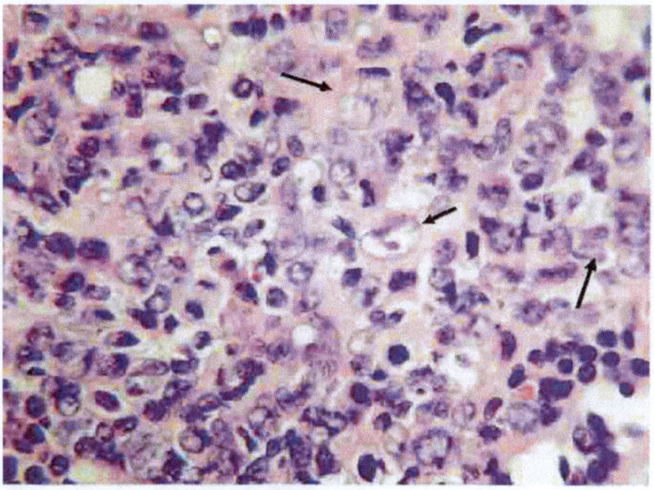

Fig. 5.97. The germinal center contains prominent FDC (*arrows*), small lymphocytes, and scattered centroblasts and plasma cells.

endocrinopathy, monoclonal gammopathy, and skin glomeruloid hemangiomas) occurs in about 60% of cases with MC and is thought to be the result of the production of autoantibodies and cytokine abnormalities.

Histologically, MC is similar to PC. With progression, both these variants develop into a burnt-out phase with severe hyalinization of vascular germinal centers that can be difficult to separate from HV (**Table 5.25**).

Syphilis Lymphadenopathy

Lymphadenopathy is due to continuous antigenic stimulation of B and T cells by the persistence of *Treponema pallidum* in the

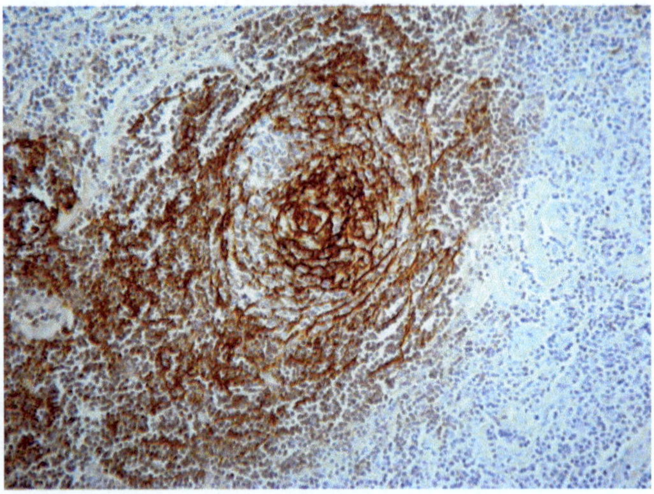

Fig. 5.98. The proliferation of FDC is highlighted by CD21 and shows extension into the interfollicular areas.

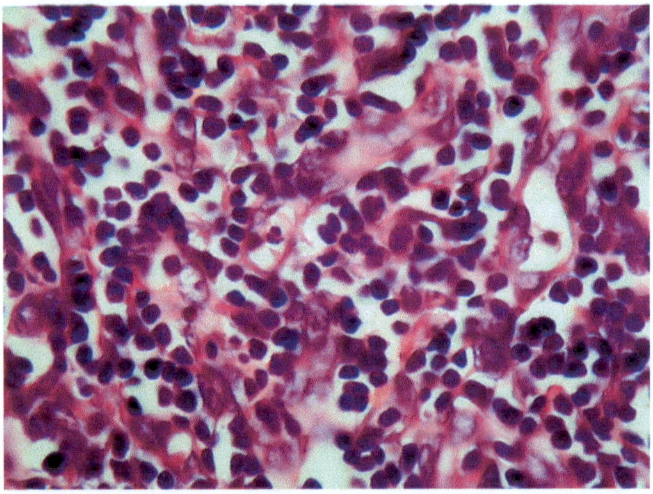

Fig. 5.99. Interfollicular areas are populated by prominent high-endothelial vessels and groups of small lymphocytes and plasma cells.

lymph nodes and occurs through all stages of the disease. There is marked follicular hyperplasia that extends throughout the lymph node and this is accompanied by prominent paracortical hyperplasia. There is also marked fibrosis of the capsule which can extend into the node and is associated with arteritis and phlebitis of the numerous vessels that occur in the capsule and perinodal tissues. These vessels are characterized by the presence of a prominent cuff of plasma cells and lymphocytes, and plasmacytosis is also prominent in the medullary cords. Small non-caseating granulomas may be seen in the paracortex with single so-called naked

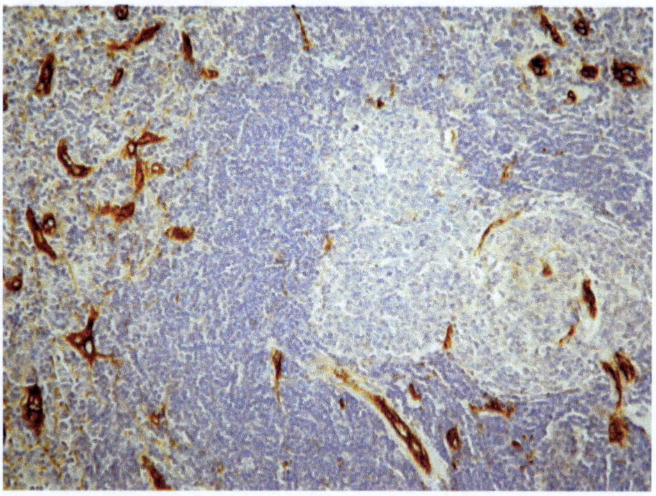

Fig. 5.100. High-endothelial vessels in the interfollicular areas are highlighted by CD34. The germinal center present is dumb-bell shaped, and sometimes more than one germinal center may be present within the same follicle.

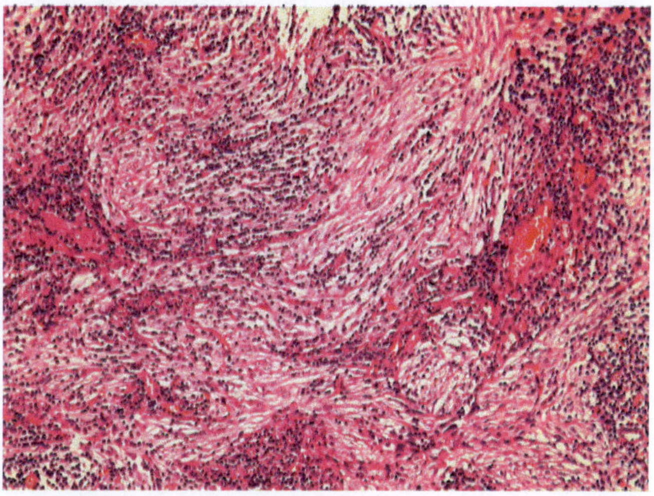

Fig. 5.101. FDC sarcoma in the nose of a Chinese male, at the site of previous excision of Castleman disease, HV, 3 years previously.

giant cells. Silver stains reveal the spirochetes in the walls of the vessels especially in the paracortex in all stages of the disease.

Kikuchi Disease

Kikuchi disease, also known as Kikuchi–Fujimoto disease and histiocytic necrotizing lymphadenitis, was first described in Asia but is now recognized to occur in the rest of the world, albeit, less frequently. It occurs predominantly in adolescent and young adult females. The disease is of unknown etiology and is self-limiting, presenting as one or more painful enlarged nodes in the

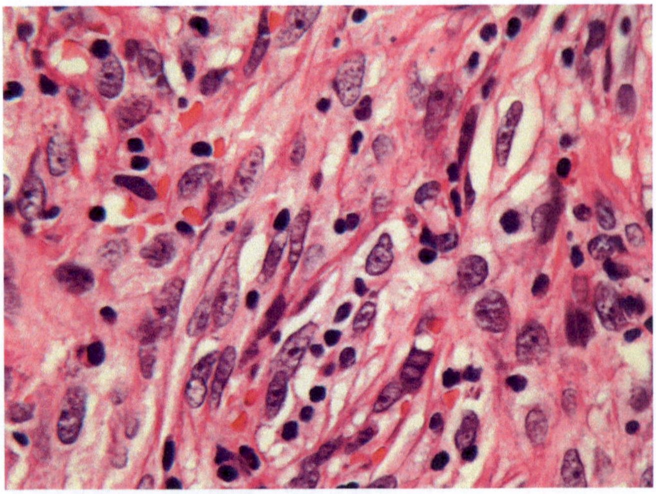

Fig. 5.102. Spindled tumor cells showing pleomorphic vesicular nuclei with eosinophilic nucleoli and occasional mitosis. They have moderate quantities of cytoplasm.

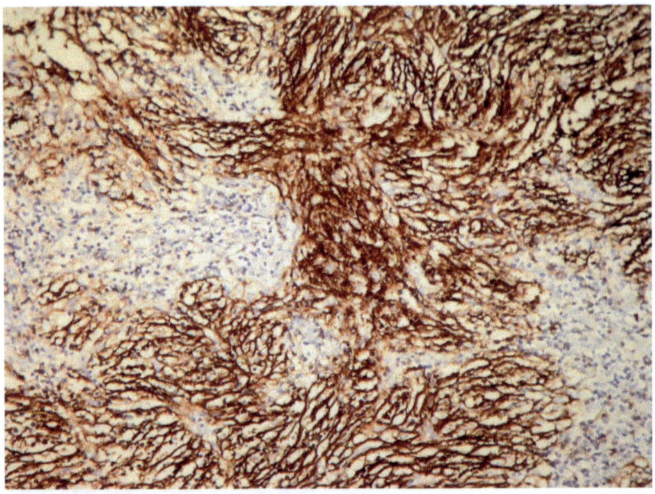

Fig. 5.103. The spindled tumor cells stain for CD21.

neck. There is accompanying fever and systemic symptoms. Other superficial nodes may be involved but with lesser frequency.

The early lymph node changes are those of a non-specific lymphoid hyperplasia with follicular hyperplasia and expansion of the paracortex that contains stimulated B and T-blast cells, plasmacytoid monocytes, and histiocytes. Apoptosis may be prominent in the paracortex. With progression, apoptosis becomes localized and distinct areas of tissue breakdown are evident. Such areas have been regarded as representing necrosis but are more likely localized areas of apoptosis. The so-called "necrotic" foci are surrounded by histiocytes and plasmacytoid monocytes but not

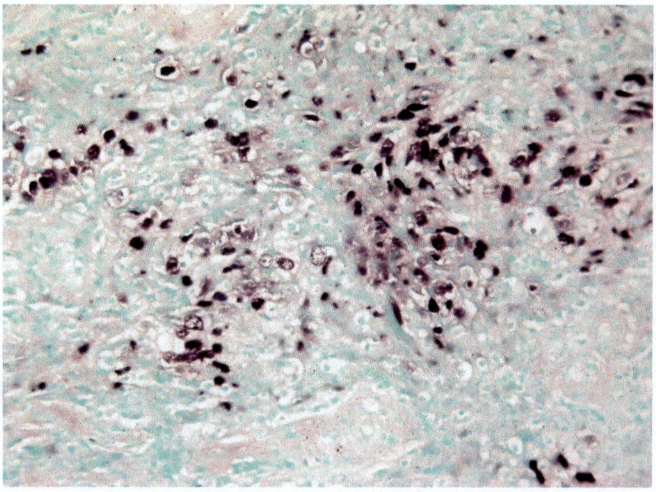

Fig. 5.104. Dendritic cell sarcoma stained for Epstein–Barr virus by EBER in situ hybridization.

neutrophils. Plasmacytoid monocytes have basophilic cytoplasm and eccentric nuclei that are pale staining and have inconspicuous nucleoli. The histiocytes often contain phagocytic nuclear debris or apoptotic particles and may display crescent-shaped nuclei resembling signet ring cells. Mixed with the histiocytes are small lymphocytes and activated cells, mostly CD3+ and fibrinoid deposits may be occasionally seen. When blast cells are abundant in Kikuchi disease, malignant lymphoma may be simulated but the heterogeneity of the infiltrate and the intact nodal architecture distinguish Kikuchi disease from lymphoma. Infectious mononucleosis can also mimic the early phase changes of Kikuchi disease. When the areas of apoptosis are large, their changes can be mistaken for cat-scratch disease and other necrotizing granulomatous lymphadenitis, but the absence of neutrophils and eosinophils is an important distinguishing feature in Kikuchi disease.

Histiocytes will stain with CD163, CD68, Mac387, and other histiocyte markers, and plasmacytoid monocytes will be labeled by CD74 (LN2), whereas CD15 will show that neutrophils are invariably absent in this lesion (**Table 5.26**; **Figs. 5.105**, **5.106**, **5.107**, **5.108**, and **5.109**).

Kikuchi disease requires differentiation from other conditions with focal necrosis. Systemic lupus erythematosus lymphadenopathy is an important distinction and is recognized on clinical grounds and by the presence of a plasma cell infiltrate, hematoxylin bodies, vasculitis, and basophilic DNA deposition on blood vessels. Necrotizing lymphadenitis of syphilis is usually accompanied by perivascular plasma cell infiltrates, *Yersinia* infection by the presence of eosinophils, and bacterial infections by accumulations of neutrophils. Cat-scratch disease, tuberculosis,

Table 5.25
Castleman disease – clinical and morphology

Hyaline vascular variant (HV – solitary
• Benign, cured by excision
• Solitary peripheral node, mostly mediastinal or extranodal tissue
• Young adults, asymptomatic
• Broad mantle zone with "onion skin" appearance
• Mildly enlarged follicles with collagenized vessels in germinal centers
• Penetrating collagenized vessel imparts "lollipop" appearance, twinning of germinal centers
• Interfollicular thick vessels, small lymphocytes, plasmacytoid, and plasma cells
• Plasmacytoid monocytes may be prominent
• May be associated with FDC tumor
Plasma cell variant (PC) – localized
• Systemic symptoms
• Abnormal laboratory tests: anemia, raised ESR, hypergammaglobulinemia, bone marrow plasmacytosis
• Associated with raised serum IL-6
• Wide age range
• Localized lymphadenopathy, abdominal nodes most commonly involved
• Follicular hyperplasia with thin mantle zones
• Prominent interfollicular plasma cells
• Progressive vessel hyalinization can resemble HV variant
• One-third shows light-chain restriction (Igλ)
Multicentric variant (MV)
• Older age group
• May be associated with HIV/AIDS and other diseases
• EBV seldom associated unless in HIV infected patients
• Multicentric
• Histology similar to PC variant
• Overproduction of endogenous interleukin-6 or from human herpes virus-8 (HHV-8)
• 60% cases associated with POEMS syndrome (polyneuropathy, organomegaly, endocrinopathy, monoclonal gammopathy, skin lesions (glomeruloid angioma)
• Progression to burnt-out phase where morphology similar to HIV lymphadenopathy
• Associated with plasmablastic lymphoma, effusion-associated DLBCL, and vascular tumors

histoplasmosis, and leprosy show characteristic proliferations of epithelioid cells and giant cells and discrete granuloma formation. Epstein–Barr virus lymphadenitis is accompanied by lymphocyte depletion and occasional hemophagocytosis by histiocytes, and tests for antibodies to viral-specific antigens are positive; in herpes simplex lymphadenitis, neutrophils and viral inclusions are also present, and unlike in Kikuchi disease, the histiocytes in herpes

Table 5.26
Kikuchi disease – clinical and morphological features

• Occurs mostly in adolescent and young adult Asian females
• Painful enlarged nodes in the neck
• Associated fever and systemic symptoms
• Self-limiting disease, etiology unknown
• Early phase changes non-specific lymphoid hyperplasia
• Paracortical B and T cell blasts prominent
• Focal areas of apoptosis
• Apoptotic areas surrounded by plasmacytoid monocytes and phagocytic histiocytes with crescentic nuclei
• Absence of neutrophils; plasma cells uncommon

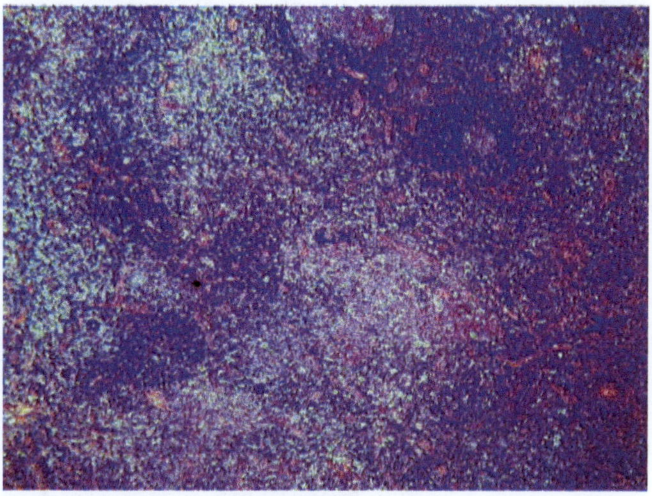

Fig. 5.105. Kikuchi disease. Early phase changes showing expanded paracortex with a mottled appearance due to the abundant immunoblasts. There are also reactive follicles present and a focus of necrosis lies below the center of the field.

lymphadenitis and granulomatous lymphadenitis are myeloperoxidase negative. Rarely Kikuchi disease may be mistaken for malignant lymphoma because of abundant stimulated cells but lymphoma cells can be detected in the non-necrotic areas of the node (**Table 5.27**).

Systemic Lupus Erythematosus

Lymph node biopsy as a method to diagnose systemic lupus erythematosus (SLE) is rare and the diagnosis is established by other manifestations of the disease. The histologic changes in SLE lymphadenopathy are very similar to those of Kikuchi disease and are distinguished by the presence of plasma cells, vasculitis, and the occurrence of hematoxylin bodies comprising amorphous

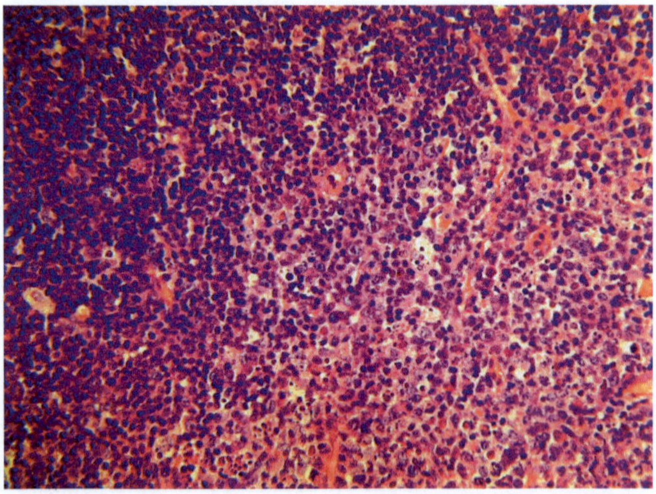

Fig. 5.106. An area of so-called "necrosis" with abundant apoptotic bodies clearly demarcated from the surrounding paracortex in the upper left field.

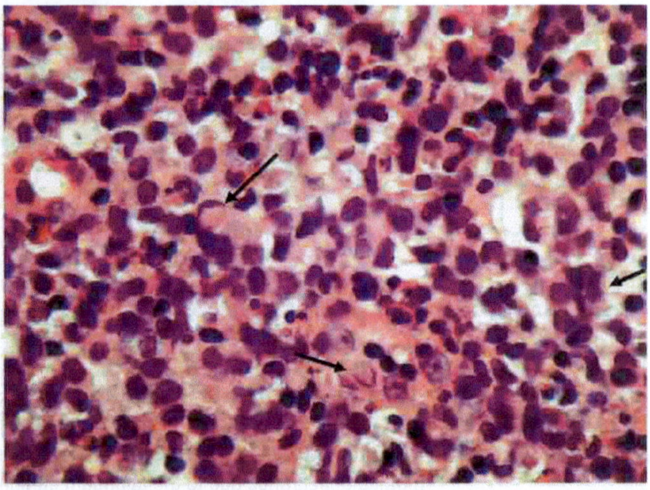

Fig. 5.107. Apoptotic bodies are scatted in the paracortex and phagocytic histiocytes with crescent-shaped nuclei are present (*arrows*).

aggregates of degenerate DNA and anti-DNA antibodies and DNA deposition on blood vessels. Hematoxylin bodies are found in necrotic areas and at their edges, and within sinuses, but they are often not present. With the advent of steroid, and other immunomodulating and immunosuppressive therapies, the classical picture of lupus lymphadenitis is seldom encountered in routine practice (**Figs. 5.110** and **5.111**).

Infectious Mononucleosis Lymphadenopathy

Infection with the Epstein–Barr virus (EBV) stimulates a vigorous humoral and cellular immune response in the acute phase.

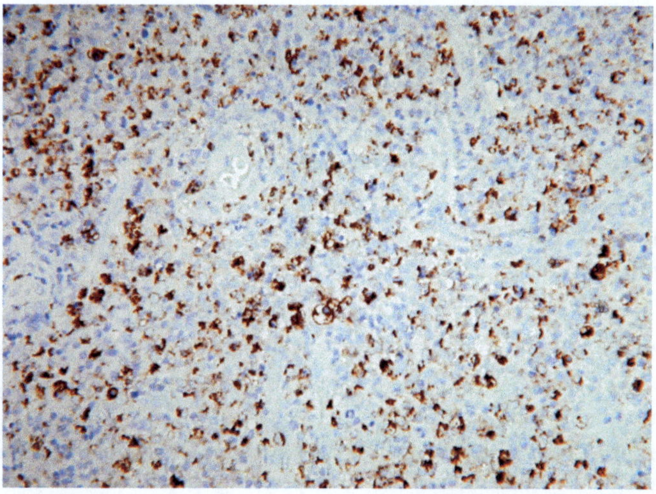

Fig. 5.108. Numerous CD68+ histiocytes are present around and within the areas of "necrosis."

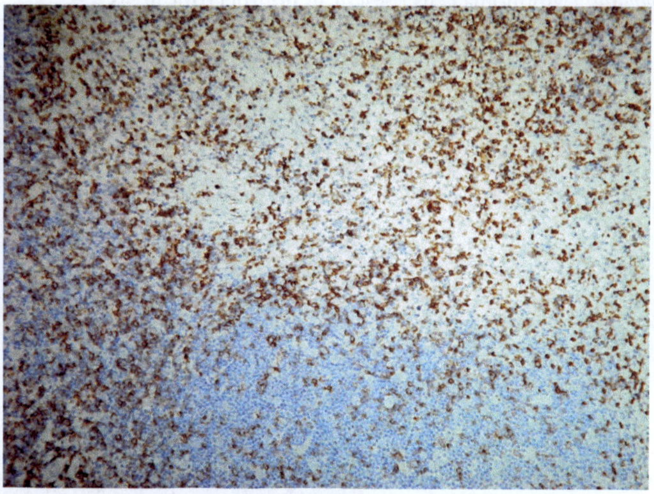

Fig. 5.109. Numerous CD3+ T cells are present within the "necrotic" areas.

The virus infects lymphoid cells in the oropharynx and persists as a latent virus throughout life. In infants and children, the infection is often trivial but in older persons the disease can be severe and persistent, sometimes simulating lymphoma. As with most viral lymphadenopathies, the histologic changes vary from a mild non-specific follicular hyperplasia to a proliferation that suggests a lymphoma. Generally, paracortical hyperplasia is more marked than follicular hyperplasia. There is a characteristic proliferation of immunoblasts of both B and T cell types that produces a mottled appearance to the paracortex. Mitotic figures are seen among these transformed lymphocytes and there may be small

Table 5.27
Distinguishing features of lymphadenitis with focal necrosis

Kikuchi disease: Abundant apoptosis, histiocytes, plasmacytoid monocytes, and absence of neutrophils and eosinophils, plasma cells infrequent
SLE: Clinical history, presence of hematoxylin bodies, numerous plasma cells, vasculitis, and DNA deposits in vessel walls
Syphilis: Perivascular plasma cell infiltrates
Yersinia and other bacteria: Neutrophils and eosinophils
Herpes simplex: Neutrophils and viral inclusions. Histiocytes are myeloperoxidase negative
Ebstein–Barr virus: Lymphocyte depletion and occasional hemophagocytosis by histiocytes. Tests for antibodies to EBV-specific antigens are positive.
Other viral lymphadenitis: Paracortical expansion with variable follicular hyperplasia. Specific diagnosis made by demonstration of the corresponding specific viral antigen by immunohistochemistry.
Tuberculosis, leprosy, and cat-scratch disease: Discrete granulomas of proliferating epithelioid histiocytes and giant cells. Etiologic agent may be identified by special stains.
Allergic reactions: Necrosis surrounded by plasma cells and eosinophils.
Lymphoma: Lymphoma cells present in non-necrotic areas.

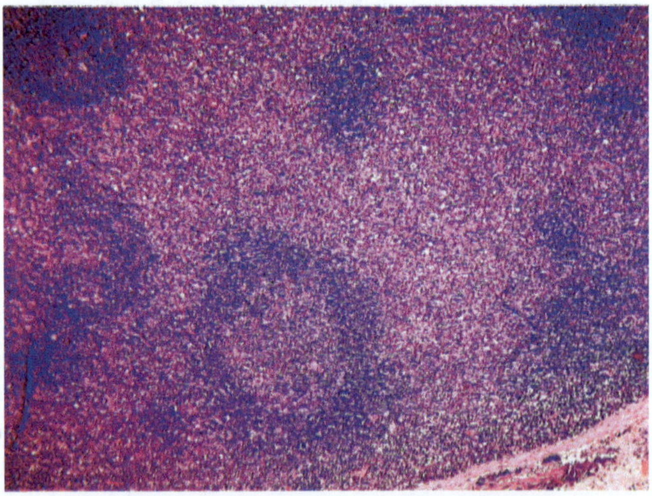

Fig. 5.110. SLE. Follicles are hyperplasic and paracortex is expanded by a dense plasmacytoid and plasma cell infiltrate as suggested by the purple hue.

groups of immunoblasts, plasmacytoid, and plasma cells within intact sinuses. Occasional large atypical and Reed–Sternberg-like cells may be seen. Monocytoid cells may also be present among the polymorphous infiltrate which extends into the capsule and trabeculae. Vascular proliferation and high-endothelial vessels are always present. The changes are not specific for EBV infection and reflect those generally seen in viral lymphadenopathies. Antibodies to the latent membrane protein are available and EBV-RNA

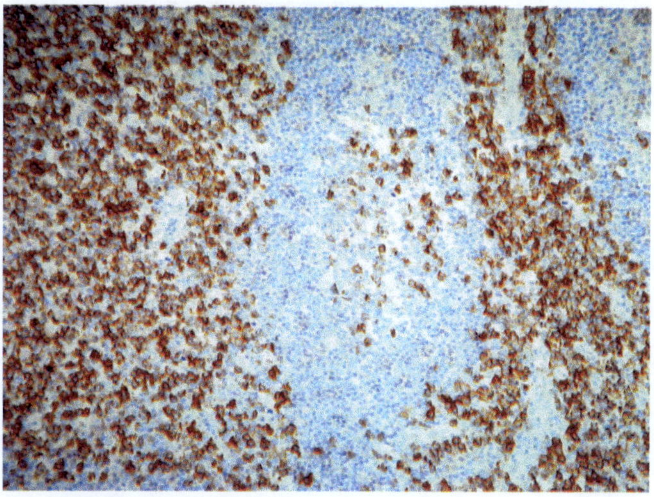

Fig. 5.111. CD38 staining reveals an abundance of plasma cells in the paracortex with a few cells within the germinal center.

Table 5.28
Infectious mononucleosis – morphology

- Non-specific reactive histology
- Mild follicular hyperplasia
- Marked paracortical hyperplasia
- Paracortex expanded with mottled appearance due to immunoblast proliferation
- Immunoblasts of B- and T cell origin mixed with plasmacytoid and plasma cells
- Monocytoid B cells in nodal sinuses
- Large atypical and Reed–Sternberg-like cells present
- Vascular proliferation
- Latent membrane protein detected by immunohistochemistry
- EBV-RNA (EBER) detected by in situ hybridization

(EBER) can be detected by in situ hybridization (**Table 5.28**; **Figs. 5.112**, **5.113**, **5.114**, **5.115**, **5.116**, and **5.117**).

Other Viral Lymphadenopathies

Measles virus, a paramyxovirus, produces a marked generalized lymphoid response as the virus replicates in macrophages and lymphocytes in the unimmunized individual. The lymphadenitis that follows vaccination with live attenuated virus is similar to those seen with many other viruses. There is follicular hyperplasia and expansion of the paracortex by a marked proliferation of immunoblasts, the latter producing a characteristic mottled

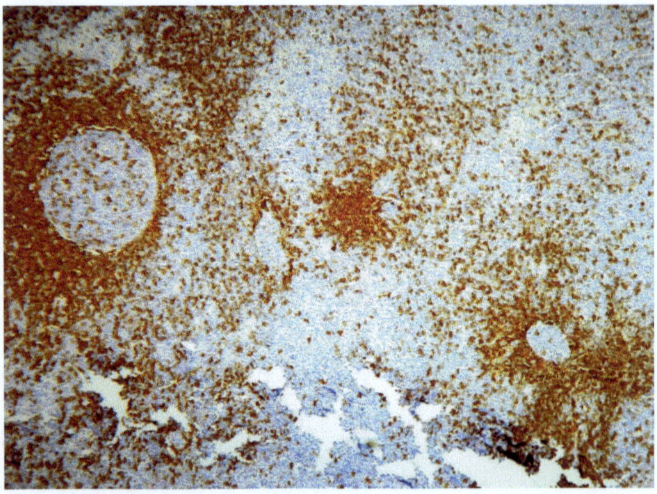

Fig. 5.112. Infectious mononucleosis showing markedly expanded paracortex with two widely separated follicles, one hyperplastic (CD20 stain).

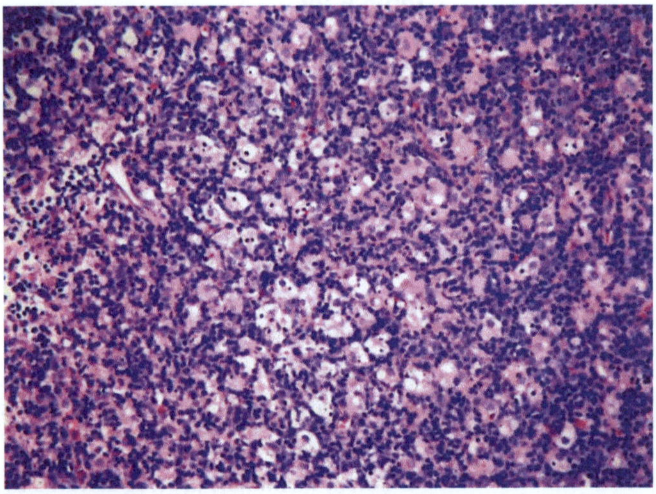

Fig. 5.113. Mottled appearance of expanded paracortex due to proliferation of immunoblasts.

appearance. Scattered in the paracortex are giant cells of the Warthin–Finkeldey type which are also seen in other hyperplastic lymph nodes especially during the prodromal stage of infections. These are large syncytial polykaryocytes, 25–50 μ in diameter and with as many as 50 nuclei.

Lymphadenopathies may be due to infection with cytomegalovirus, *Herpes simplex, Herpes zoster*, and vaccinia. The reaction is largely one of paracortical hyperplasias with less

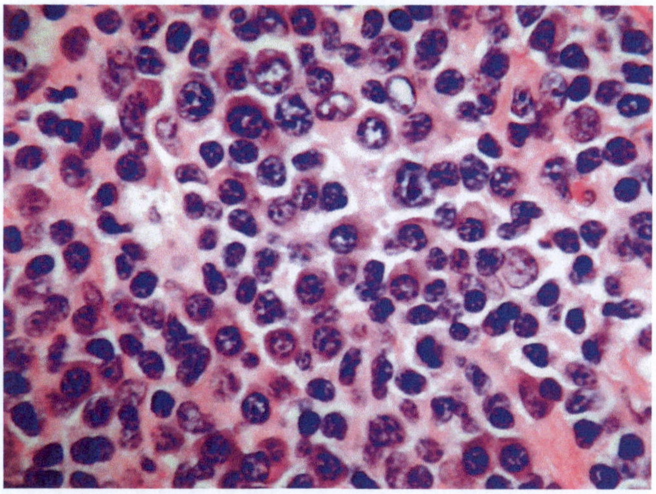

Fig. 5.114. A polymorphous infiltrate of small lymphocytes, plasmacytoid, and plasma cells is present in the paracortex.

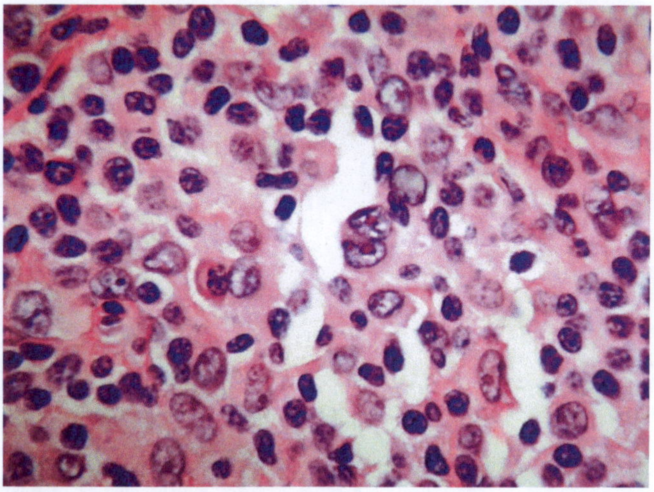

Fig. 5.115. Large transformed cells including a Reed–Sternberg-like cell are seen in the paracortex.

prominent follicular hyperplasia associated with focal monocytoid B cell hyperplasia and foci of necrosis at some stages of the infection. Antibodies to cytomegalovirus, Herpes simplex virus, and Herpes zoster virus are available for staining in paraffin-embedded sections.

Cytomegalovirus lymphadenitis presents as enlarged tender lymph nodes with effacement of architecture by a diffuse paracortical immunoblastic hyperplasia and variable follicular hyperplasia. The immunoblasts may be Reed–Sternberg-like and

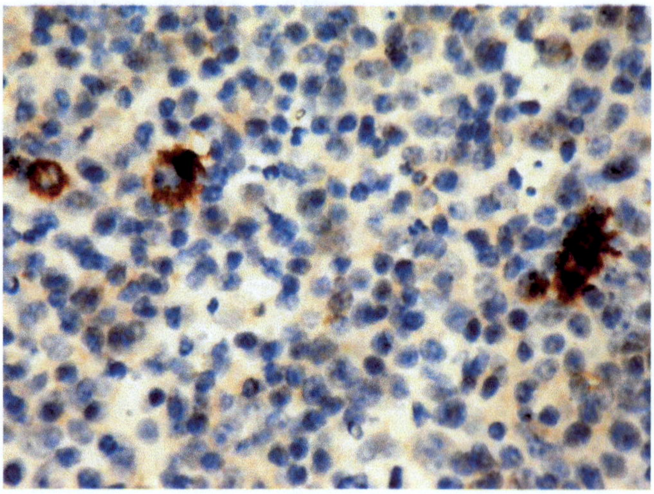

Fig. 5.116. Immunostain for latent membrane protein-1.

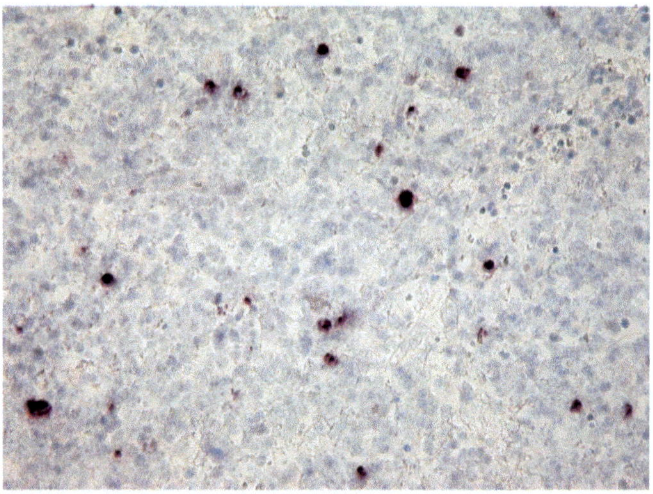

Fig. 5.117. In situ hybridization for EBV-RNA (EBER).

diagnosis is made through the identification of large intranuclear viral inclusions surrounded by a clear halo and basophilic cytoplasmic inclusions stained by the appropriate antibodies. The virus specifically infects T cells of both CD4+ and CD8+ subsets.

Most viral lymphadenitis shows paracortical hyperplasia with varying degrees of follicular hyperplasia. The relative prominence of the two components is often in a dynamic state and specific diagnosis can be made only by immunohistochemical demonstration of a specific viral antigen.

Paracortical Nodules/Expansion

Paracortical expansion is the result of stimulation of T cells and seldom occurs without accompanying follicular expansion. The separation into diseases causing follicular and paracortical can therefore only be arbitrary and the division is done largely on the basis of their most prominent presenting feature. The viral lymphadenopathies are a typical example as they may be associated with both follicular and paracortical expansion. A compounding problem is the dynamic nature of the response to viral infection which results in varying prominence of the T and B cell response; as such, specific diagnoses are made on the basis of demonstration of the virus with appropriate antibodies.

Dermatopathic Lymphadenopathy (DL)

Dermatopathic lymphadenopathy (DL) typically shows marked paracortical hyperplasia with or without accompanying follicular hyperplasia. DL is a reaction of the lymph node to the drainage of cutaneous antigens and melanin from various dermatoses. There is a proliferation of interdigitating reticulum cells (DRC), Langerhans cells, histiocytes, and T cells that produce pale-staining nodules in the paracortex. DRC and Langerhans cells have grooved nuclei and moderate quantities of pale cytoplasm. Scattered foam cells and pigment-containing histiocytes may be mixed within these nodules and similar pigment-containing histiocytes may distend the subcapsular sinus, macroscopically visible as a rim of pigment beneath the lymph node capsule.

In cutaneous T cell lymphoma, nodal involvement may be difficult to distinguish from severe DL. Localized accumulation of cerebriform T cells is a pointer to the diagnosis and it may be necessary for T cell gene rearrangement studies to confirm the diagnosis of neoplastic involvement.

S100, CD1a, and langerin (CD207) stain Langerhans cells and DRC (**Table 5.29**; **Figs. 5.118**, **5.119**, **5.120**, and **5.121**).

Table 5.29
Dermatopathic lymphadenopathy (DL) – morphology

- Draining lymph node reaction to cutaneous antigens and pigment
- Subcapsular rim of pigment visible macroscopically
- Pale paracortical nodules of proliferating DRC and Langerhans cells, histiocytes, and T cells
- Sinus histiocytosis
- Foam cells and phagocytic histiocytes in the paracortex
- S100, CD1a, and langerin stain DRC and Langerhans cells

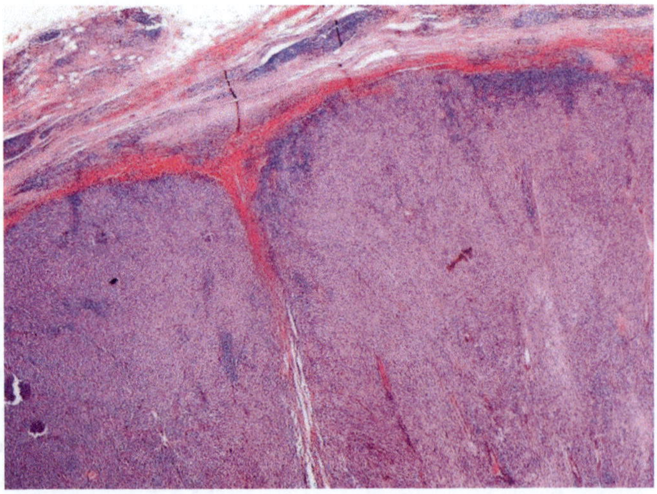

Fig. 5.118. DL. Cervical node with pale-staining areas of marked paracortical hyperplasia.

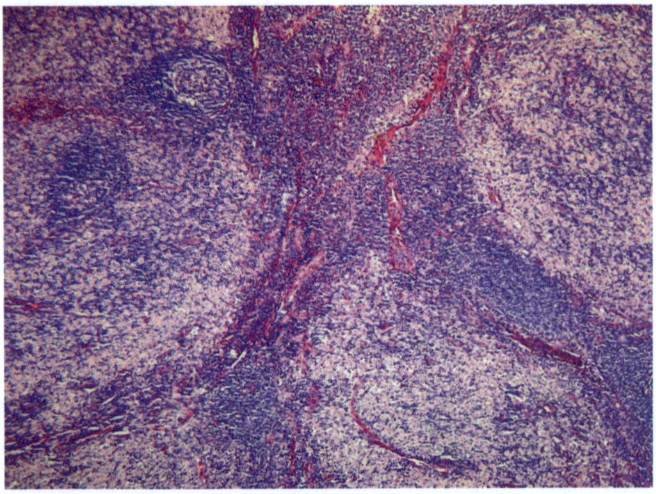

Fig. 5.119. DL in an axillary node. The nodules of pale-staining paracortex are strongly contrasted against the background of small dark lymphocytes.

Drug-Induced Lymphadenopathy

Hypersensitivity to anticonvulsant drugs including Dilantin, carbamazepine, and phenytoin may result in paracortical expansion from an infiltrate of B and T immunoblasts, small lymphocytes, histiocytes, neutrophils, and eosinophils. The immunoblasts are seldom atypical. The lymphadenopathy is generalized and typically associated with fever, skin rash, and peripheral blood eosinophilia, and can also occur with hypersensitivity to other drugs. Lymph node changes regress following drug withdrawal.

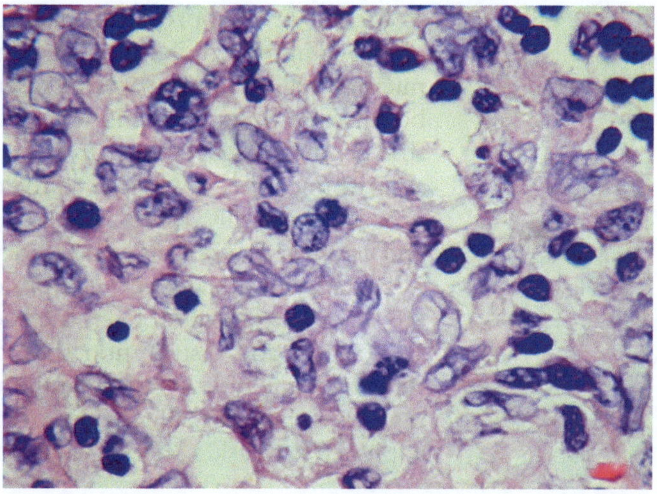

Fig. 5.120. DRC have abundant pale cytoplasm, distinct nuclear membranes that are folded, and irregular vesicular nuclei and indistinct nucleoli.

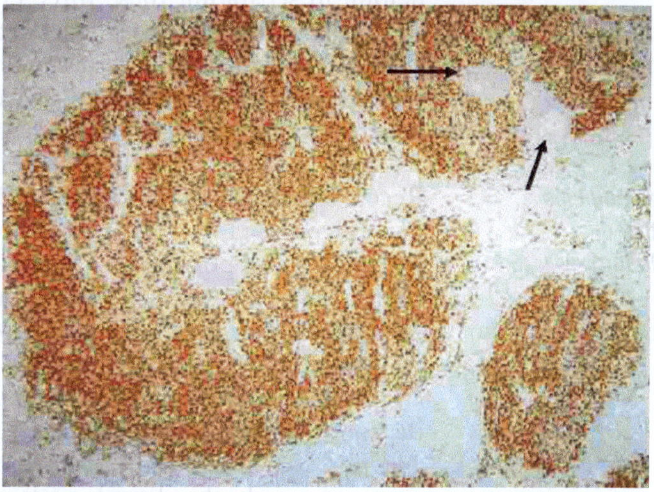

Fig. 5.121. S100 stains the paracortical DRC and residual follicles are indicated by the arrows.

The Diagnostic Approach to Nodular Infiltrates in Lymph Nodes

Despite the great interest in biological neural networks and the extensive research in artificial intelligence and cognitive modeling, we remain far from understanding how the brain functions to formulate histological diagnoses. Clearly it involves the processing and integration of a variety of factors that include pattern recognition and domain-specific knowledge. Having discussed the entities that produce a nodular pattern of infiltration, it is appropriate to formulate an approach to diagnosing the histological changes observed in the lymph node. The simplest approach is an algorithmic one achieved by answering a series of questions that needs to be sufficiently comprehensive to give consideration to all entities that produce the specific pattern of infiltration observed. Such an algorithmic process will lead to the diagnosis through a deductive process, especially when aided by immunohistochemical stains and other investigations as necessary.

Firstly, localized accumulations of distinctly different cells that are sharply demarcated from the background and display variable size, shape, and distribution should not be regarded as nodular infiltrates, and non-lymphoid infiltrates need to be excluded. Having determined that the pattern of infiltration is truly nodular, one approach is to ask a series of questions:

Are They Follicles or Nodules?

Stains for FDC will confirm the nature of true follicles, which will be associated with proliferating meshworks of FDC as in FL, MCL, and MZL. The pattern of proliferation of FDC can be helpful in separating these three entities. In FL, the meshworks tend to be expanded, sharply defined, dense, thick, and frequently confluent. In contrast, the meshworks in MCL tend to be loosely arranged and ill-defined although expanded; whereas in MZL, the meshworks are expanded but tend to be disrupted.

Are the Follicles Reactive or Neoplastic?

Reactive follicles can be very irregular and vary in size, with areas of confluence. However, they tend to retain a distinct mantle zone and may show polarization within the germinal centers. Polarization can be confirmed by the presence of a dense meshwork of FDC in the light zone compared to the dark zone, as well as by staining for Ki67, and there is a uniform distribution of CD3+ T cells in the light zone and the interface with the mantle zone. There are numerous apoptotic bodies, mitotic figures, and tingible-body macrophages present in reactive follicles. The paracortex and other lymph node compartments tend also to be expanded in reactive conditions.

Neoplastic follicles of FL are crowded and lie back-to-back, are mostly uniform in composition, and have rounded shapes. A mantle rim is often absent or attenuated. There is extension of neoplastic cells into the interfollicular regions, and similar follicles may be present in the surrounding extranodal tissue. Bcl2 and MT2 are very often positive in neoplastic follicles, and there is compression of surrounding reticulin.

Are Follicles Infrequent and "Constricted"?

MCL shows a thick rim of intermediate-sized lymphoid cells around constricted germinal centers. MCL can be identified by the FDC meshwork, and the constricted germinal centers can be displayed with stains for Ki67 and/or Bcl6. MCL are cyclin D1+/CD43+/CD5+. The follicles have two distinct layers, the germinal center and a thick surround rim of mantle cells that may merge with adjacent follicle. In contrast, cells of MZL have larger quantities of pale cytoplasm, produce a distinctive pale rim around germinal centers or an inverted follicular pattern, and are cyclin D1-/CD43– and usually CD5–.

Are the Follicles Exceptionally Large?

In progressive transformation of germinal centers, one or more follicles may be massively enlarged to four or more times greater than normal germinal centers. They show an expanded mantle zone with inward migration of mantle cells into the germinal center, breaking it up into clusters of centroblasts. Reactive follicles may be present in the background. In contrast, the neoplastic nodules of NLPHL replace the normal lymph node architecture; some of the nodules show the appearance of progressive transformation. LP cells are rosetted by CD57+/PD-1+/CD4+ follicle helper T cells and lend a mottled appearance to the nodules.

Do the Enlarged Germinal Centers Contain Atypical Cells?

The presence of homogenous clusters of atypical cells within enlarged germinal centers suggests colonization by lymphoma cells and in particular raises possibilities of FL and MZL.

Are the Nodules Homogenous or Heterogenous in Composition?

Nodules are generally poorly defined. They can be homogenous or heterogenous in composition.

Homogenous Nodules

Distension of lymph node sinuses by leukemic infiltrates produce poorly defined homogenous nodules outlined by normal reticulin. Immunophenotyping is required. The lymphoblastic leukemias/lymphomas express TdT and the corresponding lineage-specific markers. MCL and MZL produce homogenous nodules that surround constricted germinal centers.

Heterogenous Nodules

T cell hyperplasia in the paracortex is nodular. It is associated with distinctive hyperplasia of DRC which have very irregular nuclei, folded nuclear membranes, and small eosinophilic nucleoli. Their copious pale cytoplasm often contains phagocytosed melanin pigment. The T cells are intermixed with DRC and occasionally contain entrapped follicles. DRC stain with S100, CD1a, and langerin (CD207).

Proliferation or growth centers of CLL/SLL are ill-defined nodules of pallor compared to the dark blue of surrounding small lymphocytes. The nodules are heterogenous and composed of prolymphocytes, paraimmunoblasts, and small lymphocytes. The proliferation centers are not outlined by reticulin. CD23 positivity confirms the diagnosis, and there are no FDC within growth centers.

Lymphoplasmacytoid lymphoma (LPL) distends sinuses to produce heterogenous nodules comprising a mixture of plasmacytoid and plasma cells that stain for CD38 and CD138 and show light-chain restriction.

When defined by surrounding fibrosis, *Hodgkin lymphoma and nodular sclerosis* need exclusion. Lacunar cells are CD15+/CD30+/CD45–. They are present in a milieu of small lymphocytes, epithelioid histiocytes, plasma cells, and eosinophils.

If There Is Marked Follicular Hyperplasia, Can a Specific Diagnosis Be Made?

Follicular and paracortical hyperplasia tend to overlap, varying at different stages of the disease, especially in viral infections. Features that help identify specific diagnoses are as follows:

Toxoplasma lymphadenitis: Granulomas scattered throughout the node and impinging on hyperplastic germinal centers, associated with monocytoid B cell hyperplasia.

HIV/AIDS lymphadenitis: Pronounced follicular hyperplasia that coalesces, subsequently involutes, and ultimately shows lymphocyte depletion. Prominent monocytoid B cells in early stages with Warthin–Finkeldey polykaryocytes.

Kimura disease: Florid germinal center hyperplasia with focal necrosis, eosinophil microabscesses, proliferation of high-endothelial vessels, fibrosis, and occasional Warthin–Finkeldey cells.

Castleman disease: "Lollipop" germinal centers with hyalinization and proliferation of FDC, "twin" germinal centers within a common mantle zone, and stimulated cells in interfollicular areas. Prominent plasmacytoid monocytes in hyaline vascular variant.

Syphilis lymphadenitis: Combined follicular and paracortical hyperplasia, pronounced capsular fibrosis, arteritis, and phlebitis with cuffing of by plasma cells.

Kikuchi disease: Combined follicular and paracortical hyperplasia with prominent B and T blasts, areas of apoptosis surrounded by plasmacytoid monocytes and crescentic phagocytic histiocytes but no neutrophils and rare plasma cells.

Systemic lupus erythematosus: Combined follicular and paracortical hyperplasia that mimics Kikuchi disease but shows prominent plasma cells and vasculitis with occasional hematoxylin bodies.

Drug hypersensitivity: Follicular and paracortical hyperplasia with immunoblasts, small lymphocytes, histiocytes, neutrophils, and eosinophils with occasional atypical immunoblasts.

Viral lymphadenitis: Paracortical and follicular hyperplasia. Search for viral inclusions and employ antibodies to specific viral antigens.

Other conditions that produce *lymphadenitis with focal necrosis: Yersinia* and other bacteria, Herpes simplex virus, Epstein–Barr virus, tuberculosis, leprosy and cat-scratch disease, allergic reactions, and lymphoma (mostly large cell type). Histochemical stains are available for cat-scratch disease, tuberculosis, and leprosy, and immunostaining with antibodies to cytomegalovirus, Herpes simplex virus, and Epstein–Barr virus can be performed for specific identification of causative organism.

Do the Vague Nodules Represent Paracortical Nodules?

Use a reticulin stain to help localize the nodular expansions. If localized to sinuses, exclude leukemic infiltrates and metastatic processes.

Use S100 to confirm the presence of DRC in dermatopathic lymphadenopathy and involvement by cutaneous T cell lymphoma.

Clearly, the *differential diagnosis of reactive lymphoid hyperplasia* is extensive. An alternative approach to that suggested is through the identification of defining features which is discussed in greater detail in **Chapter 8**.

Briefly, *granulomatous lymphadenitis* can be due to tuberculosis and other infections including brucellosis and fungi, leishmaniasis, sarcoidosis, berylliosis, and may be seen in node draining Crohn's disease, primary biliary cirrhosis, and tumors. *Suppurative granulomatous lymphadenitis* may result from cat-scratch disease, lymphogranuloma venereum, Yersinia infection, fungi, atypical mycobacteria, lepromatous leprosy, typhoid fever, Kikuchi's lymphadenitis, SLE, and Kawasaki's disease. *Marked necrosis* in the lymph node may be seen in infarction, malignant lymphoma, SLE, Kawasaki's disease, pneumocystis carinii lymphadenitis, and the causes of suppurative granulomatous lymphadenitis. *Prominent interfollicular immunoblasts* and other large lymphoid cells should raise the possibility of viral infections such as EBV, herpes zoster and herpes simplex, post-vaccinial and drug reactions, Kikuchi's lymphadenitis, and angioimmunoblastic T cell lymphoma. *Expansion of the lymph node sinuses,* except for Whipple's disease, are generally not related to infectious conditions and should suggest the possibility of a non-specific sinus histiocytosis, sinus histiocytosis as a reaction to tumor in the draining area, Rosai Dorfman disease, reactive hemophagocytic syndrome, reaction to foreign materials, lymphangiographic contrast media, and storage diseases like Niemann–Pick and Gaucher's diseases. When lymph nodes are hypocellular with lymphoid depletion late-phase HIV-associated lymphadenopathy, primary immunodeficiencies, reactive hemophagocytic syndrome, angioimmunoblastic T cell lymphoma, and proteinaceous lymphadenopathy should be excluded (**Table 5.30**).

Table 5.30
Suggested approach to follicular and nodular infiltrates

Are they follicles or nodules?
Stain for FDC
If they are follicles, are the follicles reactive or neoplastic?
Examine for polarization, mitosis, apoptosis, tingible-body macrophages, and cellular composition Stain for bcl-2, MT2
Follicles are infrequent and small/regressed
Exclude MCL, MZL, CHL.
MCL: CD20+/cyclinD1+/Bcl2+/CD43+/CD5+/CD23–/Bcl6–/CD10–
MZL:CD20+/CD79a+/Bcl2+/CD5–/CD10–/Bcl6–/cyclinD1–, variable CD43+
CHL: RSC are CD15+/CD30+/CD45–, variable CD20+
How many layers are there in the follicle?
Two layers – MCL; three layers or inverted follicular pattern – MZL
Are the follicles exceptionally large?
Distinguish PTGC from NLPHL
PTGC: one or more PTGC mixed with enlarged germinal centers
NLPHL: closely packed nodules replace node with hyperplastic follicles compressed to periphery; LP cells CD20+/CD45+/Bcl6+/OCT2+/BOB.1+ variable EMA+; spontaneous rosetting T cells are CD3+/CD4=/PD1+
Do the enlarged germinal centers contain atypical cells?
Exclude MZL and colonization by large B cell lymphoma
Are the nodules homogenous or heterogenous in composition?
Homogenous nodules
Distending sinuses: LBL, MCL, MZL
Heterogenous nodules
– Distending sinuses: LPL
– In cortex: growth centers of CLL/SLL
– In paracortex: T cell nodules/hyperplasia
– CHL
If there is marked follicular hyperplasia, can a specific diagnosis be made?
Examine for viral inclusions, granulomas, necrosis, monocytoid B cells, Warthin–Finkeldey cells, plasma cells, neutrophils, eosinophils, mast cells, crescentic histiocytes, and "lollipop" germinal centers. Stain for organisms.
Non-neoplastic granulomatous: tuberculosis, other infections including brucellosis and fungi, leishmaniasis, sarcoidosis, berylliosis, and in nodes draining Crohn's disease, primary biliary cirrhosis, and tumors.
Suppurative granulomatous lymphadenitis: cat-scratch disease, lymphogranuloma venereum, Yersinia infection, fungi, atypical mycobacteria. Lepromatous leprosy, typhoid fever, Kikuchi's lymphadenitis, SLE, and Kawasaki's disease.
Marked necrosis: infarction, malignant lymphoma, SLE, Kawasaki's disease, pneumocystis carinii lymphadenitis, and suppurative granulomatous lymphadenitis.

Table 5.30 (continued)

Prominent interfollicular large lymphoid cells: viral infections such as EBV, herpes zoster and herpes simplex, post-vaccinial and drug reactions, Kikuchi's lymphadenitis and angioimmunoblastic T cell lymphoma.

Sinus expansion: Whipple's disease, non-specific sinus histiocytosis, sinus histiocytosis as a reaction to tumor in the draining area, Rosai Dorfman disease, reactive hemophagocytic syndrome, reaction to foreign materials, lymphangiographic contrast media, and storage diseases like Niemann–Pick and Gaucher's diseases.

Hypocellular with lymphoid depletion: late-phase HIV-associated lymphadenopathy, primary immunodeficiencies, reactive hemophagocytic syndrome, angioimmunoblastic T cell lymphoma, and proteinaceous lymphadenopathy.

Chapter 6

Diffuse Lymphoid Infiltrations

Key words: B cell neoplasms, T cell neoplasms, chronic lymphocytic leukemia, small lymphocytic lymphoma (CLL/SLL), lymphoplasmacytic lymphoma (LPL), diffuse large B cell lymphoma (DLBCL), Burkitt lymphoma (BL), extranodal lymphomas, T cell lymphoblastic lymphoma/leukemia (T-LL), peripheral T cell lymphoma, angioimmunoblastic T cell lymphoma, anaplastic large cell lymphoma (ALCL), adult T cell leukemia/lymphoma, histiocytic and dendritic ell neoplasms, Hodgkin lymphoma.

The diffuse pattern of nodal infiltration occurs when there are no follicles or few residual follicles present and the infiltrative process involves the node diffusely with complete or partial obliteration of normal architecture. While it is the most common pattern of infiltration encountered in the lymph node, it is estimated that not more than 10% of lymph node biopsies show complete architectural effacement by a diffuse infiltration. All non-Hodgkin lymphomas other than follicular lymphomas can produce a diffuse pattern, but again, a pure diffuse pattern is seen only in about 20% of lymphomas. The diffuse pattern is most common in small lymphocytic lymphoma and lymphoblastic lymphoma both of which have a more homogenous infiltrate compared to the other lymphomas. Diffuse lymphomatous infiltrates tend to uniformly involve a part, if not all of the lymph node. In contrast, infiltration by leukemias, which represents spillover from the peripheral blood, tends to involve the lymph node focally and often in a patchy manner in its early stages. Mixed cellularity and lymphocyte-depleted Hodgkin lymphoma may also produce a diffuse pattern but the infiltrate is heterogenous. Metastatic tumors produce a diffuse pattern that often spares parts of the lymph node. Benign diseases which are much more common than the lymphomas rarely produce a completely diffuse pattern. More characteristically, they produce small and multiple changes in different compartments of the lymph node such as in infectious mononucleosis, systemic lupus erythematosus, phenytoin

A.S.-Y. Leong, *A Pattern Approach to Lymph Node Diagnosis*,
DOI 10.1007/978-1-4419-7176-0_6, © Springer Science+Business Media, LLC 2011

hypersensitivity, and other infectious conditions where there are both follicular and paracortical hyperplasia and often also sinus dilatation and engorgement. As will be discussed in the relevant sections, staining for FDC with CD21, CD35, or D2-40 can be very useful for the demonstration of residual nodal architecture which may be masked by the infiltrative process.

Diffuse infiltrates can be B cell lymphomas, T cell lymphomas, histiocytic neoplasms, classical Hodgkin lymphoma, mixed cellularity, leukemias, and some reactive conditions. Hodgkin lymphoma, leukemias, and the reactive conditions are discussed in other chapters as many display defining features that reflect their identity. Several T cell lymphomas that are primary extranodal in origin may also involve lymph nodes and these are only briefly discussed (**Table 6.1**).

Table 6.1
Diffuse pattern of infiltration

B cell neoplasms
Chronic lymphocytic leukemia/small lymphocytic lymphoma (CLL/SLL)
Lymphoplasmacytic lymphoma (LPL)
Diffuse large B cell lymphoma (DLBCL)
Burkitt lymphoma
Nodal involvement by primary extranodal lymphoma and leukemias: MALT lymphoma, myeloid leukemia, lymphoblastic lymphoma, hairy cell leukemia, pro-lymphocytic leukemia (*see* Chapter 8)
T cell and NK cell neoplasms
T cell lymphoblastic leukemia/lymphoma
Peripheral T cell lymphoma
Angioimmunoblastic T cell lymphoma
Anaplastic large cell lymphoma
Adult T cell leukemia/lymphoma
Nodal involvement by extranodal lymphoma and leukemia; nodal involvement by cutaneous T cell lymphomas; others discussed in Chapter 8
Histiocytic and dendritic cell neoplasms
Histiocytic sarcoma
Langerhans cell histiocytosis
Interdigitating dendritic cell (IDC) sarcoma
Follicular dendritic cell (FDC) sarcoma
Classical Hodgkin lymphoma, mixed cellularity

B Cell Neoplasms

Chronic Lymphocytic Leukemia/Small Lymphocytic Lymphoma (CLL/SLL)

Chronic lymphocytic leukemia (CLL) and small lymphocytic lymphoma (SLL) refer to the same disease represented by different manifestations. The term “SLL” is applied when the neoplasm involves lymph nodes without leukemic manifestations and

"CLL" is used when presentation is primarily that of lymphocytosis. However, SLL patients also often develop lymphocytosis and bone marrow involvement, and lymphadenopathy is common in CLL.

CLL is the most common leukemia of adults in Western countries, the incidence increasing with age; 65 year being the mean age at diagnosis. The male:female ratio is about 1.5:2.1. The incidence is low in Eastern countries and this low incidence is maintained in migrant populations. Sites of involvement by CLL include blood and bone marrow, with lymph nodes, spleen, and liver also typically involved. Involvement of other extranodal sites is less frequent. Most patients are asymptomatic but presentation can be variable as is the course and outcome. A small IgM paraproteinemia may be found in some patients corresponding to the immunoglobulin expressed by the malignant lymphocytes. CLL/SLL is thought to be closely related to memory B cells.

Two clinical staging systems are used to define disease extent and prognosis. The Rai system employs five stages: 0 = lymphocytosis in blood and bone marrow only; I = lymphocytosis with enlarged lymph nodes; II = lymphocytosis with enlarged nodes and splenomegaly or hepatomegaly; III = lymphocytosis with anemia; and IV = lymphocytosis with thrombocytopenia. Stage 0 represents low risk, stages I and II intermediate risk, and II and IV high-risk groups. The Binet system is based on the number of involved anatomical regions, namely head and neck, axillae, groins, spleen, and liver, combined with the levels of hemoglobin and platelets. In stage A and B, hemoglobin is >10 g/dL and platelets are $>100 \times 10^9$/L. In stage A, two or fewer anatomical regions are involved; in B, three or more anatomical regions are involved, and in stage C, hemoglobin is <10 g/dL or platelets are $<100 \times 10^9$/L, regardless of the anatomical distribution of the disease.

Two clinically aggressive forms of CLL/SLL may occur. Rarely, prolymphocytic transformation may develop in which para-immunoblasts form the predominant cell type. This transformation is associated with worsening of clinical symptoms, although only a few cases have been studied and it is not known if prognosis is clearly different to the more usual form of CLL/SLL. This condition should not be confused with B-prolymphocytic leukemia which is clinically and phenotypically different and not associated with CLL.

Richter syndrome occurs in about 5% of CLL/SLL, usually associated with a change in pace of the disease, with B symptoms or with the development of bulky lymphadenopathy or hepatomegaly. Transformation occurs to a diffuse large B cell lymphoma (DLBCL) or, in very rare cases, to a histological appearance indistinguishable from classical Hodgkin lymphoma with Reed–Sternberg cells that are often positive for Epstein–Barr virus. Molecular studies have shown that the CLL/SLL and

Table 6.2
CLL/SLL – clinical

• Most common adult leukemia in Western countries
• Incidence increases with age, 65 years being the mean age at diagnosis
• "SLL" used when presentation is of lymphadenopathy without lymphocytosis
• SLL patients eventually develop lymphocytosis and bone marrow involvement
• "CLL" used when presentation is primarily that of lymphocytosis but lymphadenopathy is common
• May have a small component of IgM paraprotein
• Rai and Binet staging systems employed for extent of disease and prognosis
• Rarely prolymphocytic transformation with predominant para-immunoblasts
• Progression of symptoms and development of bulky lymphadenopathy with or without hepatosplenomegaly in <5% indicates Richter syndrome, i.e., transformation to DLBCL or classic
Hodgkin lymphoma

DLBCL are genetically related in 50–60% of cases. Prognosis is poor (**Table 6.2**).

Morphology

The architecture of the lymph node is obliterated by a diffuse monotonous infiltrate of uniformly small, round lymphocytes. Their condensed chromatin, inconspicuous or absent nucleoli, and scanty cytoplasm impart a deep blue hue to the infiltrate. The infiltrate is striking as it is generally uniform and complete throughout the node, described as "wall-to-wall," although remnants of normal architecture may sometimes be present. Mitoses are rare. There is no evidence of plasmacytic differentiation, and intranuclear immunoglobulin inclusions are very rare. The neoplastic lymphocytes spread through the capsule into the surrounding connective tissue. Paler, poorly defined nodular areas are invariably present in well-prepared sections. These are the pseudofollicles, also known as pseudofollicular growth centers or proliferation centers. They appear pale relative to the surrounding infiltrate because the cells in these proliferation centers are less-densely packed and variable numbers of larger cells are present, viz, prolymphocytes and para-immunoblasts. The former are medium sized and have dispersed chromatin and a distinct nucleolus while the latter are larger and have vesicular nuclei with a prominent central nucleolus and relatively abundant cytoplasm (so-called "baby immunoblasts"). Occasional mitosis can be found in these pseudofollicles which may vary in size and density, ranging from small and scattered to large and crowded (**Table 6.3**; **Figs. 6.1**, **6.2**, **6.3**, **6.4**, and **6.5**, **6.6**).

Table 6.3
CLL/SLL – morphology

• Diffuse monotonous infiltrate of deep blue small lymphocytes with coarsely clumped chromatin
• Remnants of normal architecture may be preserved
• Pale proliferation centers or pseudofollicles of different sizes are invariably present
• Proliferation centers contain variable numbers of larger prolymphocytes and para-immunoblasts

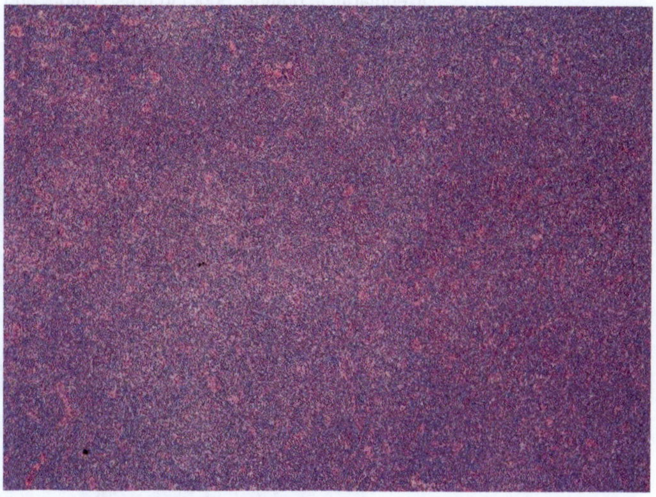

Fig. 6.1. CLL/SLL showing diffuse obliteration of nodal architecture by small round lymphoid cells with dense chromatin and scanty cytoplasm accounting for the tinctorial properties. A vague nodularity is imparted by poorly defined areas of relative pallor.

Immunohistology

The cells of CLL/SLL show weak or dim expression of surface immunoglobulin by flow cytometry. In paraffin-embedded sections with antigen retrieval in 4 M urea combined with careful proteolytic digestion, it is possible to demonstrate consistent light-chain restriction. Occasional larger cells including prolymphocytes and para-immunoblasts show cytoplasmic immunoglobulin light-chain restriction and small lymphocytes show similar in the cisternae of perinuclear endoplasmic reticulum. IgM and IgD can also be identified. Staining for FDC with CD21 or D2-40 is helpful in demonstrating residual lymphoid follicles (**Figs. 6.7** and **6.8**).

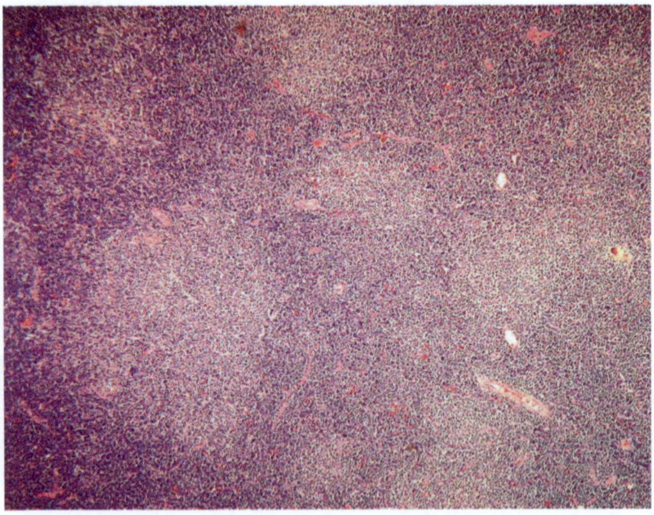

Fig. 6.2. The pale nodules are pseudofollicles or proliferation centers. They display irregularity in outline, poor circumscription, and variability in size and density.

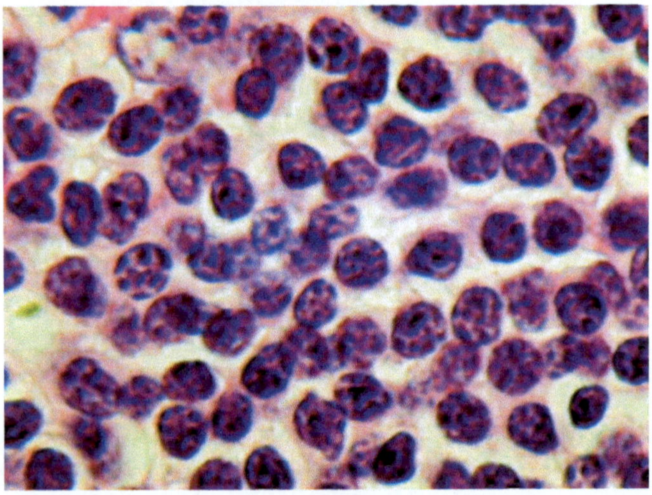

Fig. 6.3. The cells outside of the proliferation centers are mostly small round lymphocytes with coarse chromatin and scanty cytoplasm.

The B cell-associated antigens CD20 and CD79a are expressed in CLL/SLL. In addition, there is expression of CD23, CD5, and CD43. CD5 and CD43 may show variable staining in the neoplastic population. CD23 is fixation sensitive and is also a useful marker of follicular dendritic cells, allowing identification of the occasional preserved follicle in the infiltrated node. CLL/SLL cells are negative for CD10 and CD3 (**Figs. 6.9, 6.10, 6.11, 6.12**).

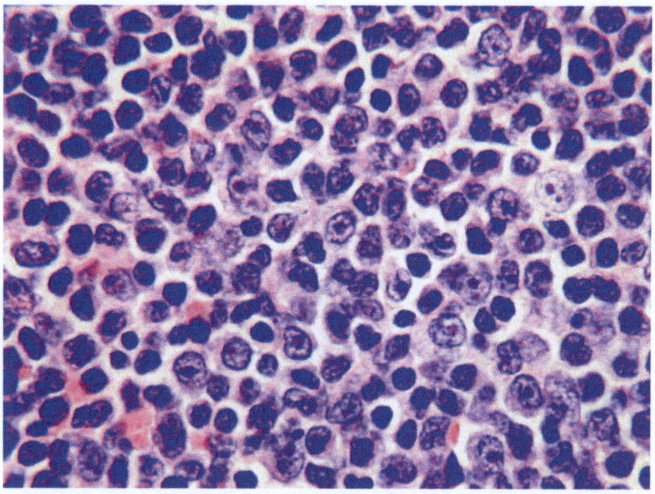

Fig. 6.4. The proliferation centers are less densely packed and made up of mostly small lymphocytes and variable numbers of larger prolymphocytes and paraimmnoblasts.

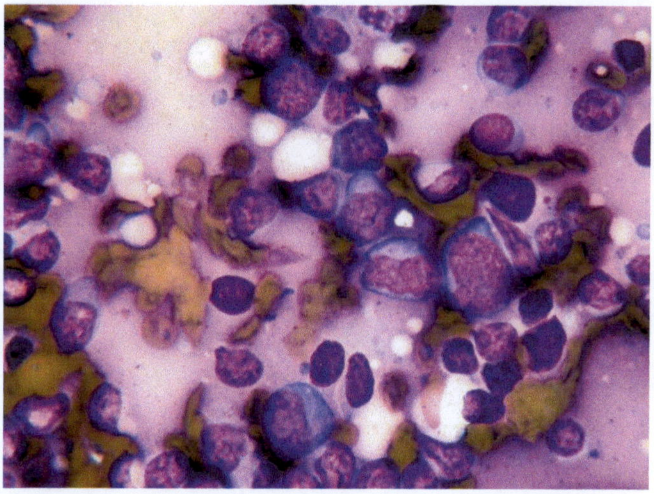

Fig. 6.5. Air-dried imprint stained with Giemsa showing a mixture of small lymphocytes and larger cells from the proliferation centers.

Genetics

CLL has the highest genetic predisposition of all hematologic neoplasms. Familial predisposition can be shown in 5–10% of patients and the overall risk is two to seven times increased for first-degree relatives of patients with CLL.

Based on DNA sequencing of the Ig genes, usually *IgH*, and comparing with germline sequences, CLL can be divided into mutated and unmutated groups (based on an arbitrary cut-off of >2%). Patients with unmutated Ig genes have a more aggressive clinical course and require therapy sooner than those with mutated Ig genes. The expression of CD38 and ZAP70

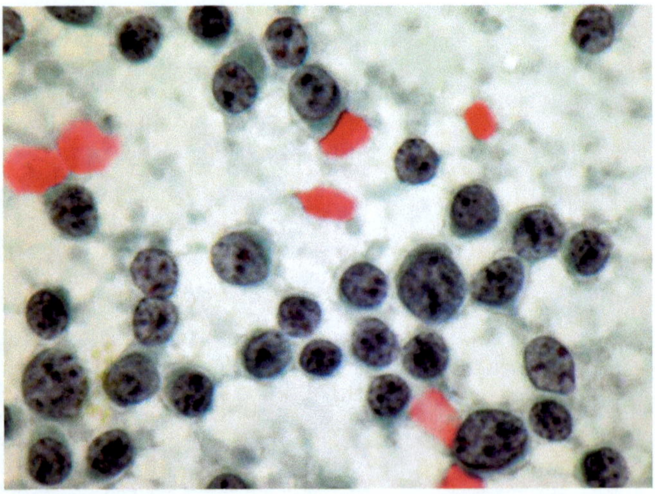

Fig. 6.6. Alcohol-fixed smear stained with Papanicolaou stain showing small lymphocytes with coarse chromatin and scanty cytoplasm typical of CLL/SLL.

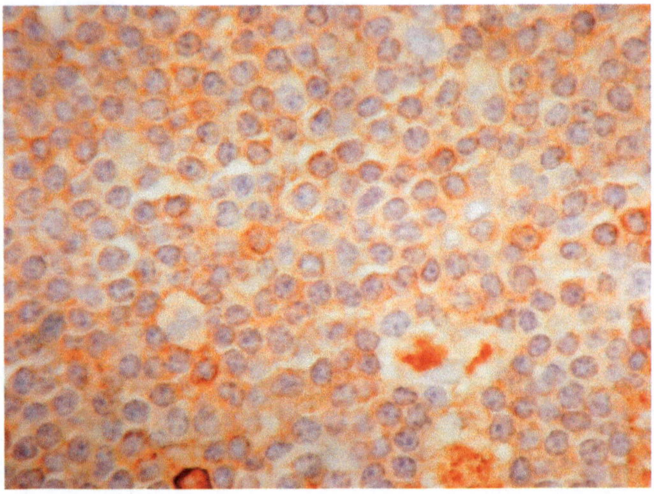

Fig. 6.7. The small lymphocytes in CLL/SLL stain for Igλ while there was no staining for Igκ.

correlates strongly, although not entirely, with unmutated Ig genes in CLL/SLL (up to 20% of cases show discordant mutational status and ZAP70) (**Table 6.4**).

With the rare conversion to diffuse large-B cell lymphoma (DLBCL), the neoplastic cells resemble the centroblastic variant of DLBCL, and a genetic relationship to the original CLL/SLL clone has been demonstrated in 50–60% of cases. In about 0.5% of cases, the transformation is to classical Hodgkin lymphoma, often positive for Epstein–Barr virus (**Figs. 6.13**, **6.14**, **6.15**, **6.16**, **6.17**, **6.18**, **6.19**, **6.20**, **6.21**, **6.22**).

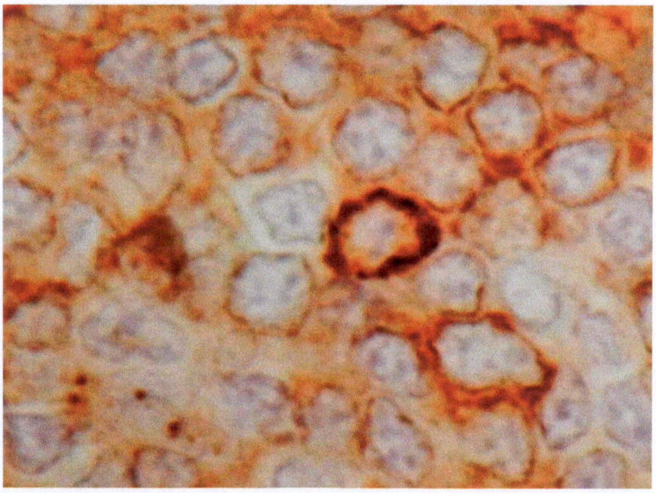

Fig. 6.8. Two cells in the field display strong cytoplasmic staining for Igλ while the other small lymphocytes show staining of cisternae of perinuclear cisternae and cytoplasm (*arrows*).

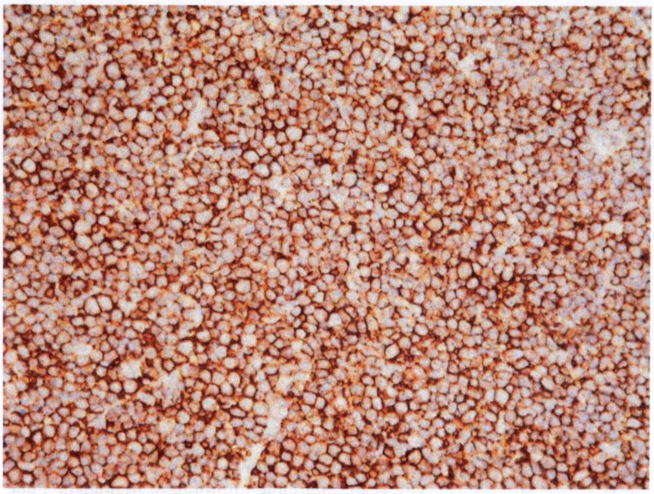

Fig. 6.9. CD20 labels the cells of CLL/SLL uniformly.

The differential diagnoses of CLL/SLL include other small cell lymphomas, namely, lymphoplasmacytic lymphoma (LPL), mantle cell lymphoma (MCL), marginal zone lymphoma, follicular lymphoma (FL), and lymphoblastic lymphoma (LL).

MCL, MZL, and FL generally produce a follicular or nodular pattern, so that the distinction from CLL/SLL is largely based on the separation of follicles from growth centers seen in the latter condition. Staining for FDC is particularly useful in this regard as growth centers are not associated with FDC. The extent of plasmacytic differentiation seen in CLL/SLL is much less that in

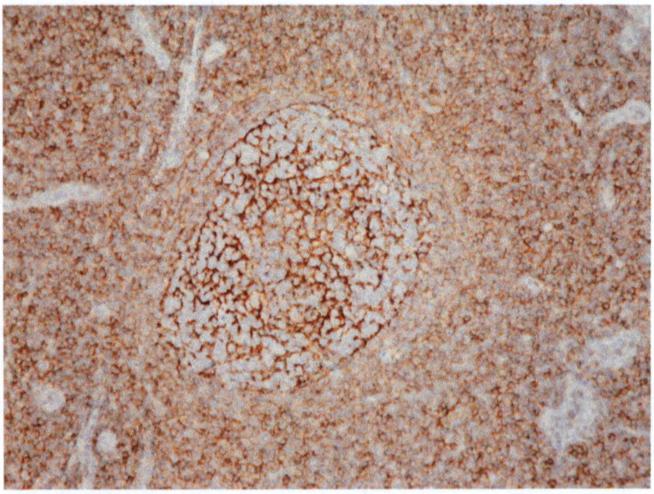

Fig. 6.10. The neoplastic cells stain with CD23, which, in this field, also stains the dendritic reticulum cells of a residual benign follicle.

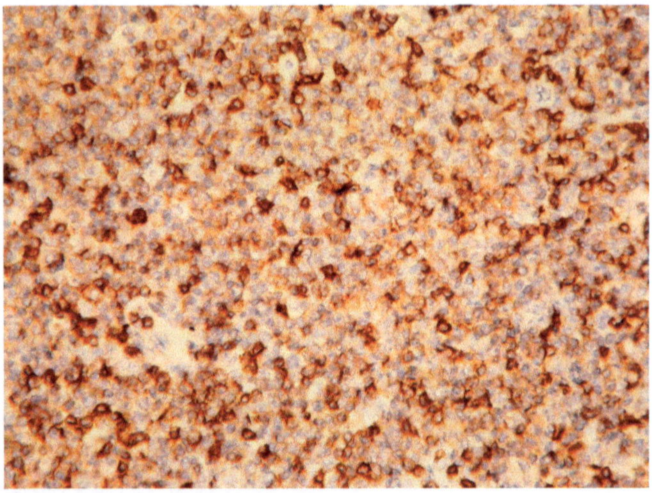

Fig. 6.11. Variable numbers of neoplastic cells stain for CD43.

LPL. Dutcher bodies and Russell bodies are rarely observed in CLL/SLL and proliferation centers do not occur in LPL. The cells of LPL are CD5–. CD38 and CD138 staining will reveal plasmacytoid cells in LPL. The neoplastic infiltrate in MCL is a monotonous population of round cells with coarse chromatin and slightly irregular nuclear outlines, and proliferation centers and para-immunoblasts are not seen. Unlike CLL/SLL cells, which are CD23+ and cyclin D1–, the cells of MCL are CD23– and cyclin D1+ and are enmeshed among proliferating FDC. The neoplastic follicles in FL are sharply circumscribed with proliferation of follicular dendritic cells and contain angulated and

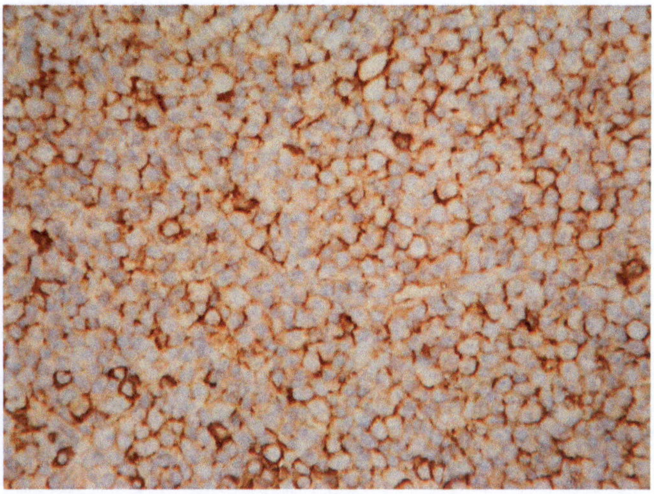

Fig. 6.12. CLL/SLL showing variable staining for CD5.

Table 6.4
CLL/SLL – immunohistology and genetics

- B cell antigens CD20 and CD79a are positive
- Weak (dim) staining for membranous Ig by flow cytometry
- Light-chain restriction can be consistently demonstrated following antigen retrieval in 4 M urea at 100°C followed by proteolytic digestion
- Variable staining for CD5 and CD43
- Consistent expression of CD23 (fixation dependant)
- CD3 and CD10 are negative
- CLL/SLL with unmutated *IgH* genes have more aggressive clinical course
- CD38 and ZAP70 expression correlate strongly with unmutated genes and poorer prognosis

cleaved centrocytes and centroblasts which are different in appearance from the round prolymphocytes and para-immunoblasts of CLL/SLL. Furthermore, neoplastic follicles, unlike proliferation centers, extend into perinodal connective tissue including fat. Neoplastic follicle cells are Bcl6+, CD10+, and CD5–, whereas CLL/SLL cells are Bcl6–, CD10–, and CD5+. Unlike proliferation centers, neoplastic follicles produce compression of surrounding reticulin. The cells of LL are medium sized with blastic nuclei that show indentations or clefts, with frequent mitoses. Affected patients are young and the neoplastic cells are positive for TdT which is negative in CLL/SLL. Frequently LL is of T cell lineage and stains accordingly with pan-T markers (**Table 6.5**).

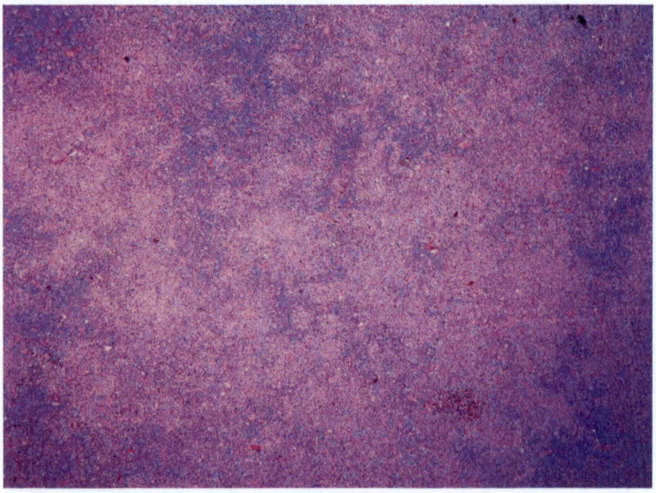

Fig. 6.13. The case shown in preceding figures developed bulky lymphadenopathy and hepatosplenomegaly 8 months after completion of treatment. Large areas of confluent proliferation centers are present representing DLBCL.

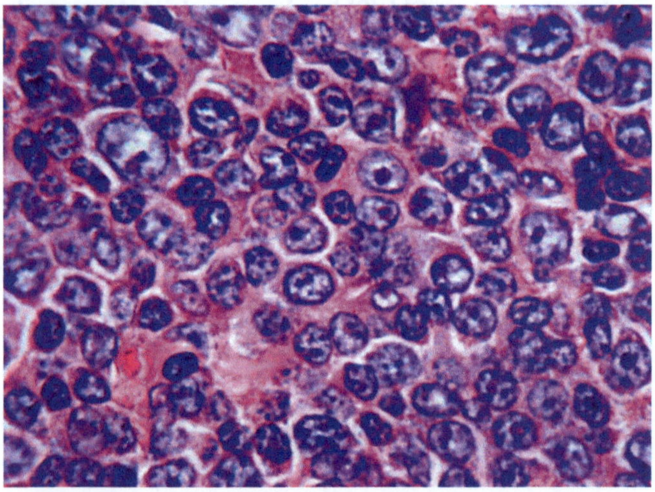

Fig. 6.14. The DLBCL is of the centroblastic type.

Lymphoplasmacytic Lymphoma (LPL)

Plasma cell differentiation may be seen in a number of B cell lymphomas. Lymphocytic tumors that are CD23+ and CD5+ and contain large numbers of immunoglobulin inclusions are now regarded as a variant of CLL/SLL, and the diagnosis of lymphoplasmacytic lymphoma is now made only in the absence of the features of other B cell lymphomas that can show plasma cell differentiation such as follicular lymphoma and marginal zone lymphoma (MZL). Mantle cell lymphoma (MCL) is not associated with plasma cell differentiation. The distinction may not always be clear-cut and some cases may need to be labeled as small B

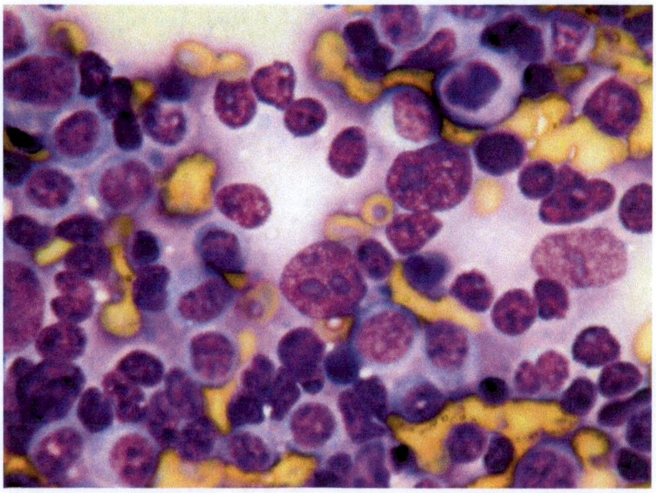

Fig. 6.15. Giemsa-stained imprint showing centroblasts with large vesicular nuclei, two to three prominent nucleoli and moderate quantities of RNA-rich cytoplasm.

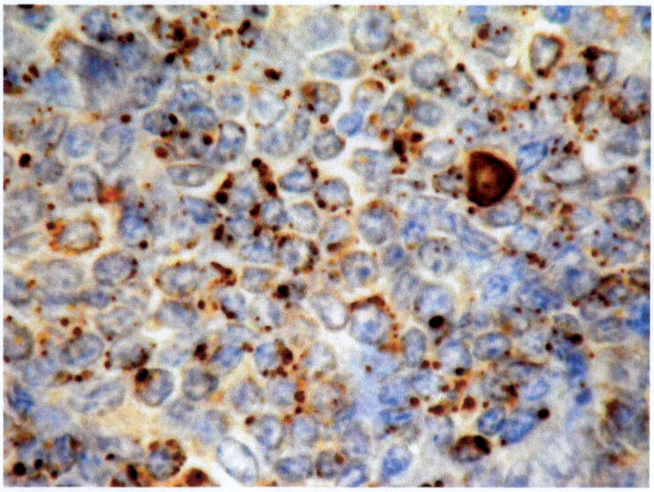

Fig. 6.16. There is prominent Igλ light-chain restriction as was in the original CLL/SLL. The centroblasts now show strong cytoplasmic staining which is both diffuse as well as globular.

cell lymphoma with plasmacytic differentiation and a differential diagnosis provided. Although often associated with a paraprotein of IgM type, this feature is not required for the diagnosis and is not specific, being also found in CLL and MZL. Waldenstrom macroglobulinemia (WM) is found in a subset of LPL cases and is defined as LPL with bone marrow involvement and an IgM monoclonal gammopathy.

LPL occurs at the median age of 65 years with a slight male predominance. A familial predisposition may exist in up to 20% of patients with WM. Hepatitis C is associated with

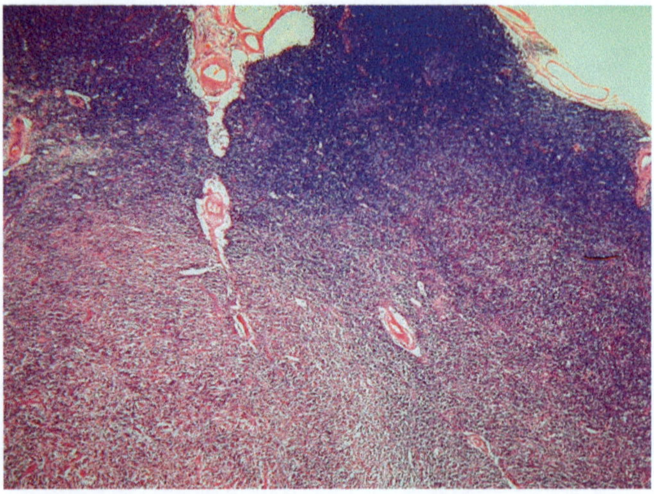

Fig. 6.17. CLL/SLL with Hodgkin disease (HD). An area of classical HD is present surrounded by CLL/SLL with proliferation centers (PC).

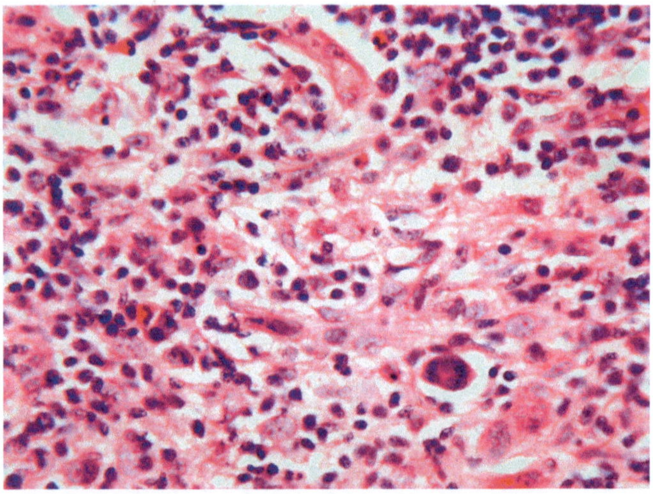

Fig. 6.18. Multilobated Reed–Sternberg (RS) cells are present mixed with small lymphocytes, eosinophils, and scattered plasma cells in the focus of HD.

a cryoglobulinemia and LPL in some series but may be non-progressive in some instances while others may behave more like CLL. LPL involves the bone marrow and in some cases lymph nodes and extranodal sites. About 15–30% of patients with WM have hepatosplenomegaly and/or lymphadenopathy. Peripheral blood may be involved. The clinical course is typically indolent, with median survivals of 5–10 years, most clinical problems developing from the paraproteinemia which causes hyperviscosity, autoantibody or cryoglobulin activity, coagulopathies, neuropathy, or deposition in the skin or gastrointestinal tract, the latter causing diarrhea.

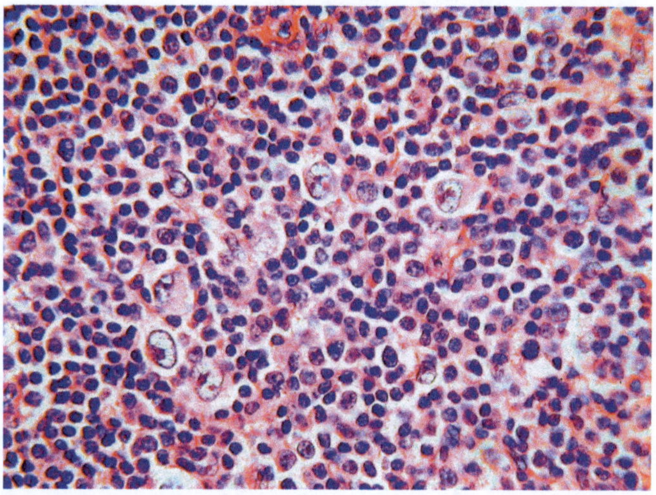

Fig. 6.19. Mononuclear RS cells are mixed with small lymphocytes and occasional plasma cells in this focus of classic HD.

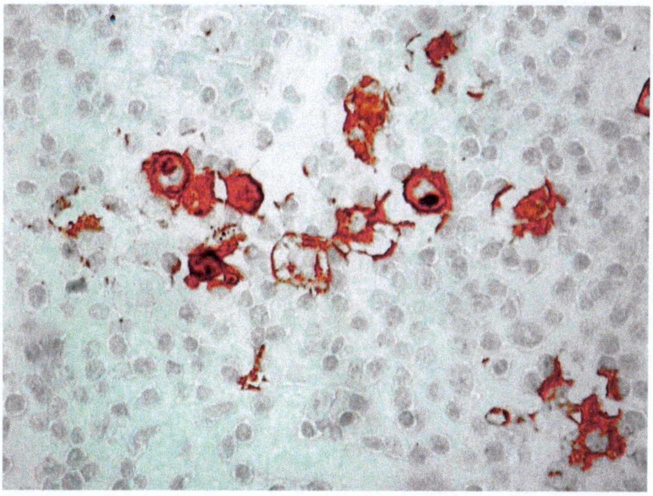

Fig. 6.20. The RS cells stain for CD15 with the characteristic pattern of membrane and Golgi staining.

Gamma heavy-chain disease is a variant of LPL. It results from the secretion of a truncated gamma chain that lacks light-chain binding sites; otherwise it usually fulfills the criteria for LPL involving lymph nodes, bone marrow, liver, spleen, and peripheral blood but can sometimes resemble plasma cell myeloma with a variable clinical course and more aggressive than that of typical IgM-producing LPL.

Alpha heavy-chain disease is another variant recognized by the presence of abnormal alpha chain in the serum. It is synonymous with immunoproliferative small intestinal disease (IPSID) which

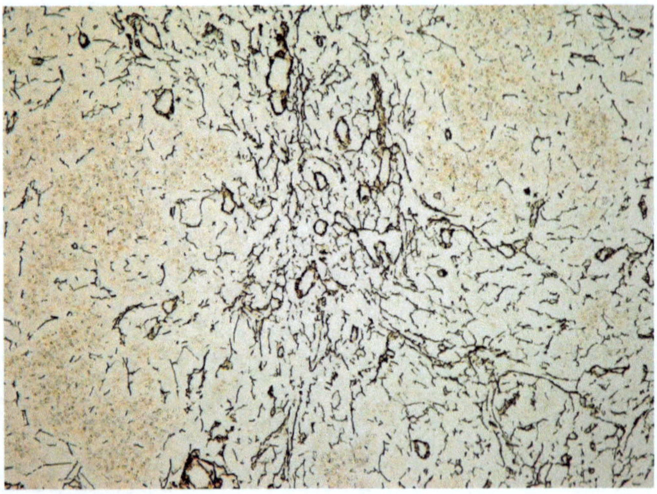

Fig. 6.21. SLL/CLL. There is no compression or displacement of reticulin fibers around the proliferation centers.

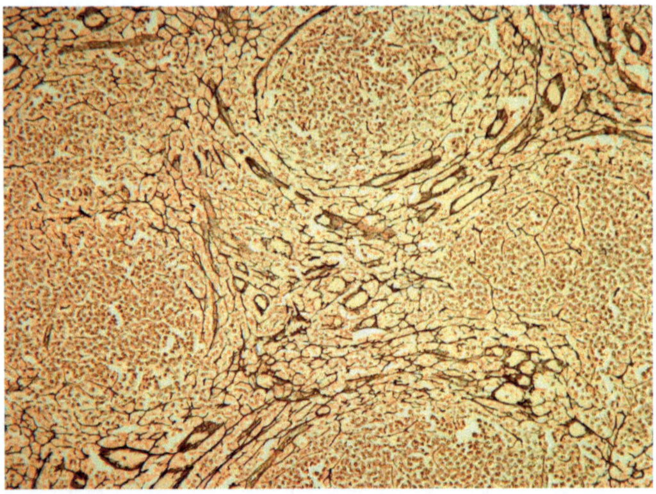

Fig. 6.22. The neoplastic follicles of FL are expansive and push surrounding reticulin and vessels aside.

is a variant of extranodal marginal zone lymphoma or MALT lymphoma which involves the small bowel (**Table 6.6**).

Morphology

Nodal architecture is often partially preserved and a monotonous population of small lymphocytes, plasma cells, and intermediate lymphoplasmacytic forms is seen alongside distended sinuses and vessels filled with proteinaceous PAS-positive material. Total replacement of the node may occur. Occasionally a vaguely follicular pattern may be imparted by the presence of more prominent residual germinal centers or a localized population of transformed

Table 6.5
CLL/SLL – differential diagnoses

- CLL/SLL: CD20+/CD79a+/CD23+/CD5+/CD43+/Bcl6–/CD10–/CD38 variable
- LPL: Plasmacytoid features, CD38+/CD138+/CD5–
- MCL: CyclinD1+/CD23–/CD5+/CD43 variable, expanded FDC meshwork
- MZL: Cyclin D1–/CD23–/CD5–/Bcl6–, residual meshwork of FDC present
- FL: Angulated cleaved centrocytes and centroblasts, CD10+/Bcl6+/CD23–lCD5– proliferation of FDC, displaces and compresses surrounding reticulin
- LL: Young patients; indented/cleaved blastic nuclei with nucleoli, frequent mitoses, TdT+, frequently of T cell lineage, CD3+/CD4+/CD8+/CD5+/CD7+

Table 6.6
Lymphoplasmacytic lymphoma (LPL) – clinical

- Median age 65 years; slight male predominance
- Diagnosis made after exclusion of other B cell lymphomas with plasmacytic differentiation
- Involves bone marrow, blood, spleen, and lymph nodes
- Most associated with IgM paraprotein (Waldenstrom macroglobulinemia), but presence of latter is not specific
- Cases with IgM paraproteinemia may manifest hyperviscosity, autoimmune and cryoglobulin activity, coagulopathy, neuropathy, and deposition in skin and gastrointestinal tract
- Clinical course indolent, median survival 5–10 years
- Variants: gamma-chain disease and alpha-chain disease (IPSID)

plasmacytoid and plasma cells. Clusters of epithelioid histiocytes may be mixed with mast cells and hemosiderin-containing macrophages. Dutcher bodies and amyloid may also be seen. The presence of proliferation centers suggests CLL/SLL and pale marginal zones should raise the possibility of marginal zone lymphoma (MZL). Infiltration of the capsule and perinodal tissue is common even when the node is only partially replaced (**Figs. 6.23, 6.24, 6.25, 6.26**; **Table 6.7**).

Immunohistology and Genetics

The neoplastic cells express B cell markers CD20 and CD79a, although the former may be lacking in more differentiated forms. IRF4/MUM1, CD38, and CD138 are helpful in highlighting

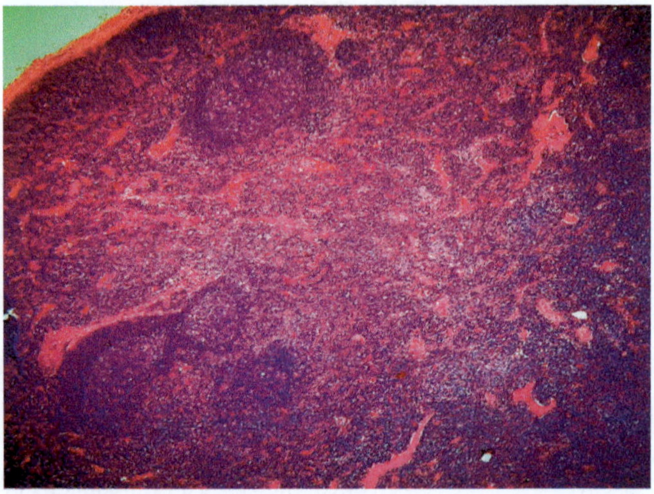

Fig. 6.23. LPL showing partial involvement of the node with preserved germinal centers. Note the dilated sinuses and vessels filled with brightly eosinophilic proteinaceous material.

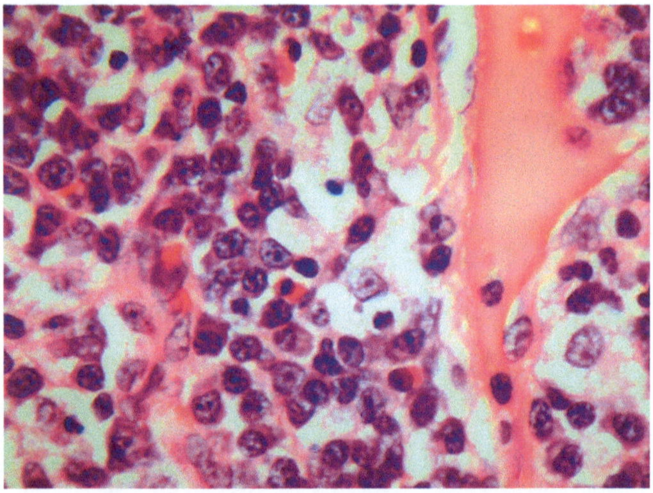

Fig. 6.24. The parasinusoidal infiltrate is a mixture of small lymphocytes, transformed cells, and plasmacytoid and plasmacytic cells. Scattered eosinophils are present and the sinus is filled with dense eosinophilic proteinaceous material.

plasma cells which may occasionally be difficult to identify. CD5, CD23, and CD10 are negative. CD43 and Bcl6 may be positive. Light-chain restriction is readily demonstrated in the plasma cells which frequently express monoclonal IgM with or without IgD and the Dutcher bodies stain for IgM.

Immunoglobulin genes are rearranged and mutated but lack the ongoing mutations that characterize post-germinal center cells. No specific chromosomal or oncogene abnormality has been recognized and little is known of the pathogenesis of LPL.

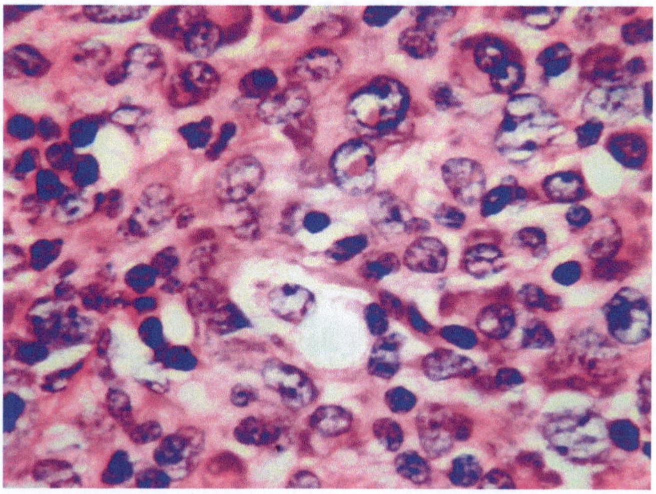

Fig. 6.25. Two Dutcher bodies resulting from nuclear invaginations of perinuclear cisternae filled with IgM are present (*arrows*).

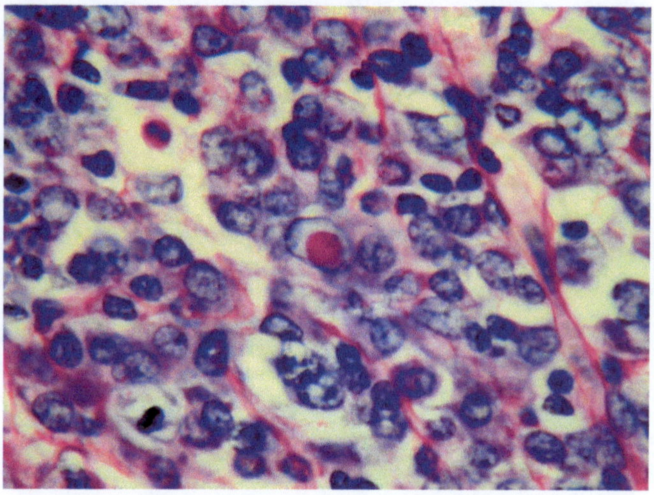

Fig. 6.26. The intranuclear pseudo inclusion of IgM stains with PAS.

Rarely some LPLs have been shown to have t(9;14)(p13;q32) chromosomal translocation that juxtaposes the PAX-6 gene with the regulatory elements of immunoglobulin heavy-chain gene (**Figs. 6.27**, **6.28**, **6.29**; **Table 6.8**).

The differential diagnoses of LPL include the other small lymphocytic lymphomas, namely, CLL/SLL, MCL, MZL, and FL. A paraproteinemia may be associated with CLL, MZL, and FL, but is not seen with MCL. **Table 6.9** shows the antibodies that are helpful in separating these five entities.

Table 6.7
Lymphoplasmacytic lymphoma (LPL) – morphology

• Diffuse or partial involvement of lymph node with involvement of perinodal tissue
• When partially infiltrated, germinal centers may be preserved and sinuses patent
• Patent sinuses filled with protein-rich fluid
• Infiltrate of small lymphocytes and plasma cells with intermediate forms
• Infiltrate may include eosinophils, mast cells, and varying numbers of epithelioid histiocytes
• Plasmacytic and plasma cells show Dutcher bodies
• Amyloid deposition may be present

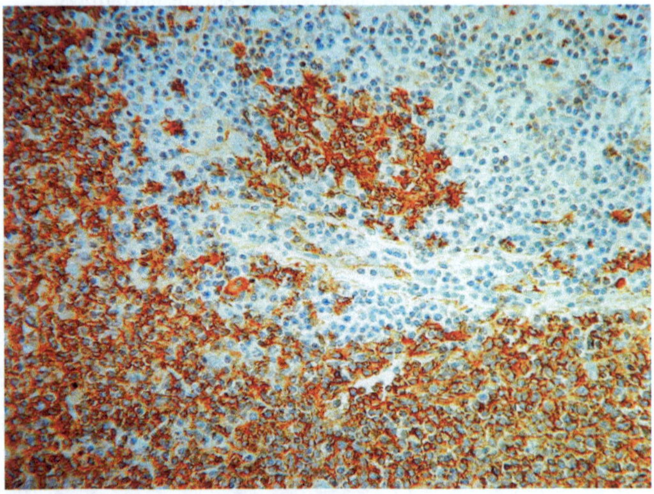

Fig. 6.27. Plasmacytic cells and plasma cells of LPL stain for CD38.

Diffuse Large B Cell Lymphoma (DLBCL)

Synonyms that have been applied to diffuse large B cell lymphoma (DLBCL) include diffuse lymphoma, large-cell, cleaved, non-cleaved and immunoblastic lymphoma; diffuse histiocytic lymphoma; diffuse centroblastic and immunoblastic lymphoma; and diffuse large-cell, cleaved, non-cleaved, immunoblastic, and polymorphous lymphoma. This lymphoma is postulated to arise from peripheral B cells of germinal center or post-germinal center (activated B cell) origin.

DLBCL accounts for 30–40% of adult non-Hodgkin lymphomas in Western countries and form a larger portion of lymphomas in less-developed countries. About 40% of DLBCLs are extranodal and account for the majority of B cell lymphomas in internal organs including the central nervous system and other

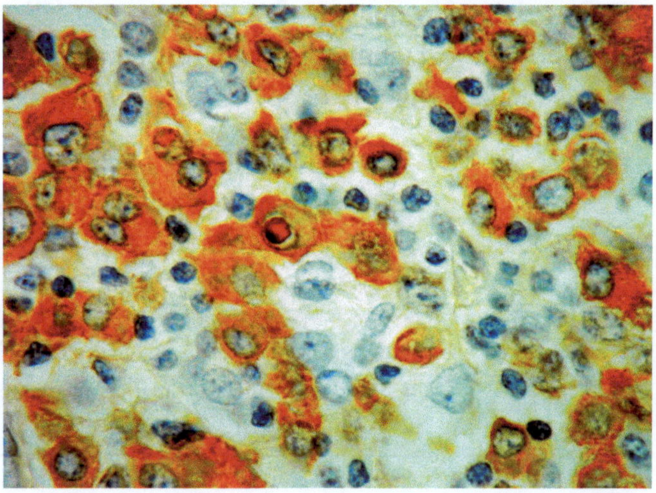

Fig. 6.28. Plasmacytic cells show Igκ light-chain restriction and two Dutcher bodies are present (*arrows*).

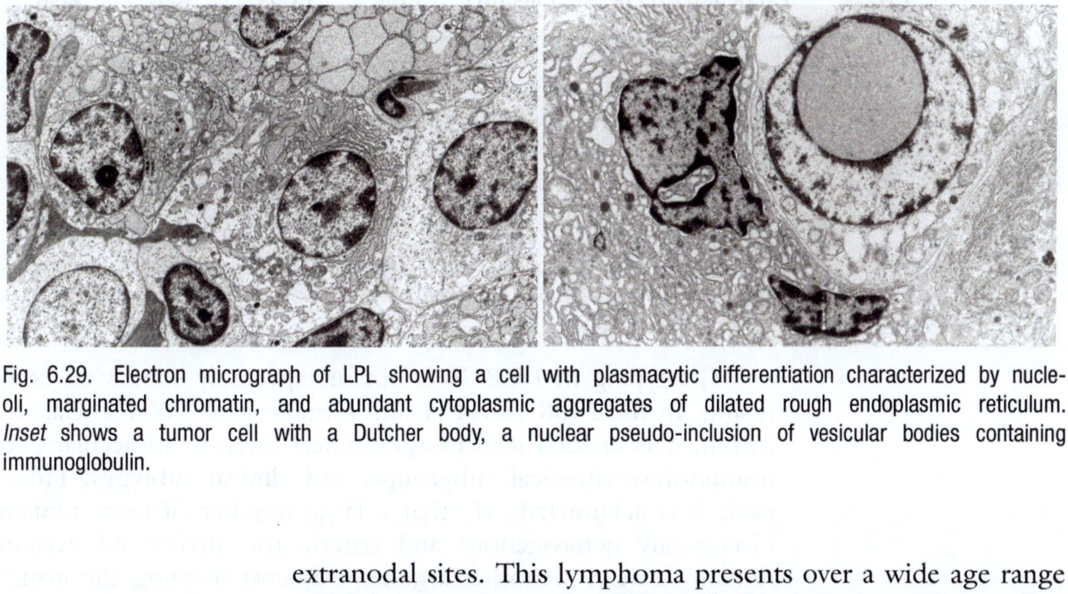

Fig. 6.29. Electron micrograph of LPL showing a cell with plasmacytic differentiation characterized by nucleoli, marginated chromatin, and abundant cytoplasmic aggregates of dilated rough endoplasmic reticulum. *Inset* shows a tumor cell with a Dutcher body, a nuclear pseudo-inclusion of vesicular bodies containing immunoglobulin.

extranodal sites. This lymphoma presents over a wide age range and is more common in adults and older persons with a median in the seventh decade, but children are occasionally affected.

By definition, DLBCL includes all B cell lymphomas with a diffuse growth pattern and neoplastic cells with nuclei that equal or exceed that of normal macrophage nuclei or are more than twice the size of small lymphocytes. However, this group of B cell lymphomas is heterogenous in clinical presentation, morphology, immunophenotype, and molecular characteristics; furthermore, they may arise *de novo* or evolve from pre-existing low-grade B cell lymphomas such as lymphocytic, follicular, marginal lymphomas, or nodular lymphocyte-predominant Hodgkin lymphoma.

Table 6.8
Lymphoplasmacytic lymphoma – immunohistology and genetics

- CD79a+, CD20–/+, CD38+, CD138+, IRF4/MUM1+
- IgM monoclonality, light-chain restriction
- CD5–, CD23–, CD10–, Bcl6+/–,
- Dutcher bodies are PAS+ and IgM+
- *IG* genes rearranged with somatic hypermutation but no ongoing mutations
- No specific chromosomal or oncogene abnormality
- Rare t(9;14)(p13;q32) reported

Table 6.9
Antibody panel to separate small lymphocytic lymphomas

	CD23[a]	CD38 and CD138	CyclinD1	CD5	CD43	Bcl2	Bcl6
CLL/SLL	+	–	–	+	+	–	–
LPL	–	+	–	–/+	+	–/+	–/+
MCL	–	–	+	+/	–	+	–/+
MZL	–	–/+	–	–/+	+/–	+	–
FL	–	–	–	–	–/+	+	+

[a]Fixation dependant. CLL/SLL, chronic lymphocytic leukemia/small lymphocytic lymphoma; LPL, lymphoplasmacytic lymphoma; MCL, mantle cell lymphoma; MZL, nodal marginal zone lymphoma; FL, follicular lymphoma.

The typing of DLBCL is not unexpectedly somewhat confusing. In the 2008 World Health Organization (WHO) classification, it is divided into morphological variants, molecular and immunohistochemical subgroups, and clinical subtypes. However, it is acknowledged "that a large number of cases remain biologically heterogenous and criteria for further subdivision remain unclear." Another argument against dividing the group of DLBCL relates to the fact that subclassification by morphology is difficult, with poor reproducibility. Importantly, the current treatment of all cases of DLBCL, regardless of nomenclature, is the same.

The International Prognostic Index based on clinical parameters is useful in prognostication. Concordant bone marrow involvement was associated with a very poor prognosis of 10% 5-year survival. Discordant involvement, however, did not influence outcome significantly. The prognostic influence of immunoblastic features is controversial and various prognostic immunohistological markers including Ki67 and the expression of Bcl6, CD10, and 1RF4/MUM1 appear to lose their influence by the addition of rituximab to multiagent chemotherapy. In any case, the use of such immunohistological markers to assign prognosis does not currently have a role in routine clinical practice.

DLBCL is a high-grade, aggressive lymphoma that is potentially curable with multiagent therapy. The long-term remission rate used to be 50–60%, but with the addition of anti-CD20 monoclonal antibody rituximab to CHOP, there has been a remarkable improvement in survival (**Table 6.10**).

Table 6.10
Diffuse large B cell lymphoma: Clinical

30–40% of adult non-Hodgkin lymphomas
Occurs at all ages; median age seventh decade
60% nodal, 40% extranodal
Heterogenous clinical subtypes
May be primary or the result of transformation of a low-grade B cell lymphoma
Divided into morphologic variants, immunophenotypic and molecular subgroups, and clinical subtypes
Treatment currently the same irrespective of variant, subgroup, or subtype
High-grade, aggressive lymphoma but potentially curable with modern therapy
Immunohistological markers for prognostication controversial
Addition of rituximab to CHOP therapy improves prognosis significantly

Morphology

The 2008 WHO classification includes, among the heterogenous group of DLBCL, four common morphologic variants and a group of rare variants. The common morphologic variants are centroblastic, immunoblastic, anaplastic, and T cell/histiocyte-rich B cell lymphomas. Rare variants include DLBCL with a myxoid stroma or a fibrillary matrix and those with pseudorosette formation, spindle shapes, or signet ring formation. Very rarely, cytoplasmic granules, microvilli, and intercellular junctions may also be seen.

Centroblastic variant: This is by far the most common variant and comprises a diffuse infiltrate of medium to large lymphoid cells with oval vesicular nuclei containing two to four nucleoli that often appear attached to the nuclear membrane. Cytoplasm is scanty and amphophilic to basophilic. The tumor may be monomorphic, composed almost entirely of centroblasts, or polymorphic when there is a mixture of centroblasts and immunoblasts, or it may have numerous cells with multilobated nuclei.

Immunoblastic variant: In this variant >90% of the cells are immunoblasts with a single central nucleolus and moderate

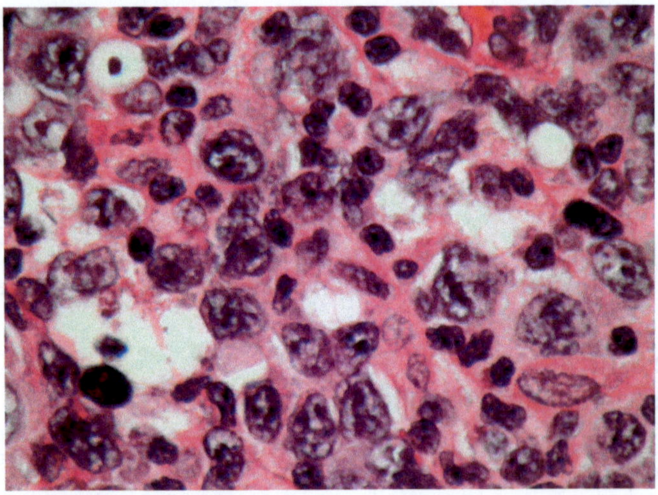

Fig. 6.30. DLBCL, centroblastic variant.

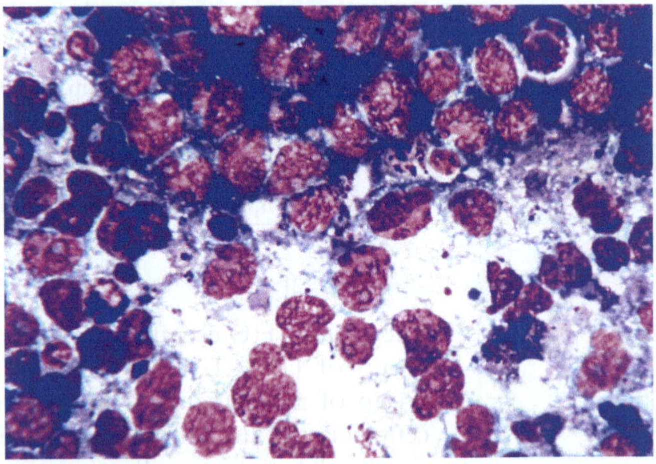

Fig. 6.31. The centroblasts have large vesicular nuclei with two or more nucleoli and moderate quantities of cytoplasm.

quantities of basophilic cytoplasm. Cells with plasmacytoid differentiation may be present.

The distinction of the immunoblastic from the more common centroblastic variant is acknowledged to show poor reproducibility (**Figs. 6.30, 6.31, 6.32, 6.33**).

Anaplastic variant: The cells of this variant are characteristically large and have bizarre pleomorphic nuclei that may resemble Reed–Sternberg cells and the cells of anaplastic large cell lymphoma. They may show a sinusoidal or a cohesive growth pattern that mimics undifferentiated carcinoma. These tumors are biologically unrelated to anaplastic large cell lymphoma of cytotoxic

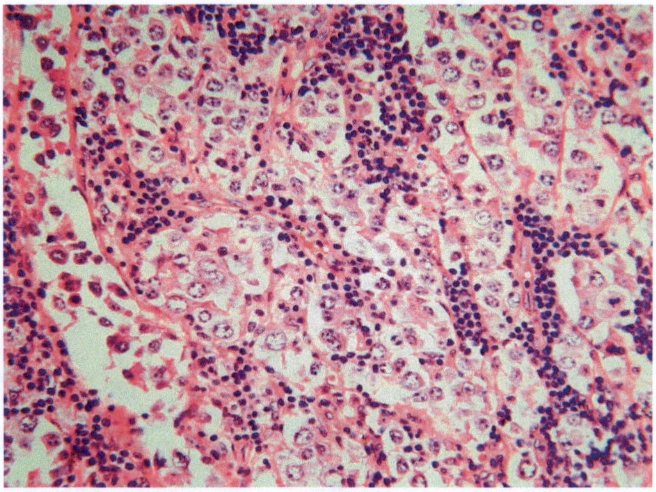

Fig. 6.32. DLBCL, immunoblastic variant showing permeation of sinuses by neoplastic cells.

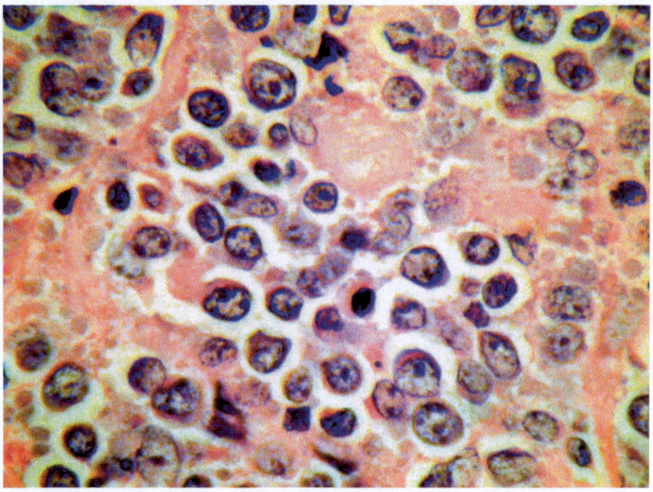

Fig. 6.33. The large cells have vesicular nuclei with prominent central nucleoli and moderate quantities of dense cytoplasm.

T cell derivation and are not related to ALK-positive large B cell lymphoma (**Figs. 6.34, 6.35**).

T cell/histiocyte-rich large B cell lymphoma (THRLBCL): This variant accounts for about 10% of all DLBCLs. It is defined as a polymorphous infiltrate that is characterized by a limited number of scattered large atypical B cells embedded in a background of abundant small T cells and often variable numbers of histiocytes. The pattern of infiltration is diffuse, less commonly a vaguely nodular pattern may be seen but the atypical cells do not form aggregates or sheets and are always dispersed, often mimicking

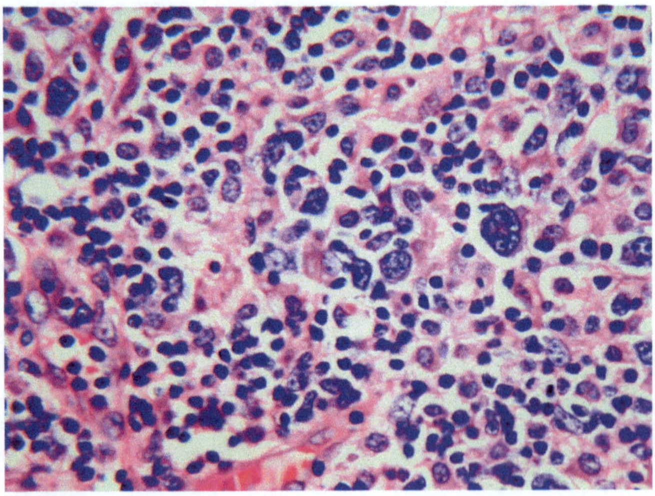

Fig. 6.34. DLBCL, anaplastic variant. An infiltrate of large cells is present with scattered multinucleated giant cells.

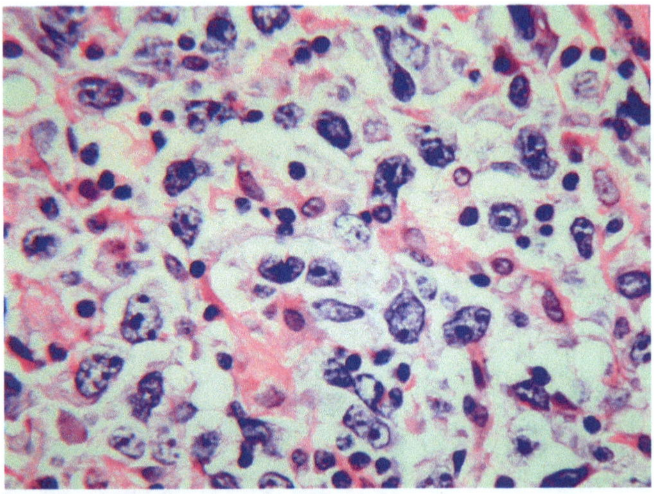

Fig. 6.35. The lymphoma cells have large irregular nuclei with prominent nucleoli and abundant pale cytoplasm.

the cells of Hodgkin lymphoma; in particular, the appearances may resemble nodular lymphocyte-predominant Hodgkin lymphoma (NLPHL) with a diffuse component. A relationship between the latter condition and THRLBCL has been postulated but the association remains controversial. The background cells comprise mostly T cells and eosinophils, and plasma cells are not found. The atypical large B cells usually lie among clusters of epithelioid histiocytes that may not be readily recognizable by conventional examination. Only cases with this typical morphology should be included as THRLBCL. Lymphomas with B cells showing a spectrum of cell size, morphology, and distribution should not be included. The demonstration of atypical cells within meshworks of FDC indicates a diagnosis of NLPHL.

The morphologic definition of this disease is accompanied by the following clinical features: presentation in middle-aged men, fever, malaise, splenomegaly, and/or hepatomegaly. Almost half the cases present at advanced stage with intermediate to high risk International Prognostic Index score and are often refractory to conventional chemotherapy.

THRLBCL is considered an aggressive lymphoma, especially those cases that contain abundant histiocytes, although there is some clinical heterogeneity.

The large atypical cells express pan-B cell markers and Bcl6. CD15, CD30, CD38, are negative. The T cells stain for CD3 and CD5. Unlike in NLPHL, the atypical cells of THRLBCL do not rosette with CD3+ or CD4+, CD57+, Bcl6+, PD-1+ T cells, are not enmeshed by FDC, and are not EBV associated (**Figs. 6.36, 6.37, 6.38, 6.39, 6.40**, and **6.41**).

Rare morphologic variants: Rarely, DLBCL may display a myxoid stroma or a fibrillary matrix. Sometimes they may show pseudorosette formation or may occasionally be spindled or display features of signet ring cells. Cytoplasmic granules, microvillous projections, and intercellular junctions have also been reported (**Figs. 6.42, 6.43, 6.44, 6.45, 6.46, 6.47, 6.48, 6.49, 6.50, 6.51, 6.52; Table 6.11**).

Immunohistology and Genetics

DLBCLs express pan-B cell markers including CD20 and CD79a. Surface and/or cytoplasmic immunoglobulin with light-chain restriction can be demonstrated, IgM being the most frequent

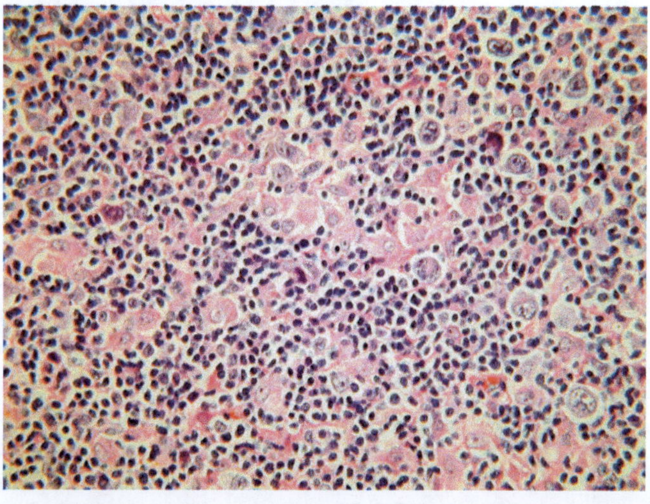

Fig. 6.36. THRLBCL composed of a polymorphous infiltrate of large atypical cells among small lymphocytes and epithelioid histiocytes.

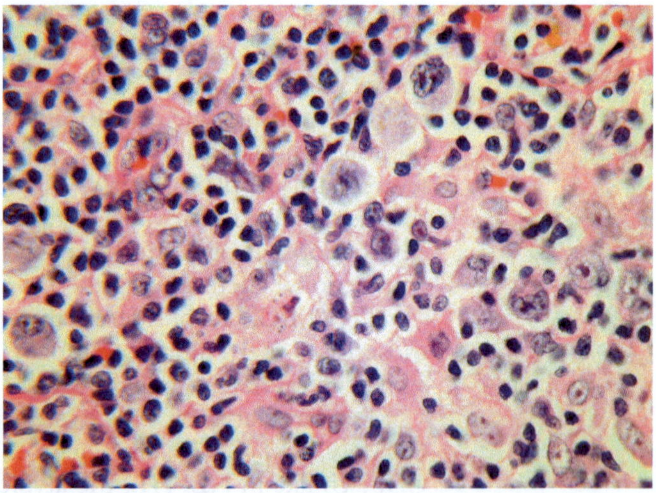

Fig. 6.37. Large atypical cells have lobated nuclei that are vesicular and contain prominent nucleoli. There are moderate quantities of amphophilic cytoplasm and some cells mimic Hodgkin cells.

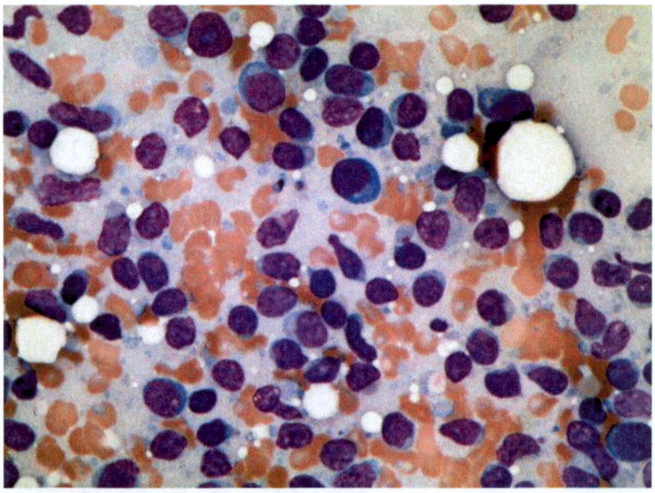

Fig. 6.38. TCRBCL, imprint. Besides the atypical cells with prominent nucleoli and basophilic cytoplasm a mixture of other cell types is present. They include small lymphocytes, stimulated cells, and plasma cells.

followed by IgG and IgA. The plasma cell markers CD38 and CD138 are rarely expressed. CD30 can be found in the anaplastic variant (**Figs. 6.53** and **6.54**).

CD5 expression seen in about 10% of cases of DLBCL signifies a poor prognosis. Such tumors usually represent *de novo* DLBCL rather than those arising from CLL/SLC. CD5-positive DLBCL can be distinguished from blastoid MCL, cyclin D1 expression being seen in the latter which is also associated with

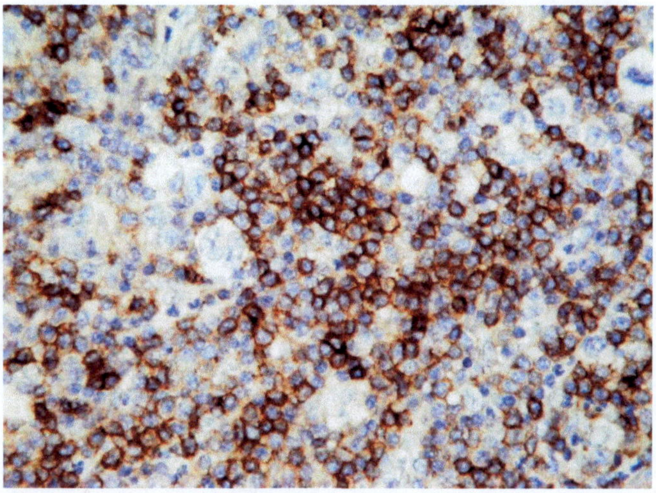

Fig. 6.39. The small T lymphocytes stain for CD3 but the large atypical cells do not.

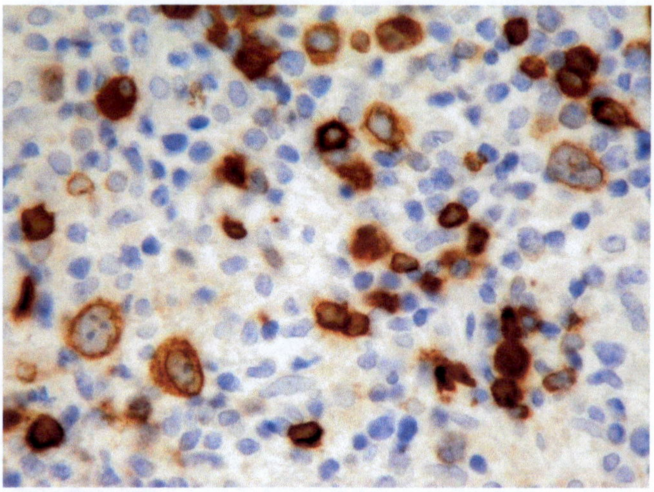

Fig. 6.40. CD79a labels the atypical cells as well as plasma cells and occasional small B cells in the field.

a proliferation of FDC. Bcl2 expression is seen in about 30–50% of cases with some studies suggesting a poorer prognosis.

The frequency of Bcl6, CD10, and IRF4/MUM1 expression varies with Bcl6 positivity being the most frequent (in up to 90%), and CD10 and IRF4/MUM1 each expressed in up to 60% of cases. Unlike in normal germinal-center cells, where expression of Bcl6 and IRF4/MUM1 is mutually exclusive, coexpression of these proteins occurs in about 50% of DLBCLs. These immunophenotypic groups do not determine therapy, although they may reflect behavior.

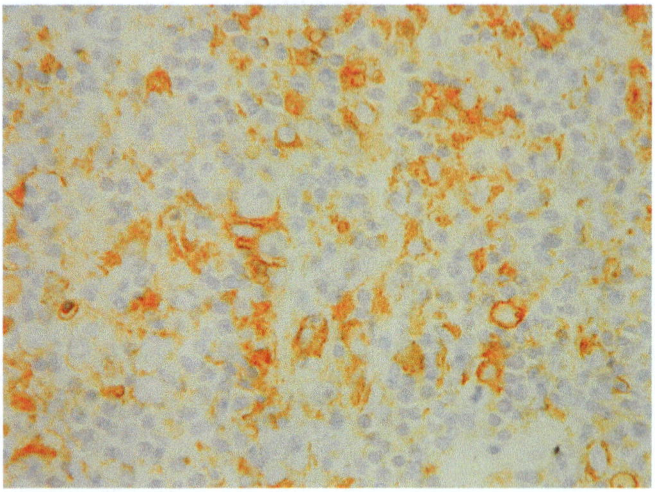

Fig. 6.41. HAM56 highlights abundant epithelioid histiocytes in the background.

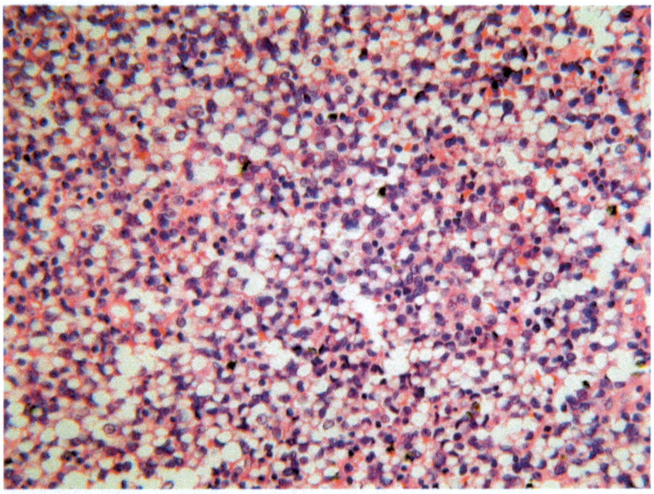

Fig. 6.42. DLBCL, signet ring type, composed of non-cohesive cells with cytoplasmic vacuoles, involving a groin lymph node.

Besides the CD5-positive subgroup, DLBCL can be divided immunophenotypically into germinal-center-like and non-germinal-center-like subgroups based on the expression of CD10, Bcl6, and IRF4/MUM1, although this subgrouping does not correlate exactly with gene expression. CD10–/Bcl6+/MUM1– as well as those with >30% of tumor cells CD10+ are regarded as germinal-center-like DLBCL. Non-germinal-center-like DLBCL are CD10–/Bcl6– or CD10–/Bcl6+/MUM1+.

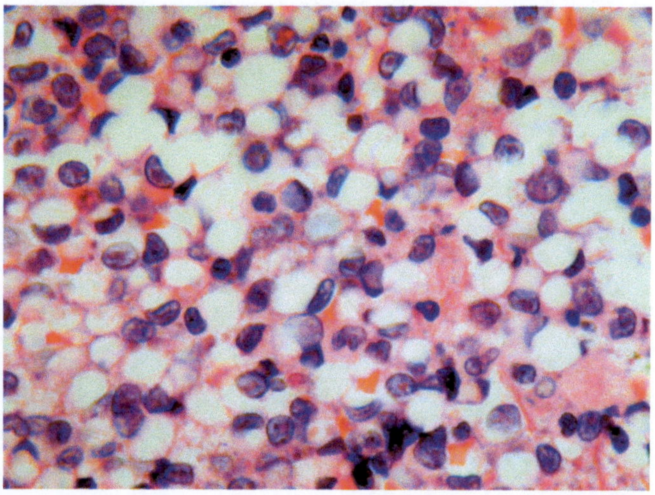

Fig. 6.43. The cells contain distinct single cytoplasmic vacuoles, often indenting the nucleus to produce a signet ring appearance.

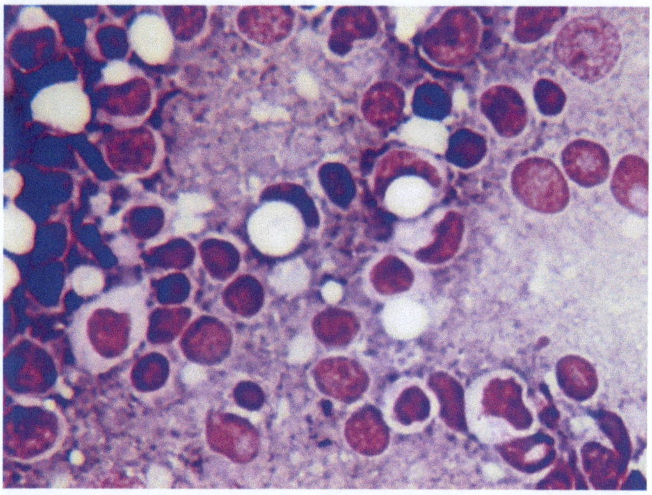

Fig. 6.44. Giemsa-stained imprint showing signet ring cells.

Ki67 shows a proliferative index of more than 40% and as high as 90% in some cases, and there is p53 expression in 20–60% of cases.

Immunoglobulin heavy- and light-chain genes show clonal rearrangement and hypermutations in the variable regions. Aberrant somatic hypermutations targeting multiple genetic loci are often encountered and may contribute to oncogenesis.

Chromosomal translocations involving the *BCL6* gene at 3q27 are most common, occurring in as many as 30% of cases. t(14;18) involving the *Bcl2* gene similar to that in FL occurs in 20–30% of cases, and in 10% *MYC* rearrangements may occur

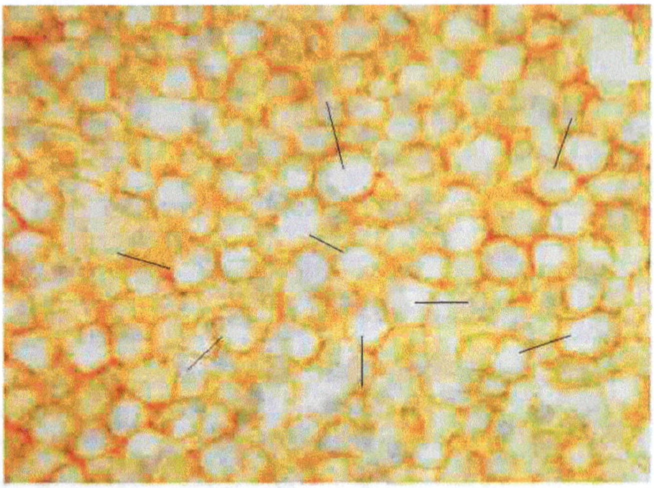

Fig. 6.45. Membranous CD20 staining is seen in the lymphoma cells including those with signet ring appearance (*arrows*).

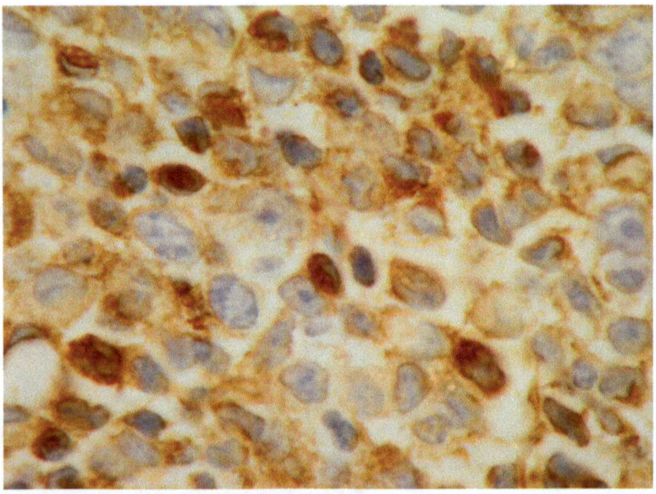

Fig. 6.46. The lymphoma cells show cytoplasmic staining for IgM (including the signet ring cells) and were labeled for CD45 (not shown) but not for IgG or IgA (not shown).

with *IG* gene or with a non-*IG* gene as the break partner. Some cases with *MYC* rearrangements may have concurrent *IGH-BCL2* translocation and/or *BCL6* break or both. Such cases usually have a proliferation index of >90% and have been called "B cell lymphomas, unclassified, with features intermediate between diffuse large B cell lymphoma and Burkitt lymphoma."

Gene expression profiling has indentified three subgroups of DLBCL. These have been termed germinal-center B cells (GCB), forming 45–50% of cases, activated peripheral B cells (ABC-like), and those that do not fit into either of these categories and do

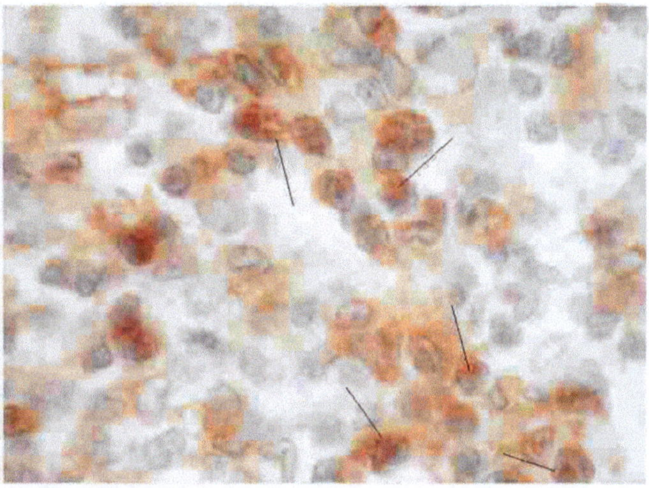

Fig. 6.47. There is Igκ light-chain restriction in the lymphoid cells as well as in the signet ring cells (*arrows*).

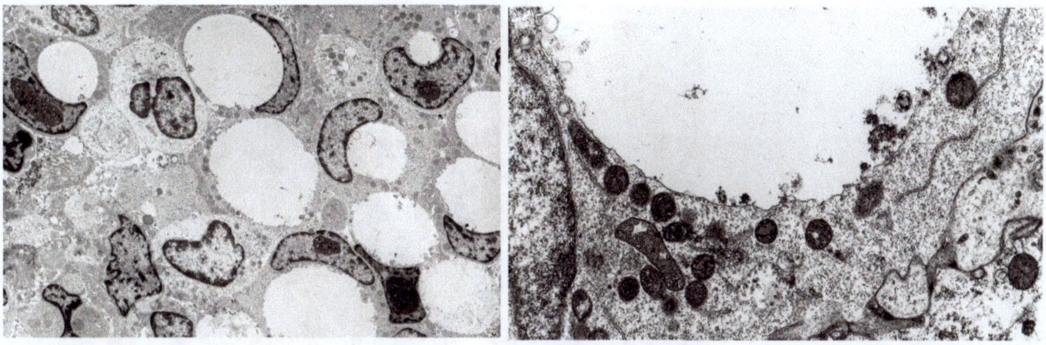

Fig. 6.48. DLBCL with signet ring change. Many cells contain cytoplasmic vacuoles that displace crescentic nuclei. *Inset* shows that the vacuoles are membrane-bound and contain peripheral microvesicles and membranous material but are otherwise apparently empty.

not represent a distinct subgroup. The former two subgroups are associated with different chromosomal aberrations but the correlation of these groups with immunophenotype is variable (**Table 6.12**).

Clinical Subtypes

The 2008 WHO classification indentifies a number of clinical subtypes of DLBCL, several of which occur in extranodal sites, namely primary DLBCL of CNS, primary cutaneous DLBCL, leg type, primary mediastinal (thymic) large B cell lymphoma, intravascular large B cell lymphoma, plasmablastic lymphoma, DLBCL associated with chronic inflammation, lymphomatoid granulomatosis, and primary effusion lymphoma. These extranodal subtypes are listed in **Table 6.13** and will not be discussed.

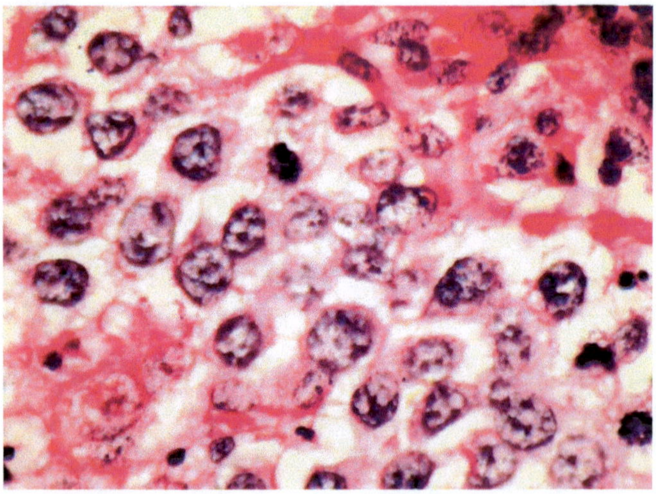

Fig. 6.49. Abdominal node with DLBCL composed of villous lymphoid cells. The noncohesive large cells have abundant pale ill-defined cytoplasm.

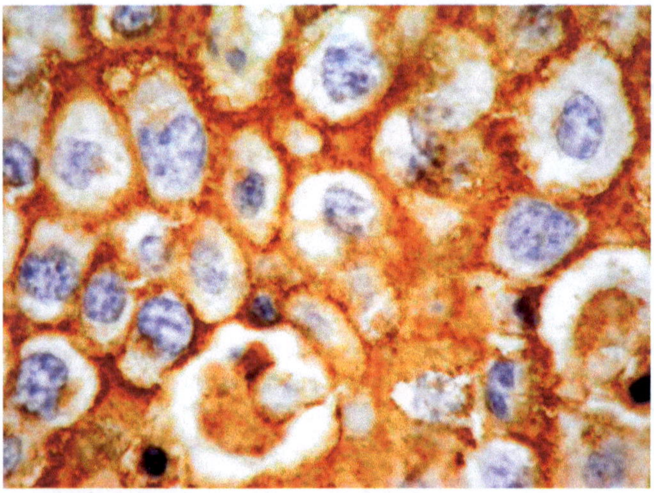

Fig. 6.50. CD45 stains the cell membranes which are fuzzy because of numerous microvillous projections.

Node-Based Subtypes of DLBCL

Subtypes of DLBCL that involve lymph nodes are EBV-positive DLBCL of the elderly, ALK-positive DLBCL, and large B cell lymphoma arising in HHV8-associated multicentric Castleman disease. While these subtypes are infrequent, they are sufficiently distinctive to be considered clinical and pathological entities. Two other unclassifiable subtypes have earned a place in the 2008 WHO classification. They are B cell lymphoma, unclassifiable, with features intermediate between DLBCL and Burkitt lymphoma, and B cell lymphoma, unclassifiable, with features intermediate between DLBCL and classical Hodgkin lymphoma. The

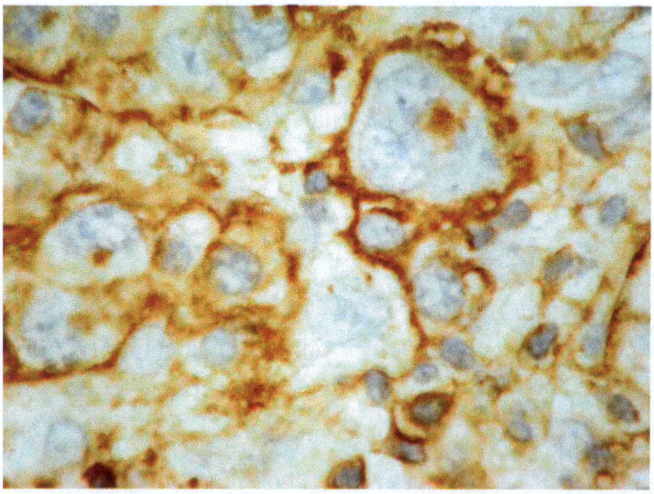

Fig. 6.51. CD20 identifies the B cell nature of the lymphoma. The stain enhances the fuzzy nature of the cell membranes. There is also staining of the Golgi.

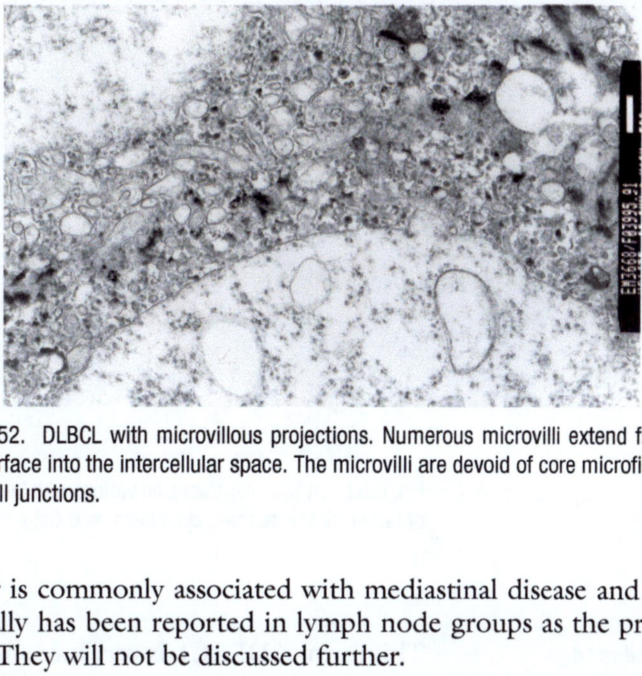

Fig. 6.52. DLBCL with microvillous projections. Numerous microvilli extend from the cell surface into the intercellular space. The microvilli are devoid of core microfilaments and cell junctions.

latter is commonly associated with mediastinal disease and occasionally has been reported in lymph node groups as the primary site. They will not be discussed further.

EBV-Positive DLBCL of the Elderly

This subtype of DLBCL is an EBV-driven B cell lymphoma thought to be related to immunological deterioration or senescence in immunity seen in the older person. It occurs in the absence of any known immunodeficiency or prior lymphoma, accounting for 8–10% of DLBCL in Asian countries. While this disease is extranodal in 70% of cases, commonly occurring in the skin, lung, tonsil, and stomach with or without nodal involvement, the remaining patients have lymph node disease alone.

Table 6.11
Diffuse large B cell lymphoma: Morphology

A group of large B cell lymphomas with heterogenous morphology, immunophenotypes, and molecular characteristics
Partial or complete effacement of nodal architecture
Sinusoidal pattern of infiltration rarely occurs
Variable sclerosis present
Tumor cells at least 2× size of small lymphocytes or the size of a macrophage
Morphological variants include centroblastic, immunoblastic, anaplastic lymphomas, THRLBCL, and other rare variants
THRLBCL distinguished from NLPHL by the absence of FDC meshwork and rosetting of atypical cells by CD4+/CD57+/PD–1+ T cells
Rare morphologic variants include spindle cell, signet ring, microvillous, pseudo-rosetting, and granular subtypes

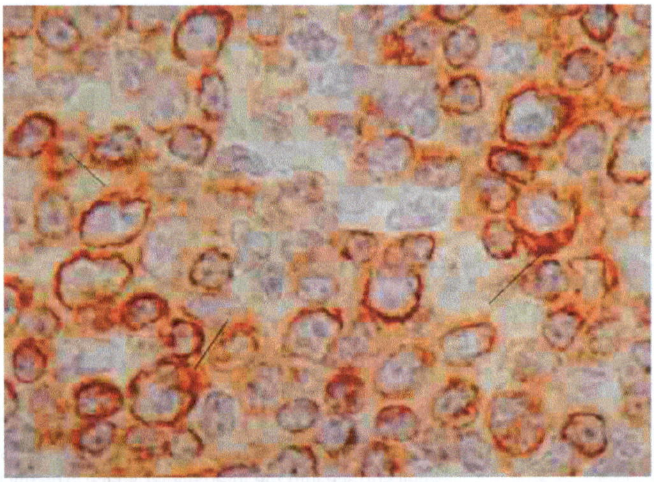

Fig. 6.53. DLBCL, centroblastic variant with Igκ light-chain restriction showing staining of perinuclear cisternae, cytoplasm, and Golgi (*arrow*).

ALK-Positive Large B Cell Lymphoma

This form of DLBCL is very rare and is made up of monomorphic large B cells with immunoblast-like and sometimes plasmablastic morphology. The infiltration is diffuse and often within sinuses. This lymphoma seems to occur in all age groups with a predisposition for males (M:F ratio 3:1). Presentation is at an advanced stage and involvement is mainly nodal, sometimes with mediastinal involvement. Extranodal sites may be involved and include soft tissue, nasopharynx, stomach, tongue, and bone.

The neoplastic cells display a strong granular cytoplasmic expression of ALK protein and few cases may show cytoplasmic,

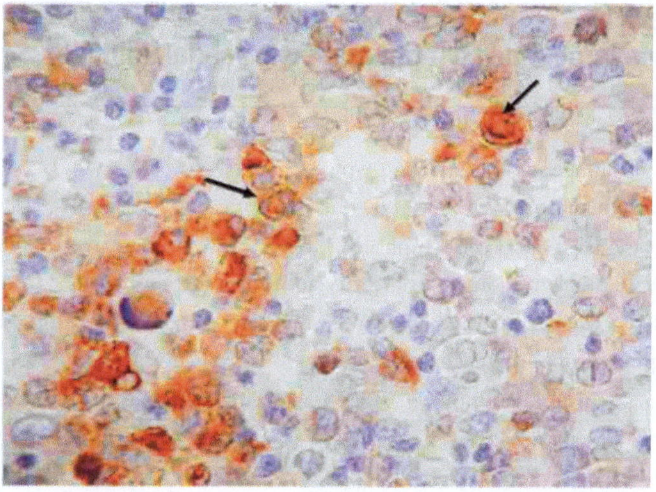

Fig. 6.54. DLBCL, immunoblastic variant with IgM restriction showing globular and diffuse cytoplasmic staining as well as staining of a Dutcher body (*arrow*).

Table 6.12
Diffuse large B cell lymphoma: Immunohistology and genetics

CD20+, CD79a+, CD30–/+, Ki67+ (40–90%)
cIgM+>cIgG+>cIgA+, cIg light-chain restriction
Bcl6+ (60–90%), CD10+ (30–60%), IRF4/MUM1+ (35–65%)
Co-expression of Bcl6 and IRF4/MUM1 in about 50%
Germinal-center-like: CD10+ or CD10–/Bcl6+/MUM1–
Non-germinal-center-like: CD10–/Bcl6– or CD10–/Bcl6+/MUM1+
Ki67 fraction high (>40%), p53+ in 20–60%
IgH and Ig light chain clonally rearranged
Somatic hypermutations in variable regions
Translocation in 3q27 involving *Bcl6* gene in up to 30%
CD5+ occurs in about 10% of cases, representing de novo DLBCL
Bcl2+ in 20–30% with some studies suggesting a poorer prognosis
Gene expression profiling divides into three groups – germinal-center B cells (GCB), activated peripheral B cells (ABC), and others

nuclear, and nucleolar ALK staining pattern associated with the NPM-ALK protein. In addition, they also strongly stain for EMA and plasma cell antigens such as CD38 and CD138 but are negative for the lineage-associated markers CD20, CD79a, and CD3. CD45 is weak or negative and the cells are negative for CD30. The tumors may be positive for CD4, CD57, IRF4/MUM1, with focal staining for CD43 and perforin.

Table 6.13
Diffuse large B cell lymphoma – extranodal subtypes

DLBCL of CNS
Primary cutaneous DLBCL, leg type
Primary mediastinal (thymic) DLBCL
Intravascular large B cell lymphoma – CNS , skin, bone marrow. Asian variant – multiple organs
Plasmablastic lymphoma – oral cavity and other extranodal sites; frequently in HIV+ patients
DLBCL associated with chronic inflammation – body cavities, long-standing pyothorax
Lymphomatoid granulomatosis – lung
Primary effusion lymphoma – HHV8 associated, often associated with immunodeficiency

Clearly, the morphologic appearances and phenotypic expression require separation form CD30+, ALK+ T/null anaplastic large cell lymphoma and often rely on the lack of expression of CD30 and staining characteristics of ALK protein which is cytoplasmic and granular. This pattern reflects the most frequent genetic abnormality which is t(2;17)(p23;q23) resulting in the clathrin–ALK (CLTC-ALK) fusion protein. Survival is not predictable and, as these tumors are usually negative for CD20, they are insensitive to rituximab.

Large B Cell Lymphoma Arising in HHV8-Associated Multicentric Castleman Disease

This highly aggressive form of lymphoma arises from a monoclonal proliferation of HHV8-infected cells that resemble plasmablasts expressing IgM. It arises in the setting of multicentric Castleman disease and is usually associated with the human immunodeficiency virus infection. HHV8 itself has 11 open reading frames that result in homologues to several human proteins including IL-6 that can stimulate transcription and cell proliferation. While the lymphoma cells resemble plasma cells with nucleoli and abundant dense immunoglobulin-rich cytoplasm, they correspond to a IgM-producing naïve plasma cell without *IG* somatic hypermutation and should be distinguished from plasmablastic lymphoma which occurs in the oral cavity and other extranodal sites in that the latter show class-switched and hypermutated *IG* genes.

Kaposi sarcoma is often present in patients with this form of lymphoma, and primary effusion lymphoma and its extra cavity counterpart may be the complications but these latter conditions are usually co-infected with EBV and the neoplastic cells do not express Ig (**Table 6.14**).

Burkitt Lymphoma

Burkitt lymphoma (BL) is a highly aggressive lymphoma with an extremely short doubling time. It often presents in extranodal sites or as an acute leukemia. The tumor cells are monomorphous medium-sized transformed lymphoid cells often with the

Table 6.14
Diffuse large B cell lymphoma – nodal subtypes

EBV-positive DLBCL of the elderly
ALK-positive large B cell lymphoma
Large B cell lymphoma in HHV8-associated multicentric Castleman disease
B cell lymphoma unclassifiable, features intermediate between DLBCL and Burkitt lymphoma
B cell lymphoma, unclassifiable, features intermediate between DLBCL and classical Hodgkin lymphoma

characteristic translocation involving *MYC* but this is not specific. In fact, one single morphologic, genotypic, or immunophenotypic parameter cannot be employed specifically for diagnosis and a combination of several is necessary. The postulated normal counterpart is germinal-center or post-germinal-center B cells.

Three clinical variants are recognized, each with different clinical presentation, morphology, and biology.

Endemic BL

Endemic BL occurs in equatorial Africa and Papua New Guinea with a correlation between the geographic occurrence and climatic factors such as rainfall, altitude, and temperature which correspond to the distribution of endemic malaria. It is the most common childhood malignancy in these regions with a peak incidence at 4–7 years of age and with a male:female ratio of 2:1. In this variant, the EBV genome is present in the majority of neoplastic cells in all patients, with a strong link with endemic malaria, the latter impacting on immunity and viral persistence. However, these two infections are not sufficient to account for the distribution of BL in these high-risk regions and it is possible that other cofactors including arboviruses and plant tumor promoters may play a role.

Sporadic BL

The sporadic variant occurs throughout the world, mainly in children and young adults, representing only about 1–2% of all lymphomas. The median age of presentation in adults is 30 years and male:female ratio is 3:1. Both endemic and sporadic variants occur in North Africa and South America. EBV may be detected in about 30% of sporadic BL.

Immunodeficiency-Associated BL

This variant is seen as the initial manifestation of the acquired immunodeficiency syndrome (AIDS), in association with HIV infection. EBV is identified in 20–40% of these cases.

Clinical

The clinical presentation varies according to the epidemiologic variant. Extranodal sites are most often involved in all variants with CNS involvement common to all variants. The jaws and facial bones including orbit are involved in about 50% of cases of endemic BL, with the distal ileum, caecum and/or omentum, gonads, kidneys, long bones, thyroid, salivary glands, and breasts as other common sites. The bone marrow may be focally involved but a leukemic presentation is uncommon. The patients often present with bulky disease and a high tumor burden is the result of its rapid doubling time so that 70% present at advanced stage. Tumor lysis syndrome can occur when therapy is instituted due to rapid tumor cell death.

Jaw involvement is uncommon in sporadic BL and the majority of cases present with abdominal masses with frequent ileo-cecal involvement. Similar to the endemic variant, the ovaries, kidneys, and breasts are also frequently involved. Breast infiltration in sporadic BL is often bilateral and massive and occurs during onset of puberty, pregnancy, or lactation. Lymph node involvement is seen more commonly in adults than in children, with rare involvement of Waldeyer ring and mediastinum. Retroperitoneal masses can produce spinal cord compression and paraplegia.

In the immunodeficiency-associated variant, lymph node and bone marrow localization is common.

While the tumor is highly aggressive especially in the endemic and sporadic variants, it is potentially curable. Staging is largely related to the tumor burden, identifying patients with limited-stage disease and those with extensive intra-abdominal or intrathoracic tumor. Bone marrow and central nervous system involvement, unresected tumor >10 cm in diameter, and a high LDH serum level are recognized poor prognostic factors. Intensive combination chemotherapy achieves up to 90% cure rates in those patients with limited disease and 60–80% in those with advanced stage, the results being better in children than in adults. Relapse, when it occurs, is seen within the first year after diagnosis (**Table 6.15**).

Morphology

The prototypical BL cell is seen in the endemic and sporadic variants, especially in children. The tumor cells are medium sized (about the size of histiocyte nuclei or smaller). The pattern of growth is diffuse and monotonous. The cells may surround uninvolved nodes and appear to be cohesive. Cell molding and retracted squared off cell outlines may be seen. Chromatin is finely clumped and dispersed and multiple basophilic paracentral nucleoli are present. The cytoplasm is deeply basophilic and contains vacuoles which are best visualized in imprints. These features impart a deep grey hue to the uniformly diffuse infiltrate. Mitotic activity is high and there are numerous apoptotic cells with phagocytic macrophages containing apoptotic debris imparting the characteristic "starry sky" appearance.

A florid granulomatous reaction in typically limited-stage disease signifies a better prognosis, and in some cases plasmacytoid differentiation may be observed in which the tumor cells show eccentric basophilic cytoplasm and their nuclei contain a single

Table 6.15
Burkitt lymphoma (BL) – epidemiological variants

Endemic BL • Occurs in equatorial Africa and Papua New Guinea • Corresponds to the geographical distribution of malaria • EBV detected in the majority of cells in all cases • Extranodal sites involved, including CNS • Jaws, facial bones (including orbit) involved in about 50% of cases • Other sites – distal ileum, caecum, omentum, long bones, gonads, kidneys, salivary glands, thyroid, and breasts; bulky involvement
Sporadic BL • EBV involved in about 30% of cases • Majority present with abdominal involvement of ileocaecal region, ovaries, kidneys, and breasts; jaw involvement uncommon. • Breast involvement occurs with onset of puberty, pregnancy, or lactation. • Abdominal masses can compress spinal cord to produce paraplegia • Lymph node involvement more common in adults than in children
Immunodeficiency-associated BL • EBV indentified in 25–40% of cases • More common in HIV than other forms of immunosuppression • Nodal and bone marrow involvement common

central nucleolus. The latter change occurs more commonly in immunodeficiency states. Other cases may show greater nuclear pleomorphism and more prominent but fewer nucleoli. While these used to be called "atypical BL," these morphological variants share similar gene expression profiles and are part of the same spectrum of BL (**Figs. 6.55, 6.56, 6.57, 6.58; Table 6.16**).

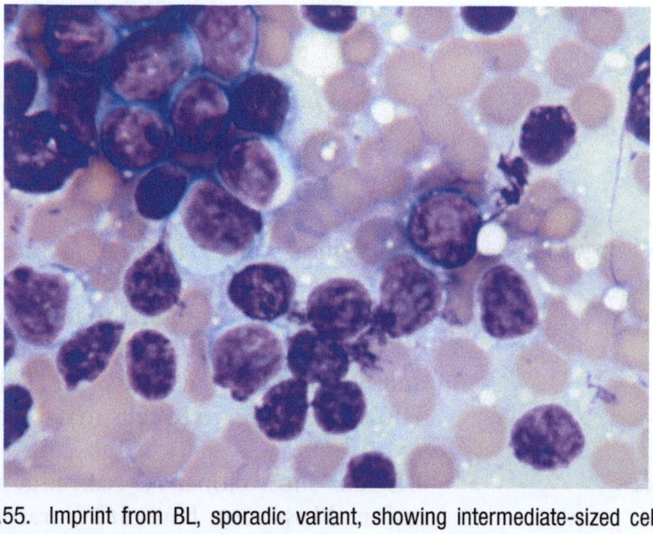

Fig. 6.55. Imprint from BL, sporadic variant, showing intermediate-sized cells with scanty basophilic cytoplasm that contains lipid vacuoles. Multiple nucleoli are present in the tumor cells.

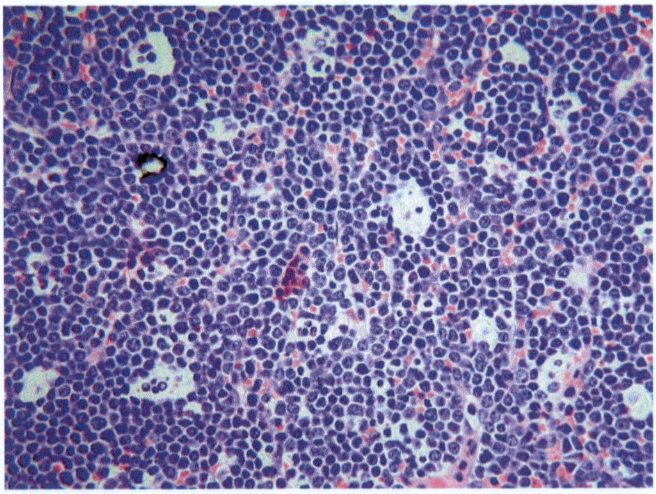

Fig. 6.56. Diffuse, monotonous infiltration of node with a starry sky pattern. The retracted cytoplasmic borders produce a "squared-off" appearance. Numerous mitotic figures and apoptotic bodies are present.

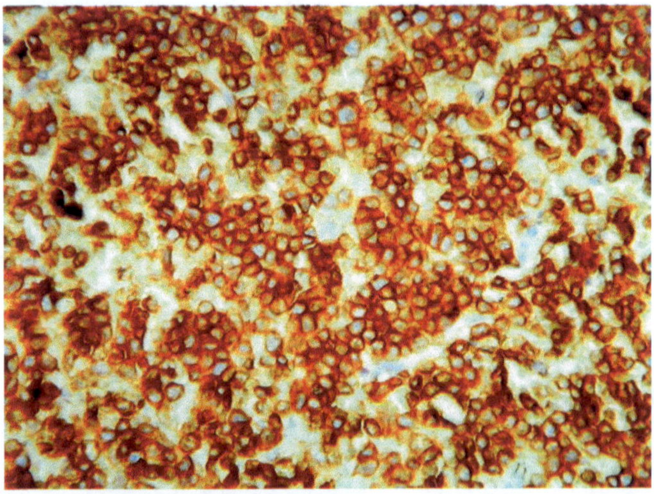

Fig. 6.57. The tumor stains for CD79a.

Immunohistology

The tumors cells express moderate to strong levels of membranous IgM with light-chain restriction. The B cell antigens CD20 and CD79a are expressed together with CD10, Bcl6, CD38, and CD43. They are usually negative or only weakly positive for Bcl2 and are uniformly negative for Tdt. The Ki67 index is close to 100% and scattered T cells may be present.

Genetics

BL cells show clonal *IG* rearrangements with somatic hypermutation. Most cases have *MYC* translocation at band 8q24 to the *IG* heavy-chain region, 14q32, or less commonly, at the lambda

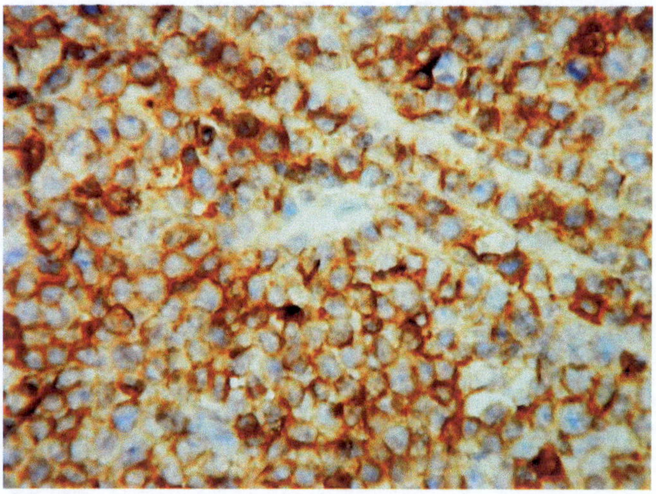

Fig. 6.58. There is strong staining for CD10 but staining for Bcl2 and TdT was negative (not shown).

Table 6.16
Burkitt lymphoma – morphology

Diffuse, monotonous deep blue/grey infiltrate with starry sky pattern
Intermediate-sized cells with dense basophilic cytoplasm
Nuclei oval, finely clumped chromatin, and multiple basophilic nucleoli
Scanty basophilic cytoplasm contains lipid vacuoles (best seen in imprints)
Cell moulding and "squared-off" retracted cytoplasmic outlines
Very brisk mitosis and numerous apoptotic bodies
Granulomatous response indicates better prognosis
Plasmacytoid differentiation more common in immunodeficiency states

22q11 or kappa 2p12 light-chain loci. As many as 10% of cases may lack *MYC* translocation by FISH. The explanation for this is uncertain; furthermore, *MYC* translocations are not specific to BL.

Gene profiling studies show a consistent gene expression signature for BL, clearly distinct from that of DLBCL (**Table 6.17**).

B Cell Lymphoma, Unclassifiable, with Features Intermediate Between DLBCL and BL

This group of diffuse B cell lymphoma shows morphological and genetic features of both DLBCL and BL; some of these cases previously classified as Burkitt-like lymphoma. The majority have morphological features intermediate between DLBCL and BL with some smaller cells resembling BL and some larger cells resembling DLBCL. A starry sky pattern is displayed as well as an

Table 6.17
Burkitt lymphoma – immunohistology and genetics

Express B cell antigens as well as CD10, Bcl6, CD38, and CD43
High Ki67 index (>90%)
Negative for Bcl2 and TdT
IG rearrangement with somatic hypermutation
MYC translocation to *IG* heavy chain region or Igκ or Igλ region
Gene expression signature of BL distinct from DLBCL

immunophenotype that is consistent with BL. Some cases resemble BL morphologically but have an atypical immunophenotype or genetic features different to BL. At present, this category is heterogenous and may include some cases of transformed follicular lymphomas. Cases of otherwise typical DLBCL with *MYC* rearrangement and otherwise typical cases of BL without demonstrable *MYC* rearrangement should not be included in this category.

Nodal Involvement by Primary Extranodal Lymphomas and Leukemias

Nodal involvement by primary extranodal lymphomas and leukemia includes MALT lymphoma, myeloid leukemia, lymphoblastic lymphoma, hairy cell leukemia, and pro-lymphocytic leukemia. These entities are described in Chapter 8.

T Cell and NK Cell Neoplasms

Pre-T cells migrate from the bone marrow and differentiate predominantly in the thymus. Early thymocytes in the thymic cortex have rearrangement of T cell antigen receptor (TCR) genes and express CD7 and subsequently CD2 (the sheep erythrocyte receptor), CD5, and CD3. CD7 persists on the mature T cell and as differentiation progresses, the thymocytes move into the thymic medulla, co-expressing CD4 and CD8 before segregating into separate CD4+ and CD8+ mature T cells. Natural killer (NK) cells are closely related and share immunophenotypic and functional similarities with T cells.

The rearrangement of the TCR chain genes is a clonal marker of T cell lymphomas. αβ T cells and γδ T cells are the two major classes, both chains consisting of an external variable (V) and a constant (C) portion. The αβ TCR is most commonly expressed in mature T cells and also represents the most common TCR in T cell lymphomas. The γδ TCR is expressed in a minority of T cell lymphomas that tend to develop in subcutaneous tissue, spleen, and liver.

The classification of B cell lymphomas, with the exception of DLBCL, is a good reflection of the maturation sequence and compartmentalization of B lymphocytes, allowing a conceptual understanding of these neoplasms and providing a guide to treatment. In contrast, the current WHO classification of T cell lymphomas is clearly less satisfactory. This is due to a number of reasons including the marked morphological variation of neoplastic T cells and the difficulty in characterizing the neoplasms according to their maturation due to the variable and aberrant expression of T cell antigens. The inability to identify clonality with immunohistochemical markers is another drawback that places a greater reliance on molecular techniques. Furthermore, the similarities between T cell neoplasms and the closely related NK cells pose added problems of identification and classification. Although NK cell lymphomas retain germline TCR genes, usually involve extranodal sites, and only rarely involve lymph nodes, some tumors exhibit combined features of T cell and NK cell tumors.

One simple way of classifying T cell neoplasms is to divide them into precursor and mature (peripheral) T cell types. Precursor T cell neoplasms derive from the bone marrow, thymus, and lymph nodes. Peripheral T cell neoplasms often occur in lymph nodes but also extranodally. This latter group of lymphomas comprises a mixture of fairly well-defined entities and neoplasms of purely descriptive terms.

T-Lymphoblastic Leukemia/Lymphoma (Precursor T Cell Lymphoblastic Leukemia/Lymphoma)

Clinical

Both T-lymphoblastic leukemia and T-lymphoblastic lymphoma are referred to as T-lymphoblast leukemia/lymphoma (T-LBL) as they are biologically very similar neoplasms. The leukemic disease is most frequent in adolescent males and comprises some 15% of childhood acute lymphoblastic leukemias (ALL) and 25% of all adult ALL. T-LBL comprises about 85–90% of all lymphoblastic lymphomas and is also most frequent in adolescent males but may be seen in any age group.

The bone marrow is involved in all cases, with >25% bone marrow blasts as the threshold definition for leukemia. The mediastinum (thymus) is frequently involved, although any lymph node (usually above the diaphragm) or extranodal site such as skin, tonsil, liver, spleen, central nervous system, and testes may be infiltrated. The mediastinal mass may often exhibit rapid growth, sometimes producing compression symptoms. Pleural effusions are common.

The clinical course is very aggressive and therapy is complex, involving multiagent chemotherapy and prophylaxis of so-called sanctuary sites that include the central nervous system and gonads. Prognosis is relatively worse in adults than in children (**Table 6.18**).

Table 6.18
T-Lymphoblastic leukemia/lymphoma – clinical

T-lymphoblastic leukemia and T-lymphoblastic lymphoma biologically very similar
Childhood and adolescent disease; male predominance
T-lymphoblastic leukemia comprises 15% of childhood ALL and 25% of adult ALL
T-LBL comprises 85–90% of all lymphoblastic lymphomas
Mediastinal mass (50–75%), supradiaphragmatic nodal involvement
Extranodal involvement and pleural effusions common
Acute lymphoblastic leukemia commonly develops
Very aggressive disease; prognosis worse in adults than in children.
Relapse in sanctuary sites: central nervous system and gonads

Morphology

The infiltrate is diffuse, often with complete replacement of nodal architecture, the uniform-appearing lymphoblasts producing an even dense blue/grey hue. In some cases there is preservation of residual follicles, so-called “naked” germinal centers in which the lymphoblasts replace mantle cells with small germinal centers remaining, with areas of residual paracortical tissue, and patent sinuses. The lymphoblasts characteristically infiltrate the lymph node capsule with extension into the perinodal tissue. The infiltration in the capsule and fibrocollagenous tissue of the lymph node is typically in a single file or a linear pattern. A starry sky pattern is present, often focally. Occasionally fibrous strands encircle nodules of lymphoblasts to produce a pseudo-nodular appearance. The lymphoblasts have smaller nuclei than histiocytes and minimum cytoplasm. The chromatin is fine and dispersed, imparting a dusty appearance, and nucleoli are absent or inconspicuous. Nuclear membranes are thin and nuclear contours are highly irregular or convoluted or indented, or they may be round or non-convoluted. The mitotic rate is high. The uniform and often complete diffuse infiltration may resemble CLL/SLL but the infiltrate is of a lighter blue grey colour and the Indian file pattern of infiltration is not seen in CLL/SLL. The clinical settings are clearly different (**Figs. 6.59, 6.60, 6.61, 6.62, 6.63; Table 6.19**).

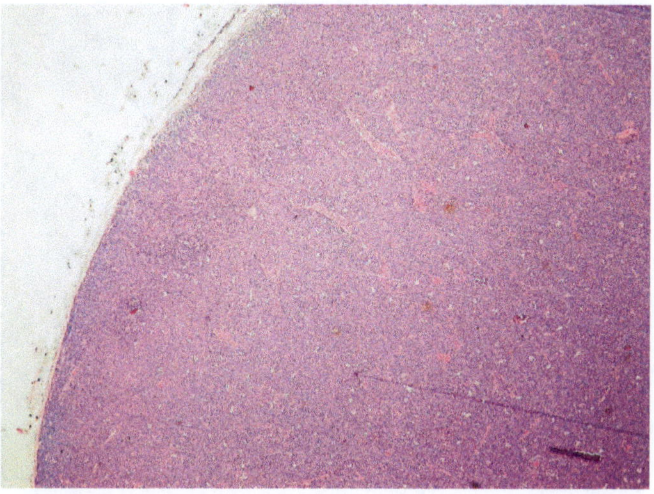

Fig. 6.59. T-LBL in cervical node. The infiltrate is diffuse and the lymphoblasts impart a dense *grey* hue.

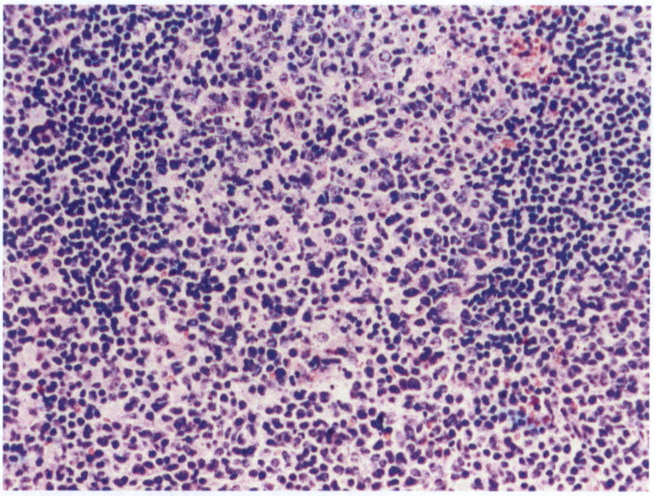

Fig. 6.60. A residual germinal center in the cortex surrounded by lymphoblasts. A thin mantle zone remains, partially eroded by neoplastic cells.

Immunohistology and Genetics

The T lymphoblasts stain with PAS, acid phosphatase, and nonspecific esterase but these are not specific and sensitive.

T-LBL cells display an immunophenotype that reflects the stages of normal T cell maturation. They express Tdt and most commonly express CD7 and cytoplasmic CD3. The expression of other T cell antigens is variable, namely, CD1a, CD3, CD4, CD5, CD7, and CD8. The co-expression of CD4 and CD8 is common or the phenotype may be CD4+/CD8–, CD4–/CD8+, or CD4–/CD8–. CD10, CD43, and CD45RO may be positive. Other markers including CD99 and CD34 may be positive, indicating

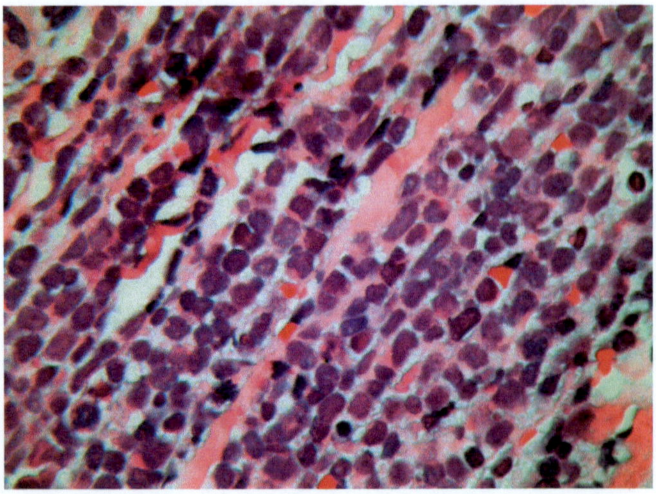

Fig. 6.61. A characteristic single file or linear pattern of infiltration is seen in the capsule of the lymph node.

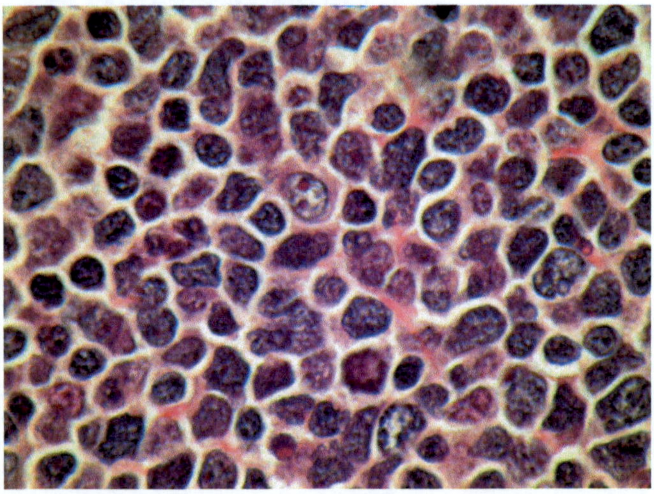

Fig. 6.62. Lymphoblasts are of small to intermediate size with a high nuclear/cytoplasmic ratio.

the precursor nature of the neoplastic cells. CD79a can be positive in about 10% of cases, and myeloid-associated markers can be expressed, reflecting lineage infidelity.

T-LBL almost always shows clonal rearrangements of the T cell receptor genes but there is simultaneous presence of *IgH* rearrangements, reflecting the lineage infidelity that is common in T-LBL. Monozygotic twins with T-AL have been shown to share the same TCR gene rearrangement, suggesting an *in utero* origin for the earliest genetic lesions (**Figs. 6.64, 6.65, 6.66**, and **6.67**; **Table 6.20**).

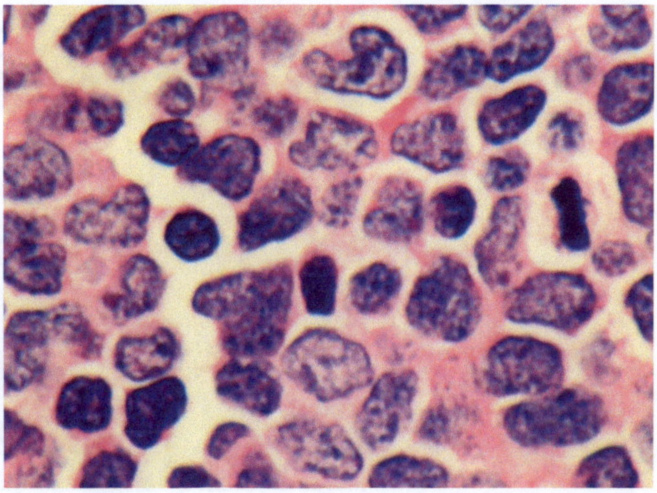

Fig. 6.63. The chromatin of the lymphoblasts is fine and dispersed, producing a dusty appearance. Nucleoli are indistinct and nuclei are convoluted with prominent irregular and indented outlines.

Table 6.19
T-Lymphoblastic leukemia/lymphoma – morphology

Diffuse infiltrate, sometimes sparing "naked" germinal centers
Monomorphous population of lymphoblasts impart a grey–blue hue to infiltrate
Indian file pattern of infiltration in capsule and fibrocollagenous tissue of lymph node
Small- to intermediate-sized nucleus, scanty cytoplasm
Convoluted and non-convoluted nuclei
Fine and dispersed chromatin produces a dusty appearance
Nucleoli indistinct
Mitosis brisk

Peripheral T Cell Lymphoma, Not Otherwise Specified (PTCL-NOS)

Peripheral T cell lymphomas represent a heterogenous category of mature nodal T cell lymphomas that does not correspond to any of the current specifically defined entities. It comprises more than one disease, some fairly well defined, and others largely descriptive and cannot be further divided based on currently available information and diagnostic tools. Synonyms have included node-based T cell lymphoma, immunoblastic sarcoma T cell type, pleomorphic small-cell lymphoepithelioid lymphoma (Lennert lymphoma), pleomorphic medium- and large T cell lymphoma, post-thymic T cell lymphoma, and mature T cell lymphoma. They account for about 30% of peripheral T cell lymphomas (PTCL) in

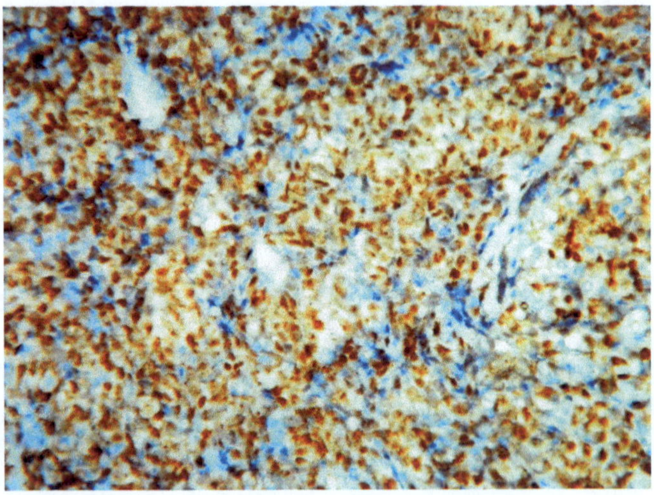

Fig. 6.64. The lymphoblasts show strong nuclear expression of Tdt.

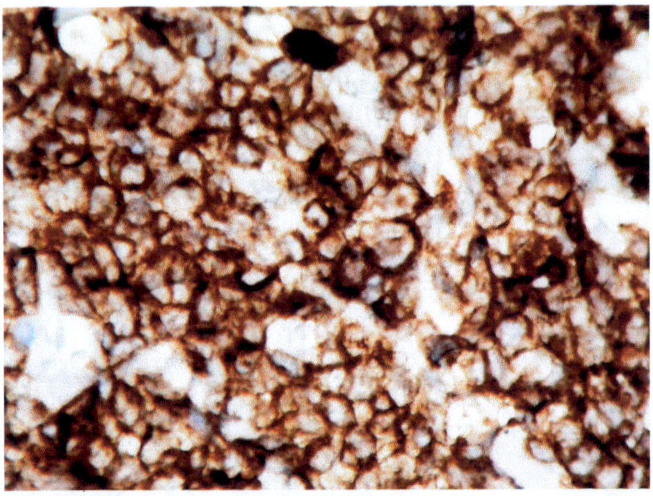

Fig. 6.65. There is distinct cytoplasmic as well as some membrane staining for CD3.

Western countries and are rarely seen in children. The postulated normal counterpart is the activated mature T lymphocyte mostly of CD4+ type.

Clinical

Peripheral lymph node involvement is the commonest presentation but any site may be affected. Bone marrow, liver, spleen, and extranodal tissue infiltration occur when the disease is generalized, with the skin and gastrointestinal tract as the most commonly affected extranodal sites. Central nervous system, salivary gland, and lung are less frequently involved. Advanced disease with B symptoms is the common presentation and there may be associated eosinophilia, pruritus, and rarely, hemophagocytic

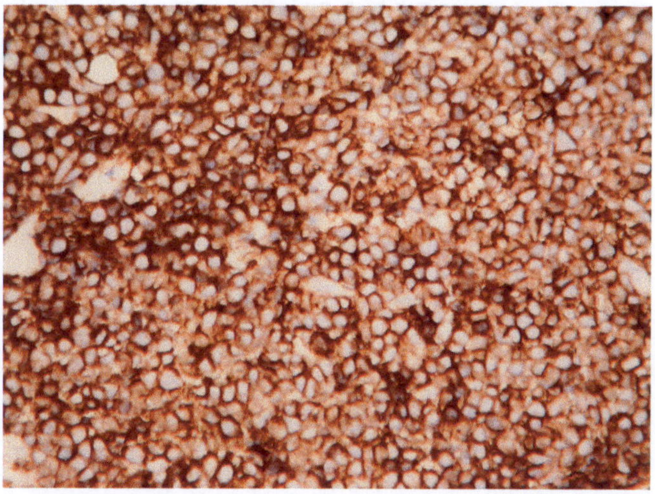

Fig. 6.66. The lymphoblasts stain for CD5. CD7 was also expressed (not shown).

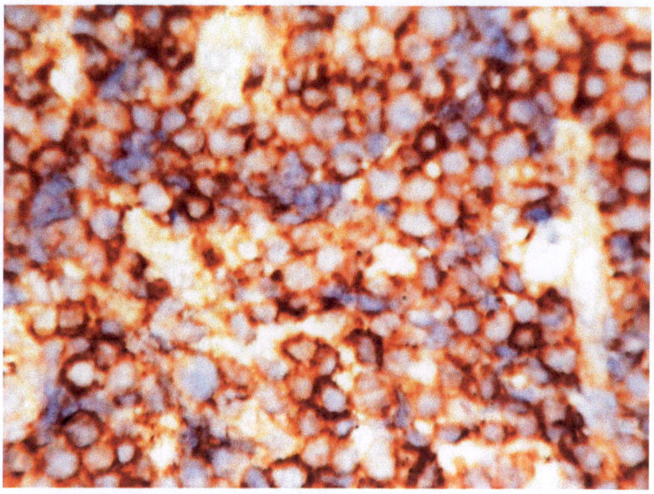

Fig. 6.67. The lymphoblasts also express CD99.

syndrome. Prognosis is invariably poor with 5-year survivals of 25–45%; age >60 years, low performance status, high serum LDH, and bone marrow involvement are recorded as poor prognostic indicators.

Morphology

The pattern of nodal infiltration is most often diffuse with effacement of nodal architecture. In a subset of cases where involvement is partial, there is preferential involvement of the T zone or paracortex, usually associated with a prominent proliferation of high-endothelial vessels. PTCL and NOS show the greatest heterogeneity among the lymphomas, attributable to both the neoplastic cells and associated changes that form the response

Table 6.20
T-Lymphoblastic leukemia/lymphoma – immunohistology and genetics

Tdt+/cCD3+/CD7+/CD5+
Variable positivity for CD1a, CD4, and CD8
Co-expression of CD4 and CD8 common, otherwise CD4+/CD8–, CD4–/CD8+ or CD4–/CD8–
Also variable positivity for CD10, CD99, CD34, CD43, and CD45RO
High Ki67 count
Lineage infidelity common, CD79a+
Monoclonal TCR gene rearrangements

to chemokines and cytokines secreted by the neoplastic T cells. The cytological spectrum of the neoplastic T cells ranges from a monomorphous to highly polymorphous infiltrate. The neoplastic cells are medium sized or large, with irregular, pleomorphic, and often bizarre nuclei that are hyperchromatic or vesicular with prominent nucleoli. The neoplastic cells have variable amounts of cytoplasm that can be eosinophilic, basophilic, or clear. Mitosis is brisk and Reed–Sternberg-like cells may be present. As a reaction to the chemokines and cytokines secreted by the neoplastic T cells, a mixture of small lymphocytes with plasma cells and stimulated B cells that may be clonal and variable numbers of eosinophils and epithelioid histiocytes are present, sometimes with sarcoid-like granulomas. A background of high-endothelial venules proliferating in an arborizing pattern is often present. In the lymphoepithelioid cell variant (Lennert lymphoma), epithelioid histiocytes may predominate but atypical or multilobated neoplastic T cells are usually not difficult to find. A small cell variant is infrequently encountered.

Three variants are recognized. The lymphoepithelioid variant or Lennert lymphoma is a diffuse growth characterized by confluent clusters of epithelioid histiocytes with intervening sheets of small neoplastic cells with nuclear irregularities. Scattered among these are larger, more atypical proliferating blasts. Inflammatory cells may be present. The neoplastic T cells are usually CD8+. The T zone variant is characterized by a perifollicular growth pattern that may be mistaken for a benign paracortical hyperplasia. The neoplastic cells are mostly small with mild cytological atypia, expressing CD3 and CD4 and show loss of CD5 or CD7. The third variant or follicular variant is very rare and consists of atypical clear cells that accumulate as perifollicular nodules that may be intrafollicular and occur in a background of progressive transformed germinal centers. They do not show the proliferation of

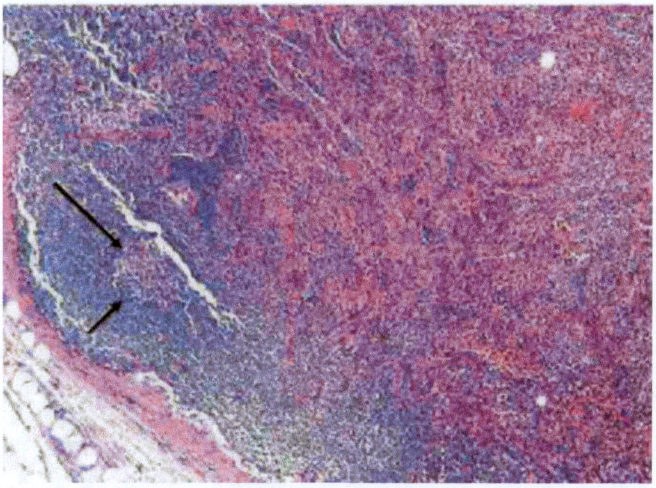

Fig. 6.68. PTCL-NOS showing partial involvement of a lymph node. A polymorphous infiltrate is present in the paracortex with preservation of a germinal center in the cortex (*arrows*). Proliferation of high-endothelial vessels is evident.

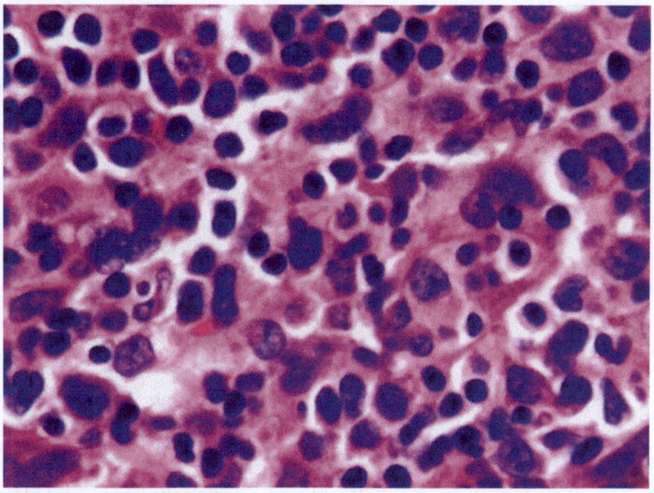

Fig. 6.69. The infiltrate is characterized by large multilobated cells with prominent basophilic nucleoli in vesicular nuclei in a background of small lymphocytes and scattered epithelioid histiocytes.

FDC associated with FL and NLPHL which they may mimic (**Figs. 6.68, 6.69, 6.70, 6.71, 6.72, 6.73, 6.74, 6.75, 6.76, 6.77, 6.78, 6.79, 6.80**).

Immunohistology

CD4+/CD8– phenotype predominates in nodal PTCL-NOS. As with most T cell lymphomas, an aberrant T cell phenotype is common with loss of CD5 and CD7. CD4/CD8 double positivity or CD4/CD8 double negativity, and expression of NK

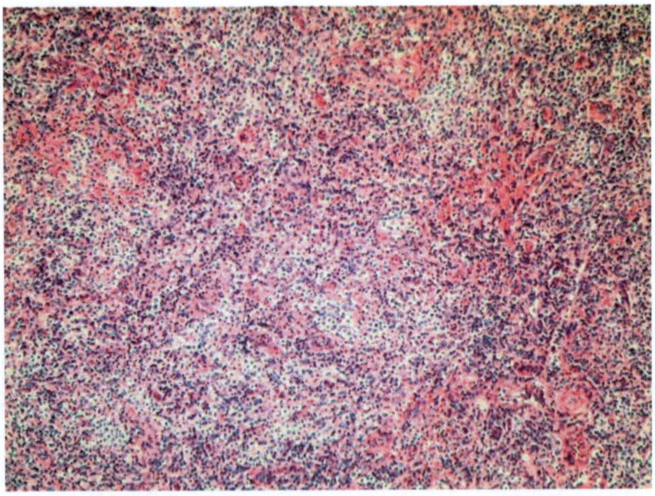

Fig. 6.70. PTCL, NOS. Medium-sized cells with clear cytoplasm infiltrate the node in a diffuse manner associated with a background of arborizing high-endothelial vessels.

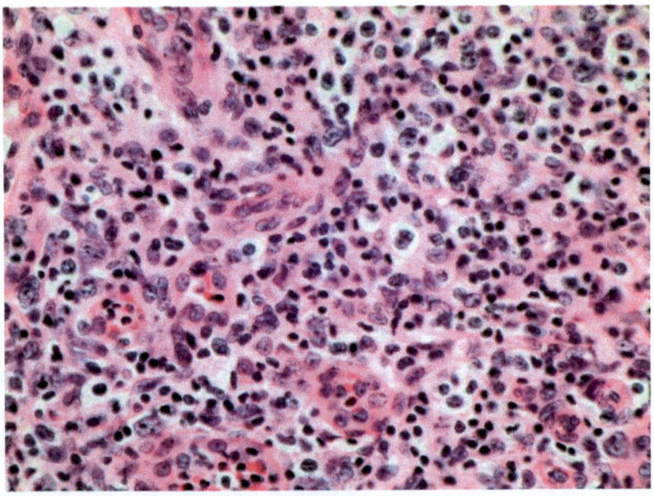

Fig. 6.71. The neoplastic cells have water-clear cytoplasm and variably sized vesicular nuclei with prominent eosinophilic nucleoli.

cell-associated antigens CD56 and CD57, and cytotoxic granule expression, commonly TIA-1, granzyme B, and perforin, may also be seen. The expression of T cell receptor β-chain (βF1) allows distinction from γδ T cell lymphomas and NK cell lymphomas. The expression of CD30, in exceptional cases together with CD15, requires separation from Hodgkin lymphoma, and aberrant expression of CD20 or CD79a may be rarely encountered. The proliferation index is usually high and a Ki67 index >70% is said to be associated with worse prognosis.

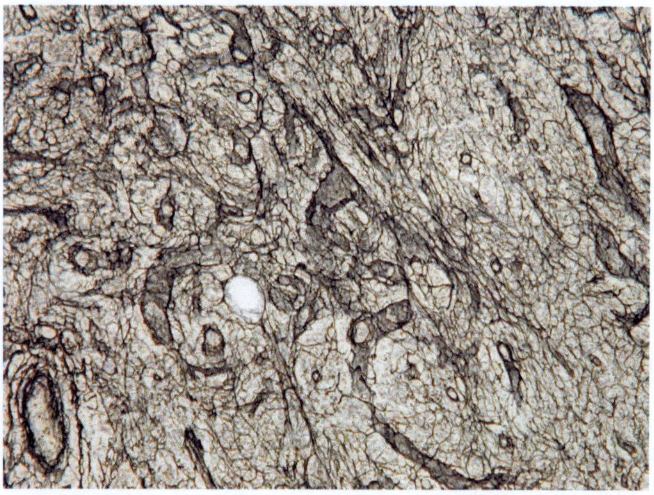

Fig. 6.72. Reticulin stain showing the arborizing post-capillary venules in the background of the neoplastic infiltrate.

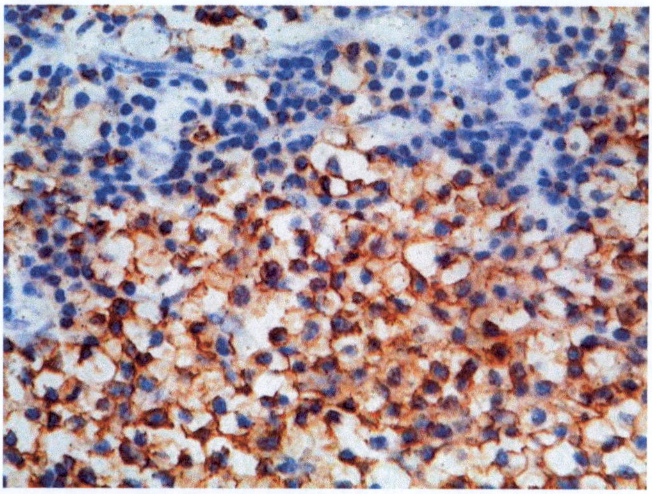

Fig. 6.73. The clear cells stain for CD3 and were CD2+/CD4+/CD8–/CD7–/CD5– (not shown).

Genetics

Most cases carry TCR gene rearrangements. The TCRβ gene is most often rearranged, followed by the TCRγ gene. The TCRδ gene is usually deleted. No recurrent molecular abnormalities have been demonstrated and gene expression profiling has produced heterogenous results (**Table 6.21**).

Angioimmunoblastic T Cell Lymphoma

Angioimmunoblastic T cell lymphoma (AITL) is a peripheral T cell lymphoma that is separately classified from peripheral T cell lymphomas, NOS in the 2008 WHO classification. This lymphoma is a systemic disease characterized by a polymorphous

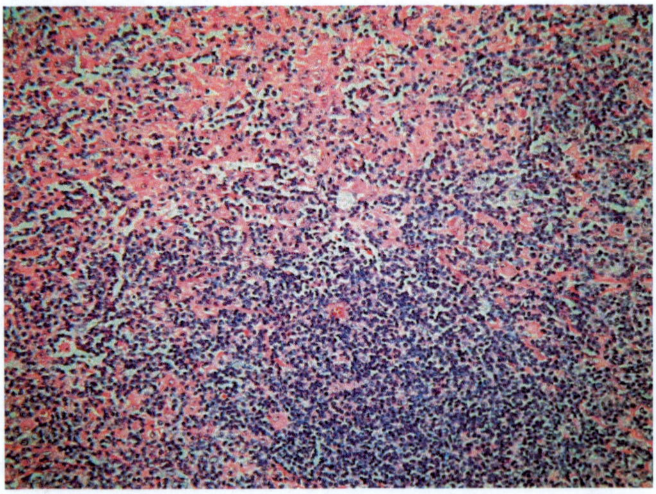

Fig. 6.74. PTCL, lymphoepithelioid variant (Lennert lymphoma). The diffuse infiltrate contains numerous epithelioid histiocytes occurring singly and in clusters.

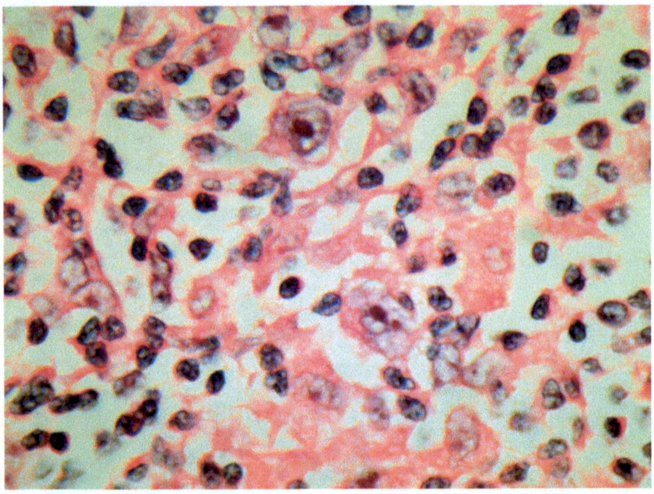

Fig. 6.75. Among the epithelioid histiocytes, small lymphocytes and stimulated cells are large atypical multilobated cells with vesicular nuclei and prominent eosinophilic nucleoli.

infiltrate involving lymph nodes, with a prominent proliferation of high-endothelial venules and FDC.

Clinical

Current evidence strongly indicates that AITL arises as a *de novo* peripheral T cell lymphoma, although the process was initially considered to be reactive with a propensity of progression to lymphoma. AITL occurs in the middle-aged and elderly, making up to 15–20% of all PTCL or 1–2% of all non-Hodgkin lymphomas. The disease is consistently associated with EBV which has a

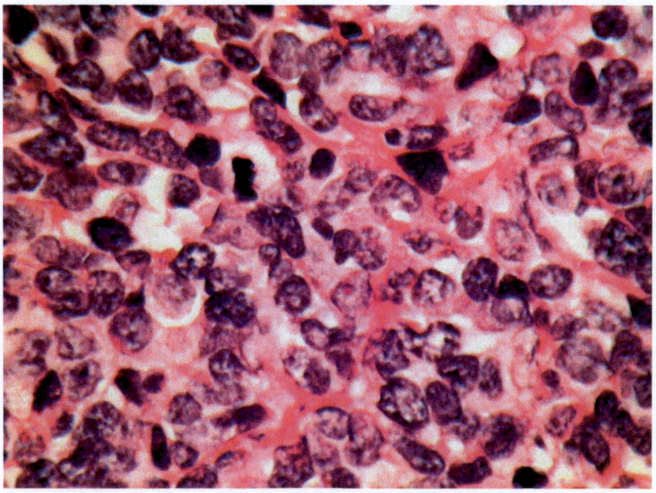

Fig. 6.76. Another example of PTCL-NOS in which the diffuse infiltrate is more monotonous and composed of large cells with vesicular irregular nuclei. Eosinophilic nucleoli are visible.

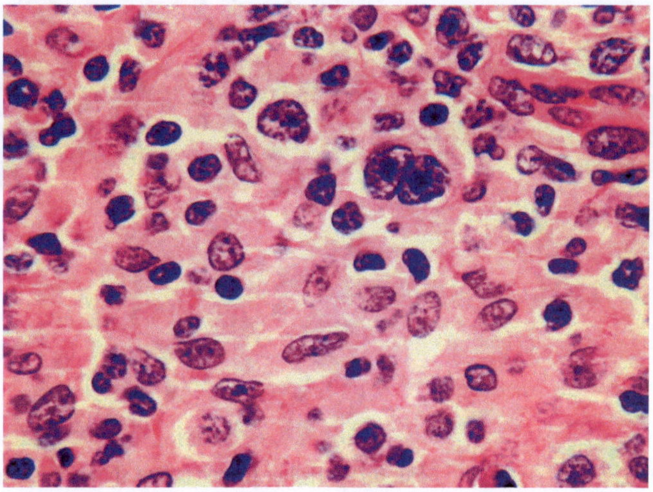

Fig. 6.77. Reed–Sternberg-like cells may be present.

suggested role in pathogenesis; however, the neoplastic T cells are negative for the virus.

In addition to generalized lymphadenopathy which is the presentation in virtually all patients, the spleen, liver, skin, and bone marrow are often involved and presentation at advanced stage is typical. Systemic symptoms and polyclonal hypergammaglobulinemia associated with a pruritic skin rash are frequent and other common findings are pleural effusion, arthritis, and ascites. There is often an accompanying immune dysfunction evidenced by the presence of circulating immune complexes, positive rheumatoid

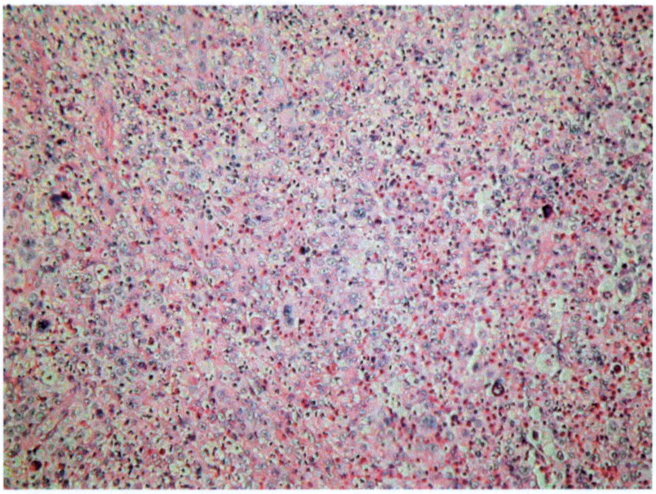

Fig. 6.78. PTCL-NOS with a marked eosinophilic infiltration. Scattered large hyperchromatic cells are visible and there is a fibrous background present.

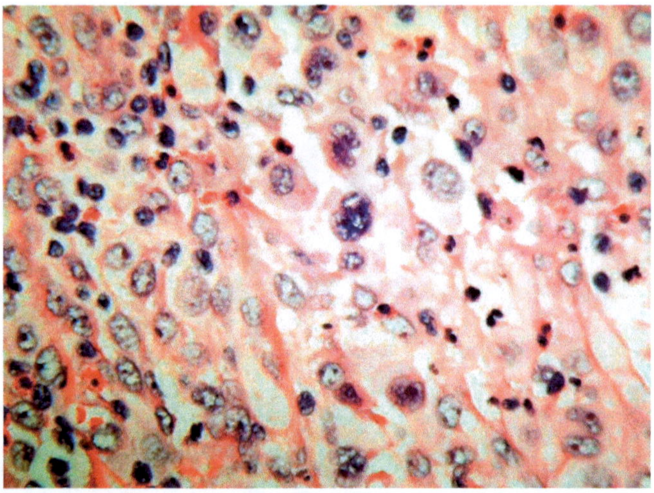

Fig. 6.79. Higher magnification shows the atypical cells with multilobated nuclei and eosinophilic nucleoli.

factor, anti-smooth muscle antibodies, and cold agglutinins with hemolytic anemia. Immune deficiency sets in with progression of the neoplastic process and expansion of the EBV-positive B cell population.

AITL is an aggressive disease with a median survival of less than 3 years; patients often succumb to infectious diseases as a result of the associated immune deficiency which makes the use of aggressive chemotherapy difficult. A supervening DLBCL can occur which is often EBV-positive (**Table 6.22**).

The postulated normal counterpart is a CD4+ follicular helper T cell.

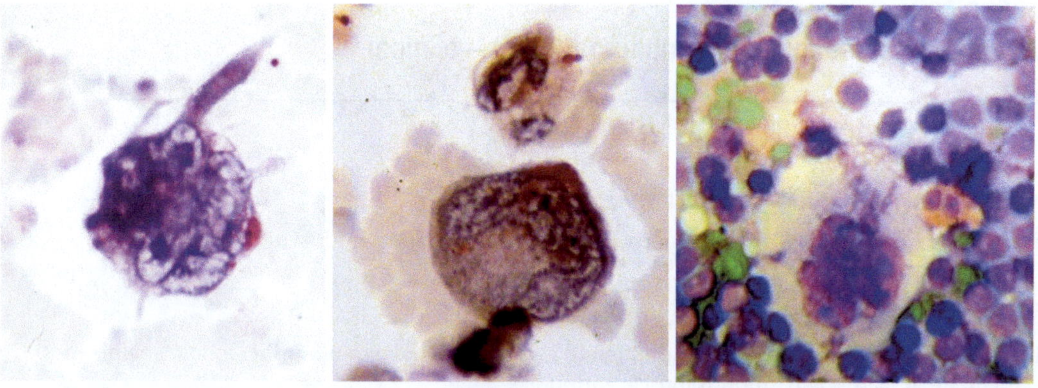

Fig. 6.80. Composite picture of large bizarre multilobated cells from different cases of PTCL-NOS. The center panel shows spontaneous sheep erythrocyte rosettes, a property of T cells, around the neoplastic cells.

Table 6.21
Peripheral T cell lymphoma, NOS – morphology and immunohistology

Morphology
Generally diffuse with destruction of nodal architecture; when partial, involves paracortex
Wide spectrum of cell types representing neoplastic as well as reactive cells
Neoplastic cells may be medium sized or large cells; small cell variant uncommon
Nuclei are often multilobated and bizarre, hyperchromatic or vesicular with prominent nucleoli
Cytoplasm is variable; may be basophilic, eosinophilic, or less frequently, clear
Background of proliferating high endothelial vessels, epithelioid histiocytes, small lymphocytes, stimulated cells, plasma cells, eosinophils, and fibrosis
Mitotic activity brisk
Three variants recognized: lymphoepithelioid (Lennert lymphoma), T zone, and follicular
Immunohistology
CD3+, CD43+, CD45RO+
CD4+/CD8–, less frequently CD4–/CD8+
Aberrant loss of a pan-T cell antigen such as CD5 or CD7
Cytotoxic proteins may be expressed, namely TIA-1, granzyme B, and perforin
CD57+ and CD56+ uncommon (<10%)
TdT–, CD1a–, CD99–
Monoclonal TCR rearrangements; no consistent molecular abnormalities demonstrated

Morphology

The spectrum of lymph node changes is remarkably variable and characterized by three common features. Infiltration is diffuse, often with perinodal involvement but sparing the peripheral cortical sinuses. There is a striking proliferation of arborizing high-endothelial venules with thick walls and hyperplastic endothelial cells in virtually all cases. The infiltrating population is highly polymorphous, with a variable number of small and large neoplastic cells mixed with numerous reactive cells that include plasma

Table 6.22
Angioimmunoblastic T cell lymphoma (AITL) – clinical

Most likely a *de novo* peripheral T cell lymphoma
Affects middle aged and elderly
Most common of all peripheral T cell lymphomas (15–20%)
Presents with generalized lymphadenopathy and advanced stage with B symptoms
Spleen, liver, skin, and bone marrow frequently involved
Other symptoms – pruritic skin rash, pleural effusion, arthritis, ascites
Immune dysfunction with circulating immune complexes, cold agglutinin hemolytic anemia, positive rheumatoid factor, anti-smooth muscle antibodies
Later develop immune deficiency with expansion of EBV+ B cells
Aggressive course, median survival <3 years
Succumb to infectious diseases due to immune deficiency
Supervening B cell proliferative diseases include DLBCL, plasmacytoma, Hodgkin lymphoma
Postulated normal counterpart is the CD4+ follicular helper T cell

cells, eosinophils, histiocytes, small lymphocytes, and follicular dendritic cells.

A merging pattern of changes is seen. This is sometimes described as comprising three phases that range from early involvement with partial preservation of nodal architecture with hyperplastic lymphoid follicles, through one where architecture is mostly effaced with small residual follicles with irregular shapes and partial disruption, to the late phase where the nodal architecture is almost completely replaced with few or no residual follicles present. The earliest phase of the disease can be difficult to diagnose. The cell population in the early phases tends to be more monotonous, and in some cases, composed of numerous atypical cells with clear cytoplasm. In the later phase, follicles may display changes of regression or appear "burnt out" and lack lymphocytes. They are composed mostly of proliferating FDC which extend to adjacent or surrounding proliferating blood vessels, a striking feature enhanced by immunohistochemical stains.

The neoplastic cells can show clear cytoplasm resulting in a distinctive appearance, and their accumulation around blood vessels produces nodules or tumor masses. Variable numbers of epithelioid histiocytes are present; they can sometimes be numerous and simulate the lymphoepithelioid variant of peripheral T cell lymphoma (Lennert lymphoma). Plasma cells can be numerous especially around vessels and associated with deposits of sludgy PAS-positive material in 20–30% of cases. Immunoblasts are present in variable numbers and irregularly shaped large cells with polylobated nuclei that simulate Reed–Sternberg cells can be seen. Mitotic figures are present in variable numbers but necrosis and fibrosis are unusual.

The peripheral blood may contain plasmacytoid lymphocytes, and plasma cells and lymphoma cells have been identified. Bone marrow involvement is variable and the infiltrate is polymorphous, composed of lymphoid cells, histiocytes, and eosinophils, clear cells being uncommonly seen (**Figs. 6.81, 6.82, 6.83, 6.84, 6.85, 6.86, 6.87, 6.88; Table 6.23**).

Immunohistology and Genetics

The neoplastic cells of AITL express markers of mature helper T cell lineage and are CD4+/CD8–. In addition, they express a

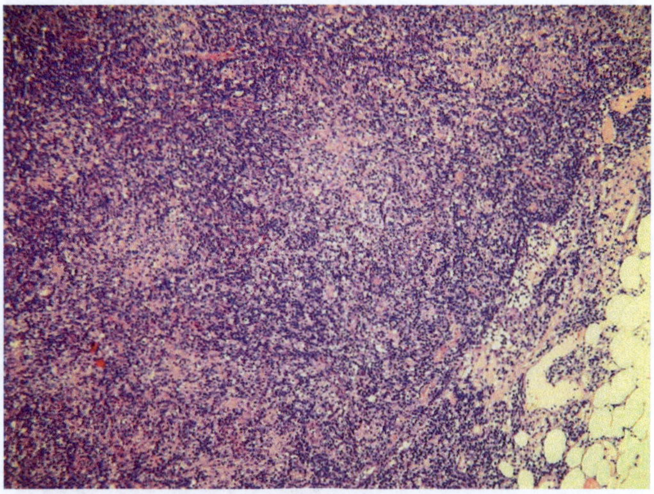

Fig. 6.81. Mid-phase AITL with effacement of lymph node architecture by a polymorphous infiltrate and spillover into perinodal tissues. Partial preservation of architecture with residual follicles was present in other areas.

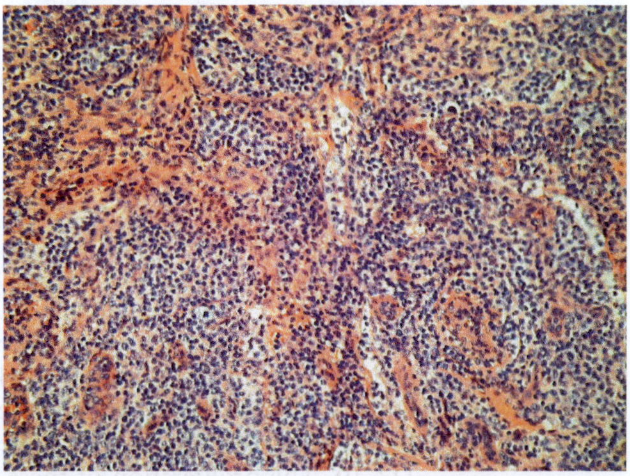

Fig. 6.82. Proliferating arborizing blood vessels are prominent.

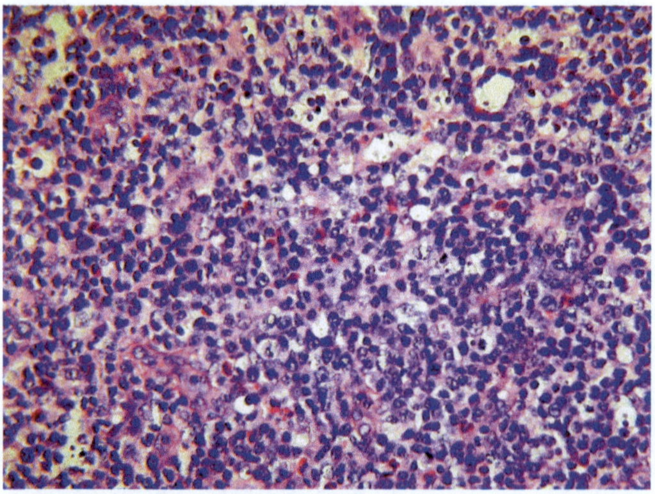

Fig. 6.83. The polymorphous infiltrate is composed of small and large cells mixed with plasma cells, eosinophils, and proliferating blood vessels.

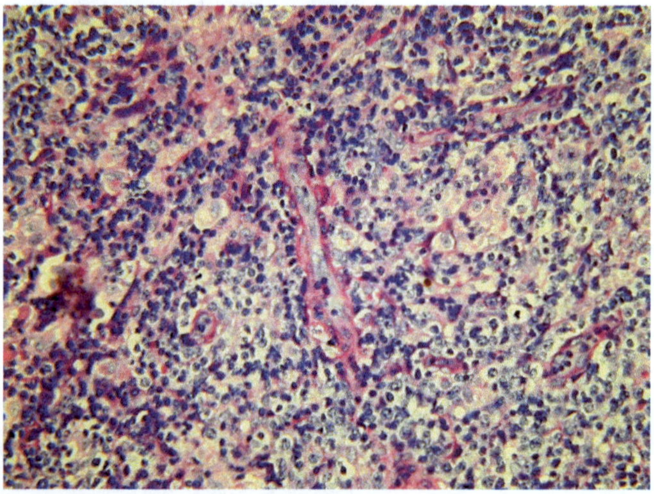

Fig. 6.84. A PAS stain highlights the blood vessels and epithelioid histiocytes are also visible in the polymorphous infiltrate.

variety of other T cell-associated antigens including CD3, CD5, CD45RO, and CD43, and may show aberrant loss of CD7. AITL also express a number of antigens expressed by reactive follicular helper T cells including CD10, Bcl6, CXCL13, and PD-1 (programmed death-1, also known as CXCR5). These T cell are also positive for CD38 and CD45 and are negative for CD8 and CD56. FDC meshworks are expanded, usually surrounding high-endothelial vessels and can be stained by CD21, CD35, and D2-40. The proliferation of these meshworks is characteristic of AITL and considered to be part of the definition of this disease,

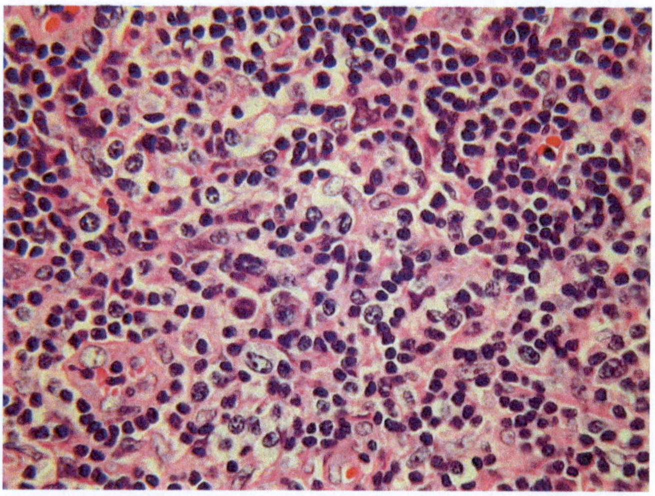

Fig. 6.85. Among the polymorphous infiltrate are seen large atypical cells with vesicular nuclei and prominent nucleoli as well as immunoblasts and plasma cells.

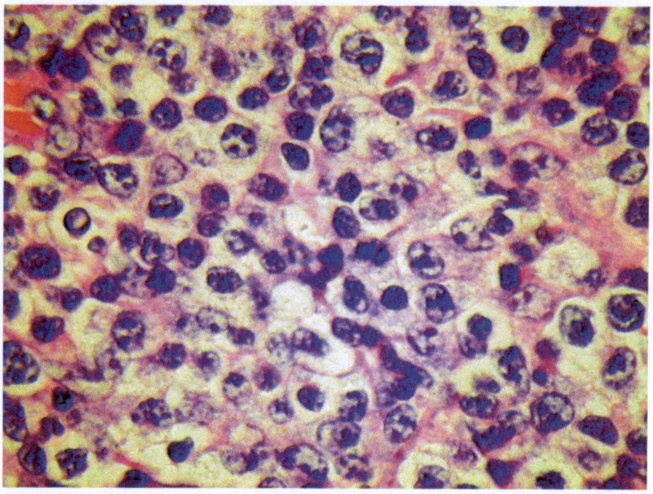

Fig. 6.86. The atypical cells are clustered around blood vessels and show moderate quantities of clear cytoplasm.

although in the early phase of the process, such meshworks may be minimal. The plasma cells and immunoblasts are polytypic, although EBV-positive B cell proliferations including DLBCL, classical Hodgkin lymphoma, and plasmacytoma may supervene. Ki67 staining may reveal a high-proliferative index as both T and B cells are proliferating.

There is clonal rearrangement of the TCR gene in the majority of cases. Clonal rearrangement of immunoglobulin genes may be found in about one-third of cases and correlate with expanded EBV+ B cells (**Figs. 6.89, 6.90, 6.91, 6.92, 6.93, 6.94**; **Table 6.24**).

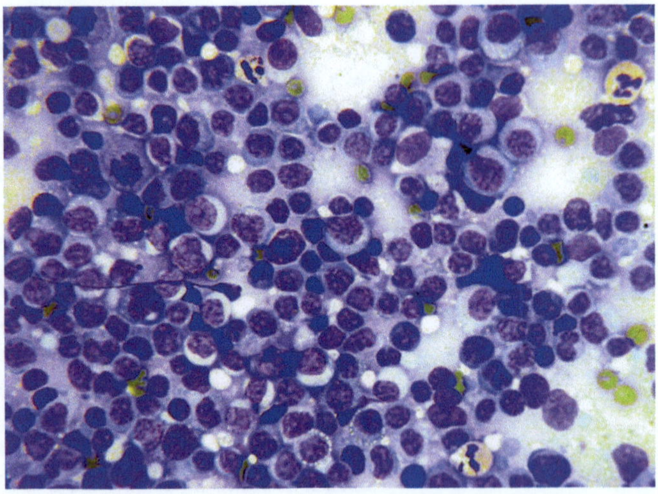

Fig. 6.87. Imprint of AITL lymph node showing sheets of the large atypical cells with moderate amounts of cytoplasm. Some cells show irregular nuclei (Giemsa stain).

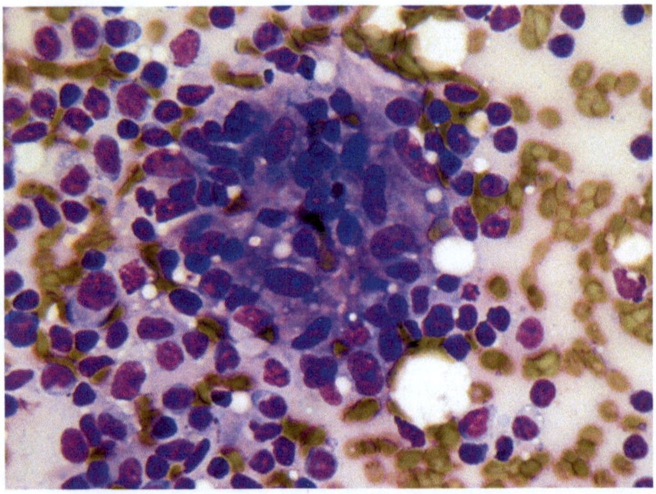

Fig. 6.88. AITL. Follicular dendritic cells with copious quantities of cytoplasm, atypical cells with pale cytoplasm, and plasma cells are present (Giemsa stain, lymph node imprint).

Anaplastic Large Cell Lymphoma (ALCL), ALK-Positive

Anaplastic large cell lymphomas (ALCL) may be anaplastic lymphoma kinase (ALK)-positive or ALK-negative. Both have comparable morphologic and phenotypic features and differ by the presence or absence of a translocation involving the *ALK* gene and expression of ALK protein and CD30. The two entities must be distinguished and also separated from primary cutaneous ALCL and other lymphomas with anaplastic features, as the prognosis of ALCL, ALK– with conventional therapy is clearly poorer than that of ALCL, ALK+.

Table 6.23
Angioimmunoblastic T cell lymphoma – morphology

Variable morphological spectrum
Diffuse process, proliferation of high-endothelial vessels, and polymorphous infiltrate of large atypical cells, FDC, immunoblasts, plasma cells, eosinophils, and epithelioid cells
Merging spectrum from hyperplastic follicles through partial effacement by more monomorphous cells with clear cytoplasm to complete effacement of architecture, nodular perivascular aggregates of atypical cells, regressed follicles, proliferation of perivascular FDC, polymorphous infiltrate, PAS+ sludge
Presence of fibrosis, blast cells and epithelioid histiocytes and atypical cells may simulate Hodgkin lymphoma and other peripheral T cell lymphomas

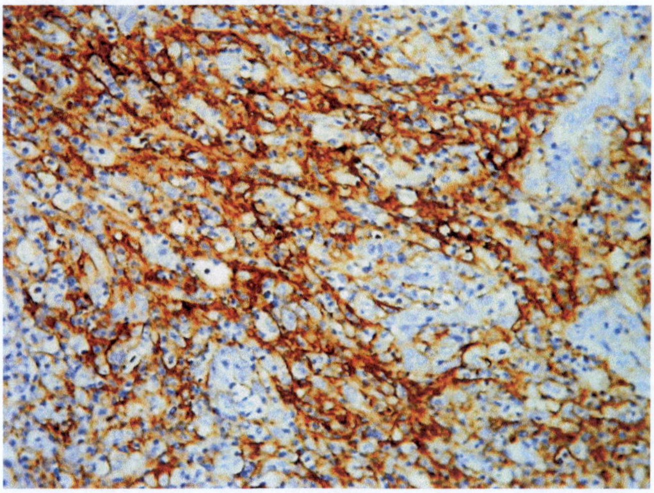

Fig. 6.89. AITL, late phase. Marked proliferation of perivascular DRCs shown by CD21 staining.

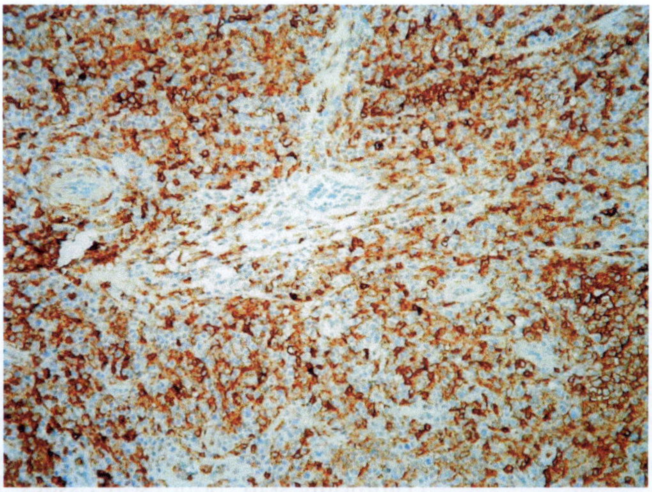

Fig. 6.90. The atypical cells, mostly perivascular in location, label for CD4.

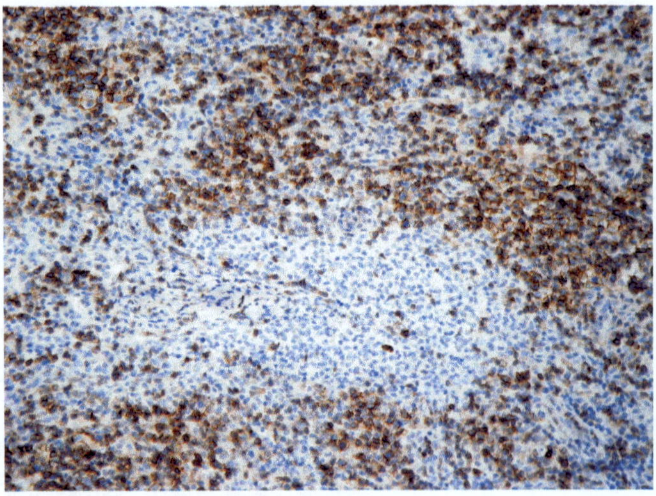

Fig. 6.91. AITL cells characteristically express CD3.

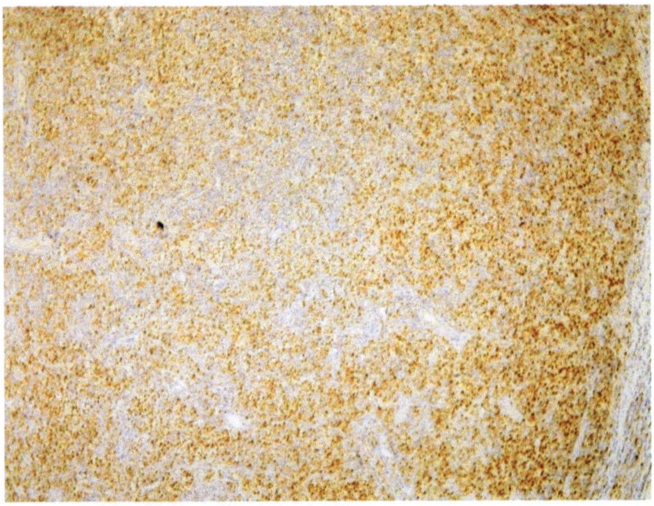

Fig. 6.92. AITL cells also express normal follicular helper T cell markers CD10 shown here as well as PD-1 and CXCL13.

Clinical

ALCL, ALK+ is a T cell lymphoma composed of large lymphoid cells with abundant cytoplasm and pleomorphic, often indented nuclei and a translocation involving the *ALK* gene on 2p23. This lymphoma accounts for about 3% of adult non-Hodgkin lymphoma and 10–20% of childhood lymphomas. It is most common in the first three decades of life. The postulated normal counterpart is the activated mature cytotoxic T cell.

The disease involves nodal and extranodal sites, the latter commonly skin, bone, soft tissues, lung, and liver. Bone marrow involvement is subtle and with immunohistochemical stains, as

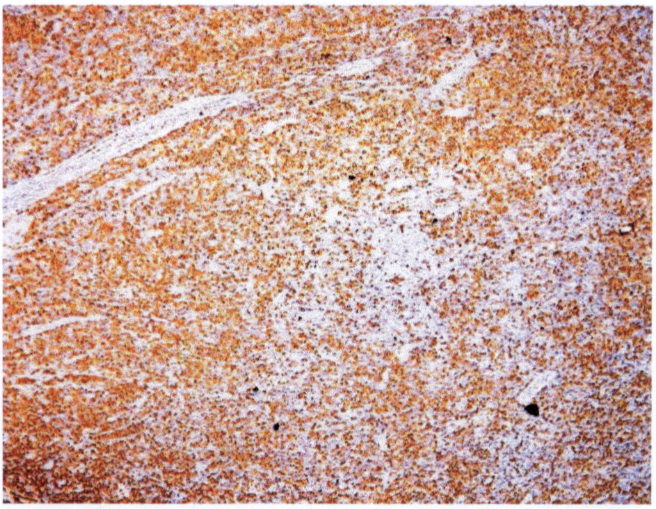

Fig. 6.93. Perivascular atypical cells stain for Bcl6 and many of the B cells in the cortex are also positive. The latter represents an expanded population of stimulated B cells that are EBV+.

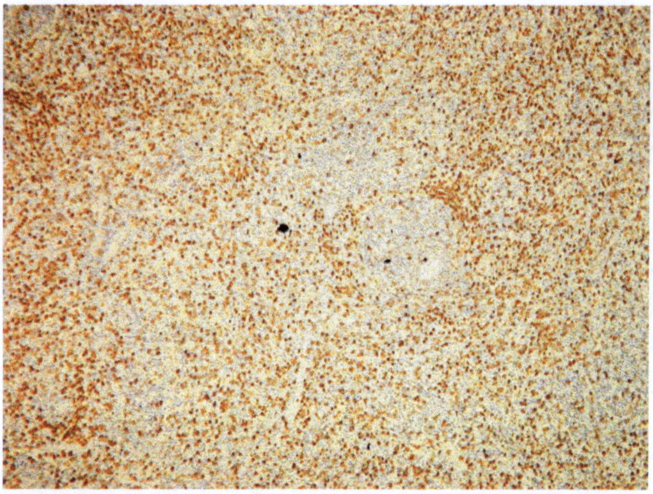

Fig. 6.94. CD79a stains the expanded population of cortical B cells but not the perivascular AITL cells.

many as 30% may be involved. Intestinal and CNS involvement is rare. The small cell variant may show leukemic involvement. The majority of patients present in advanced stage with peripheral and/or abdominal lymph node involvement and with B symptoms (**Table 6.25**).

Morphology

ALCL, ALK+ shows a wide range of appearances but the most striking characteristic is the presence of large, often cohesive, atypical, and bizarre cells with copious amounts of cytoplasm that can

Table 6.24
Angioimmunoblastic T cell lymphoma – immunohistology and genetics

Mature T cell markers – CD3+, CD5+,CD2+
Show follicular helper T cell phenotype – CD4+, CD10+, PD-1+, CXCL13+
Also Bcl6+
CD8- and aberrant loss of CD7
Marked proliferation of perivascular FDC stained by CD21, CD35, D2-40
EBV+ B cells in cortex
Monoclonal TCR gene rearrangements
May show monoclonal Ig gene rearrangements

Table 6.25
Anaplastic large cell lymphoma, ALK+ – clinical

About 3% of adult NHL and 10–20% of childhood lymphomas
Most frequent in the first three decades of life
Present as stage 3 or 4 disease with peripheral and/or abdominal lymphadenopathy
B symptoms often, especially high fever
Extranodal involvement common; sites include skin, bone, soft tissues, lung, and liver
Bone marrow involved in up to 30% when detected by immunohistochemistry
Gut and CNS involvement less common
Relatively good prognosis
Should be distinguished from ALCL, ALK–, primary cutaneous ALCL, and other anaplastic lymphomas

be eosinophilic, basophilic, or clear. These cells have pleomorphic nuclei that contain several prominent basophilic nucleoli. A variable number of cells have eccentric horseshoe-shaped nuclei, sometimes with an eosinophilic Golgi next to the nucleus. These cells are referred to as "hallmark cells" as they can be found in all variants of ALCL. The atypical cells can vary from large to small, the latter often with similar cytological features. Occasionally, tumor giant cells may be present. A variable background of small lymphocytes, stimulated cells, plasma cells, and eosinophils may be seen.

Several patterns of ALCL, ALK+ can be seen and more than one pattern may be found in a single lymph node. Relapses can show different patterns to that observed initially. In the most common pattern, the lymphoma infiltrates in a diffuse manner, obliterating nodal architecture and infiltrating nodal sinuses in cohesive chords that mimic metastatic carcinoma.

Other patterns of ALCL, ALK+ include the "lymphohistiocytic pattern" where the characteristic tumor cells are intermixed with large numbers of reactive histiocytes. In this pattern, the tumor cells tend to cluster around blood vessels. A small cell pattern has a predominant population of small- to medium-sized neoplastic cells with irregular centrally located nuclei. Sometimes the cytoplasm is pale and the tumor can be mistaken for other types of lymphoma but hallmark cells can often be found, especially around vessels. A "Hodgkin-like" pattern can also occur in which the morphological features mimic nodular sclerosis classical Hodgkin lymphoma. In less common cases, the tumor may be rich in giant cells or display sarcomatoid features or are hypocellular with a myxoid or edematous background with prominent spindle cells.

Several entities must be distinguished from ALCL, ALK+. Metastatic carcinoma is a morphologic mimic because of the severe pleomorphism and the cohesive nature of the tumor cells which infiltrate sinuses. The presence of Reed–Sternberg-like cells with a background of sclerosis and eosinophils can mimic Hodgkin lymphoma. Less commonly, metastatic melanoma, histiocytic sarcoma, DLBCL, and other peripheral T cell lymphomas can mimic ALCL. Importantly, ACL, ALK+ cannot be distinguished from ALCL, ALK– on morphological grounds and the two are separated only by the expression of ALK protein (**Figs. 6.95, 6.96, 6.97, 6.98, 6.99, 6.100, 6.101, 6.102, 6.103, 6.104, 6.105; Table 6.26**).

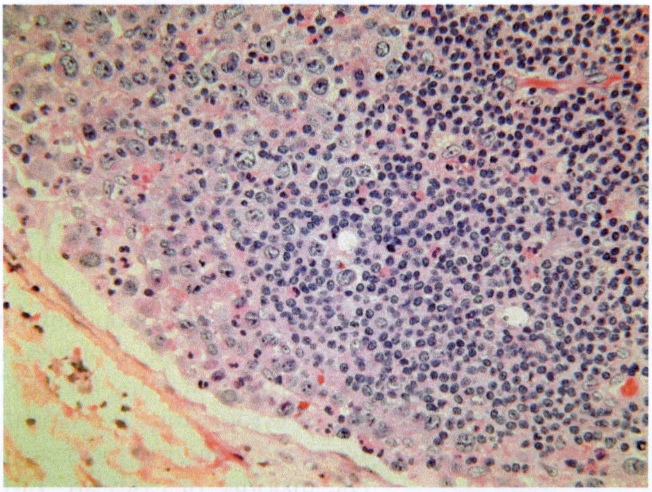

Fig. 6.95. ALCL, tumor cells distend the subcapsular sinus and infiltrate the underlying lymph node tissue as cohesive groups.

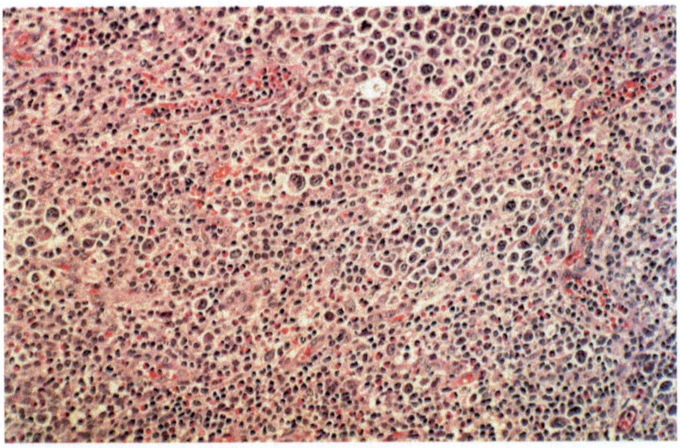

Fig. 6.96. ALCL, common pattern, shows a mixture of medium-sized and large cells percolating through the lymph node sinuses.

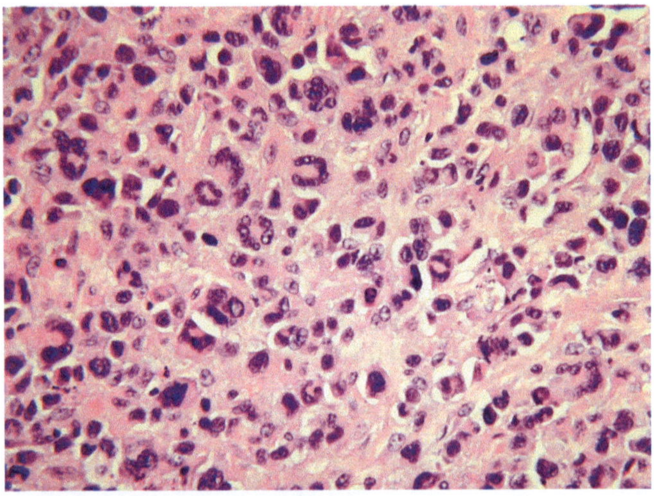

Fig. 6.97. ALCL, common pattern, composed of a mixture of pleomorphic large atypical cells, many with horse-shoe-shaped nuclei.

Immunohistology

The neoplastic cells show ALK and CD30 positivity. CD30 expression is strongest in the large cells, with staining of cell membranes and Golgi. The large lymphoma cells are often clustered around blood vessels. ALK expression is usually restricted to the nucleus, nucleoli, and cytoplasm in those tumors having the common t(2;5)/*NPM-ALK* translocation. In cases harboring variant translocations, the staining for ALK is different and may be membranous or cytoplasmic. Polyclonal antibodies can produce false-positive staining and monoclonal antibodies are preferred.

The majority of cases are EMA+ and about half the cases may be CD45–, so that ALCL should not be mistaken for metastatic carcinoma based on this phenotypic expression and the

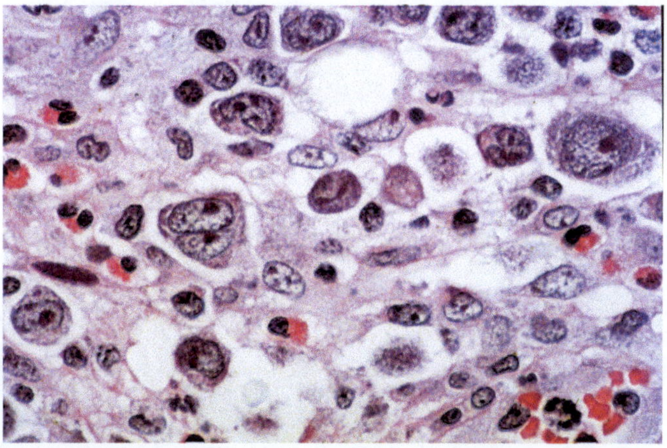

Fig. 6.98. Large atypical cells that are binucleated and contain prominent nucleoli mimic the Reed–Sternberg cells of Hodgkin lymphoma.

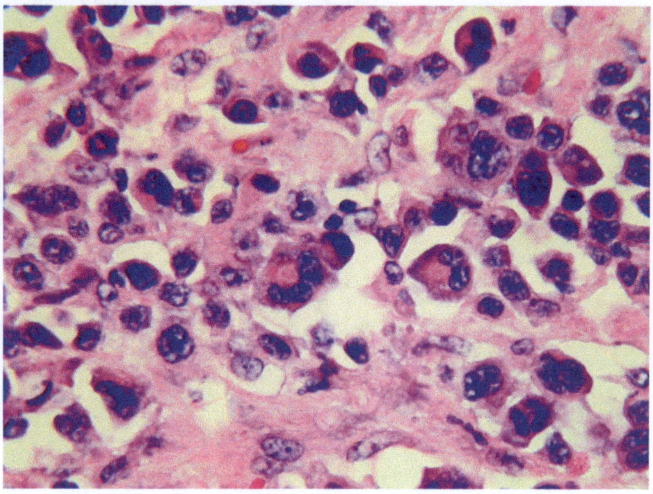

Fig. 6.99. Hallmark cells are prominent. These cells have kidney or horse-shoe-shaped nuclei and a cytoplasmic hopf is visible in several cells.

morphologic appearance. The majority of cases of ALCL, ALK+ express one or more T cell antigens, although the loss of several pan-T cell antigens may give an apparent "null" cell phenotype. Such cases of so-called "null" cell ALCL, however, show T cell lineage at genetic level and there are no other differences between the cases that express T cell antigens and those that do not. CD3 is often negative and one of the other T cell antigens such as CD2, CD5, and CD4 is positive in about 70% of cases. Positivity for cytoplasmic granules including TIA-1, granzyme B, and perforin may be found. CD8 is generally negative, CD43 and CD45RO are positive and there may be granular staining for CD68. The tumor cells are negative for Bcl2, and consistently negative for

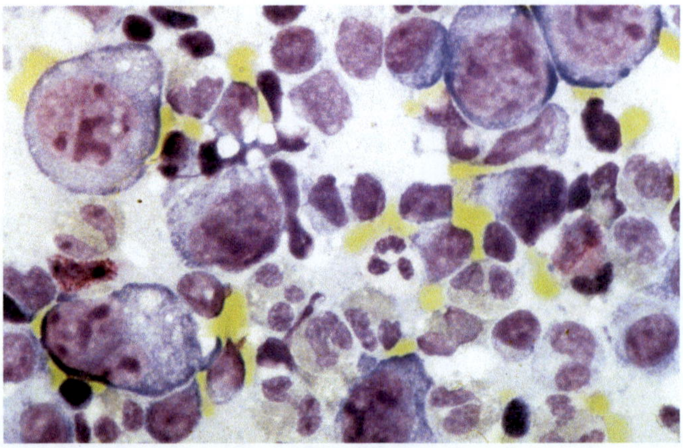

Fig. 6.100. Imprint of ALCL cells with large lobated nuclei and multiple nucleoli (Giemsa stain).

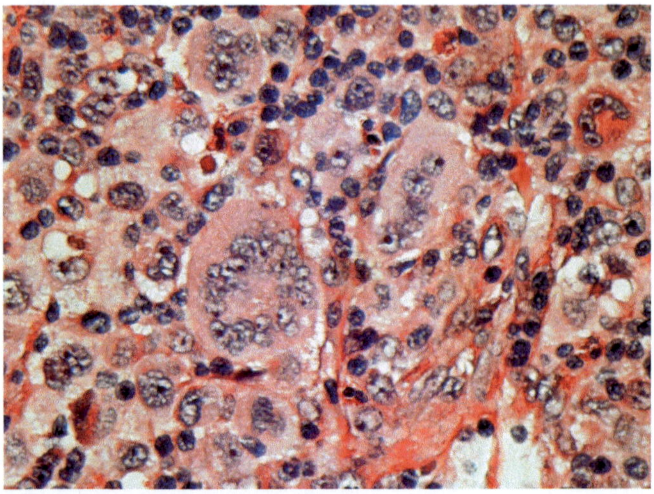

Fig. 6.101. ALCL composed of pleomorphic giant cells. Note the eosinophils in the background.

EBV (**Figs. 6.106, 6.107, 6.108, 6.109, 6.110, 6.111, 6.112, 6.113; Table 6.27**).

Genetics

The t(2;5) results in the fusion of the anaplastic lymphoma kinase (*ALK*) gene, which encodes a tyrosine kinase receptor belonging to the insulin receptor superfamily, located on chromosome 2p23 and *NPM* (nucleophosmin) gene, a housekeeping gene, on 5q35, forcing the expression of ALK. The resulting chimeric protein consists of the N-terminal portion of the NPM protein joined to the entire cytoplasmic domain of the ALK protein. The antibody ALK1 recognizes an intracellular domain of the ALK protein. With the exception of occasional cells in the central nervous

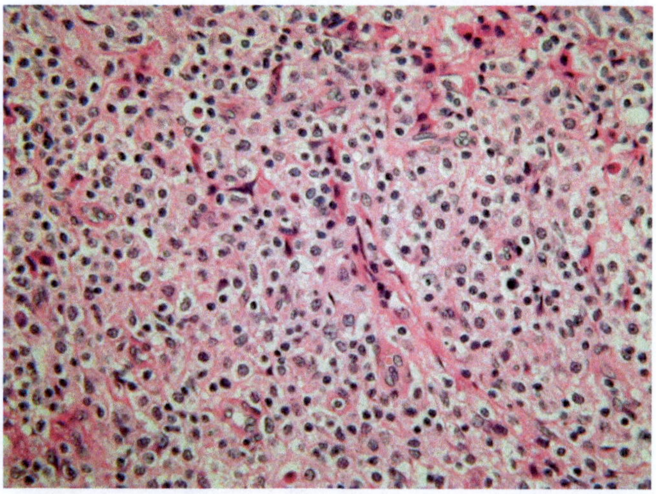

Fig. 6.102. ALCL, small cell pattern, composed of a diffuse infiltrate of small to medium-sized pleomorphic cells.

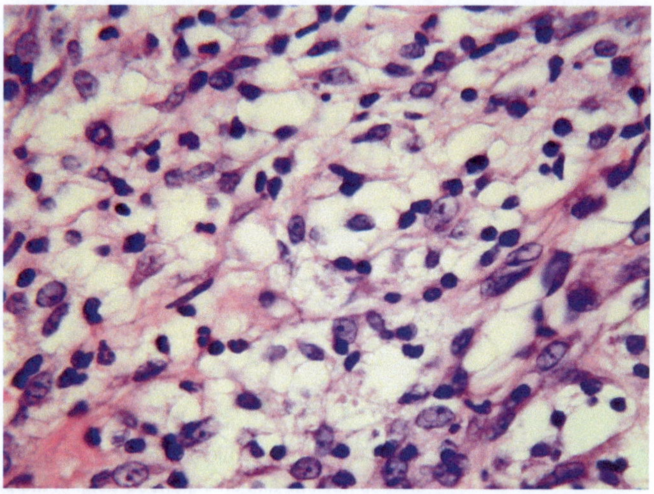

Fig. 6.103. Hypocellular ALCL. The cells have swollen clear cytoplasm and small nuclei.

system, normal cells consistently lack ALK and immunoreactivity strongly correlates with the presence of t(2;5) translocation making immunostaining the method of choice for detection of ALK protein. ALK staining is highly restricted in lymphomas and observed in ALCL with t(2;5) or variant translocations as well as a rare group of diffuse large B cell lymphoma and inflammatory myoblastic tumors. DLBCL, ALK+ usually display plasmablastic features and are CD20–, CD79a–, and CD30–, rarely having t(2;5) or t(2;17) involving the clathrin gene. ALK staining in these cases is cytoplasmic and granular.

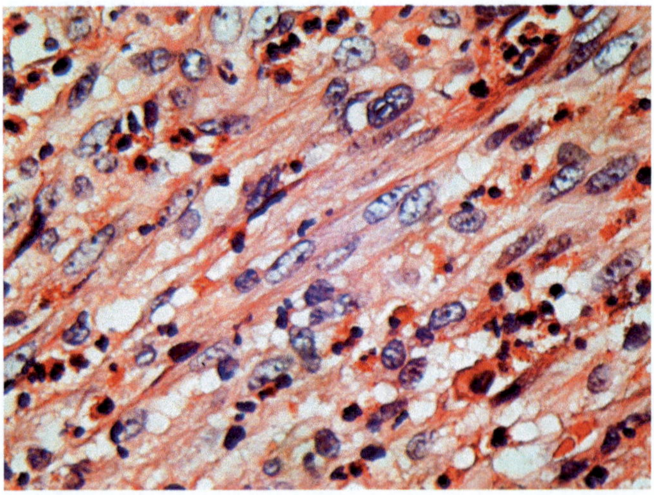

Fig. 6.104. ALCL with a sarcomatoid pattern. Other areas (not shown) contained poorly cohesive pleomorphic large cells. The spindled cells expressed CD30, ALK, and CD3.

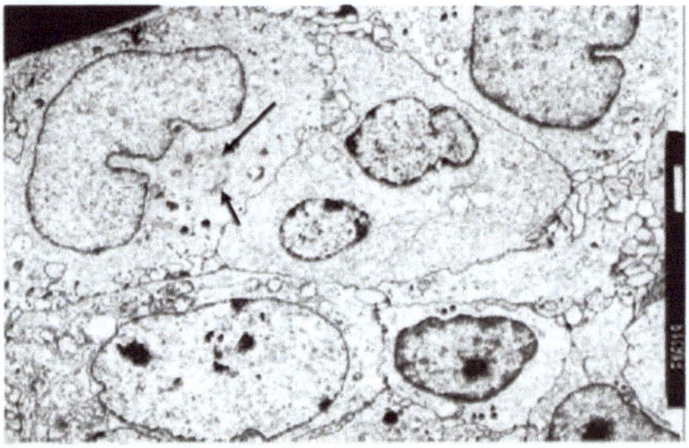

Fig. 6.105. Electronmicrograph of ALCL showing a large hallmark cell with a kidney-shaped nucleus and an expanded Golgi in the paranuclear area (*arrows*).

While the most frequent genetic alteration is the t(2;5) translocation, which occurs in about 80% of cases, variant translocations involving *ALK* and other partner genes on chromosomes 1, 2, 3, 17, 19, 22, and X also occur, producing different staining patterns for ALK. Cases of ALCL with t(2;5) show cytoplasmic, nuclear, and nucleolar staining for ALK-1 and variant translocations display cytoplasmic and/or membrane staining only. The t(2;5) can be detected by RT-PCR, but variant translocations will be negative using primers specific for *ALK* and *NPM* genes (**Table 6.28**).

About 90% of ALCL, ALK+ show clonal rearrangement of the TCR genes.

Table 6.26
Anaplastic large cell lymphoma, ALK+ – morphology

Partial or complete effacement of lymph node
Subcapsular and nodal sinuses, and paracortex infiltrated when partially involved
Most common variant composed of anaplastic large, partly cohesive cells with pleomorphic, bizarre nuclei containing prominent nucleoli.
Wreath-like, horseshoe-shaped and kidney-shaped nuclei with paranuclear hopf
Mitosis common
Other variants – small cell, lymphohistiocytic, hypocellular, sarcomatoid
Cohesive nature and infiltration of sinuses mimics metastatic carcinoma

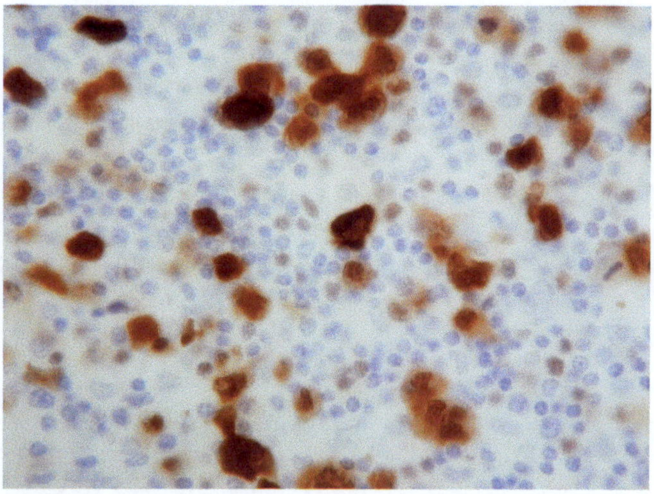

Fig. 6.106. Nuclear, nucleolar, and cytoplasmic staining for ALK in an ALCL with t(2;5) translocation.

Anaplastic Large Cell Lymphoma, ALK-Negative

ALK-negative ALCL is defined as a CD30+ T cell neoplasm that is not distinguishable from ALCL on morphologic grounds, except that it lacks the ALK protein. Similar to its ALK+ counterpart, ALCL, ALK– involves both lymph nodes and extranodal tissue, although the latter sites may be less commonly involved. Its spectrum of morphological features is very similar to that of ALCL, ALK+ with cohesive nests and cords of tumor infiltrating sinuses and T cell zones composed of multinucleated cells including hallmark, wreath-like and Reed–Sternberg-like cells.

The lymphoma cells show strong and homogenous expression of CD30 with cytoplasmic, Golgi, and membranous staining but are ALK-negative. More than half the cases express one or more T cell markers, CD3, CD2, and CD43 being the most common. CD5 and CD4 are positive in a smaller number of cases

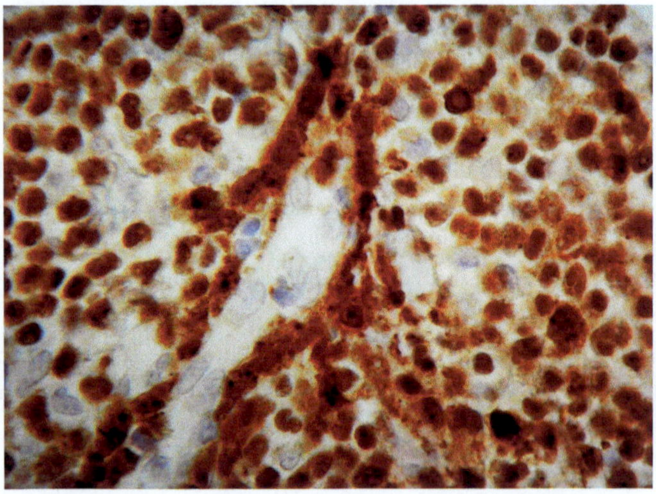

Fig. 6.107. The ALK+ tumor cells tend to cluster around blood vessels.

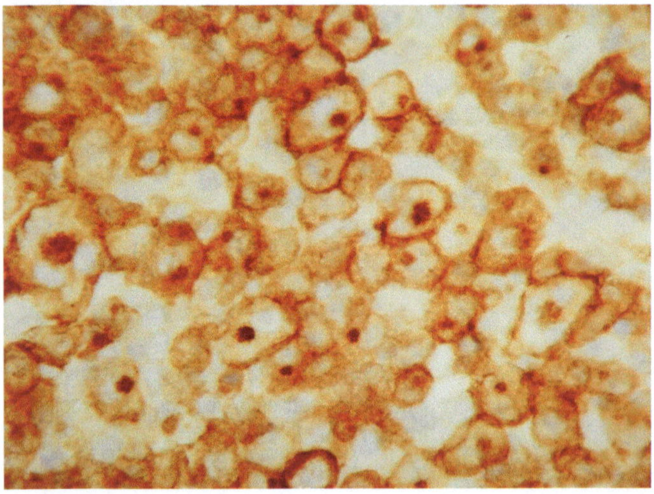

Fig. 6.108. ALCL, common variant, shows characteristic CD30 staining of cell membrane and Golgi.

and CD8 expression is rare. Cytotoxic granules and EMA may also be seen.

This disease should be distinguished from ALCL, ALK+ and primary cutaneous ALCL as its prognosis is clearly poorer with conventional therapy.

Adult T Cell Leukemia/Lymphoma

Adult T cell leukemia/lymphoma (ATLL) is a peripheral T cell neoplasm composed of highly pleomorphic lymphoid cells and is caused by the retrovirus human T cell leukemia virus type 1 (HTLV-1). This disease is endemic in several regions including Southwestern Japan, the Caribbean basin, and Central Africa

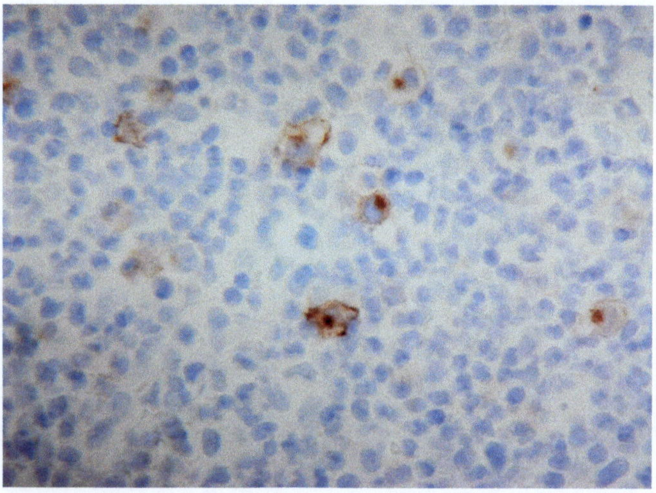

Fig. 6.109. Scattered atypical lymphoid cells stain for EMA in a membranous and Golgi pattern. CD45 was negative (not shown).

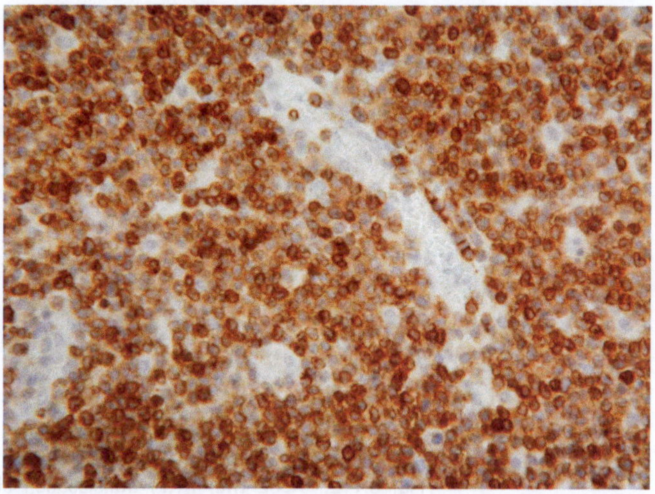

Fig. 6.110. ALCL, ALK+ showing strong staining for CD3. There was variable staining for CD4 but CD5 and CD7 were negative (not shown).

where the virus is prevalent. Sporadic cases are uncommon. The postulated normal counterpart for ATLL is the peripheral CD4+ regulatory T cell.

Clinical

Affected individuals are usually exposed to the virus early in life, the virus being transmitted in breast milk, and through exposure to peripheral blood and blood products. ATLL occurs only in adults following a long latency period, the average age of patients being 58 years. Besides infection with HTLV-1, it is likely that additional genetic alterations acquired over time are necessary for

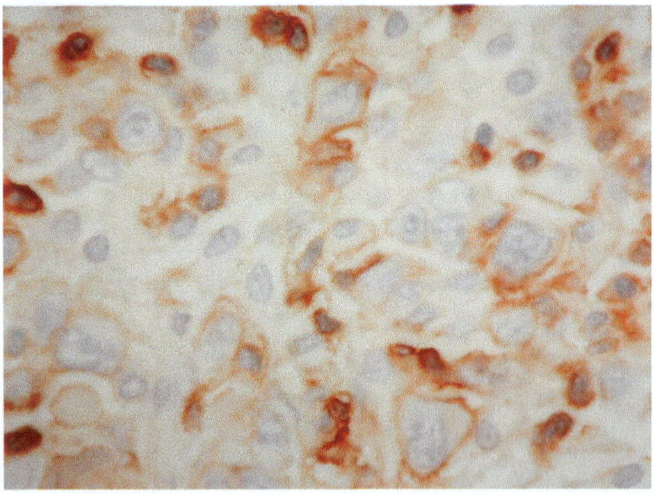

Fig. 6.111. The large atypical cells stain for CD43. There was also staining for CD45RO (not shown).

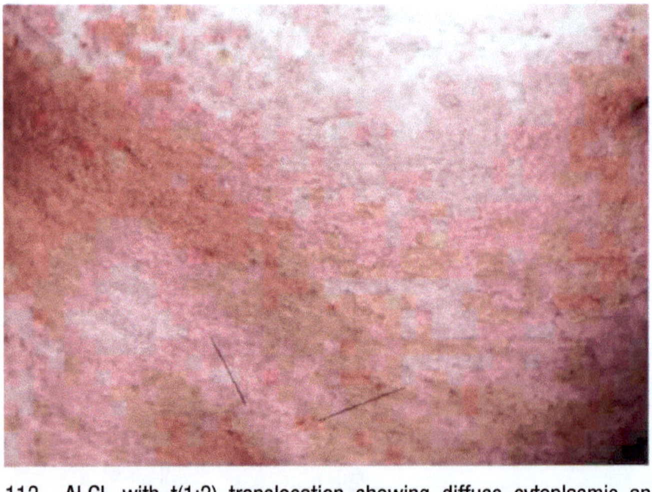

Fig. 6.112. ALCL with t(1;2) translocation showing diffuse cytoplasmic and Golgi staining for ALK protein. There is no nuclear staining in this variant translocation.

the development of the leukemia/lymphoma. HTLV-1 also indirectly causes other diseases such as a myelopathy/tropical spastic paraparesis.

Presentation of most patients is with widespread lymphadenopathy as well as involvement of the peripheral blood, with the skin as the most common extralymphatic site (>50%), particularly in Japanese patients. In addition, systemic involvement usually includes the spleen, liver, gastrointestinal tract, and central nervous system.

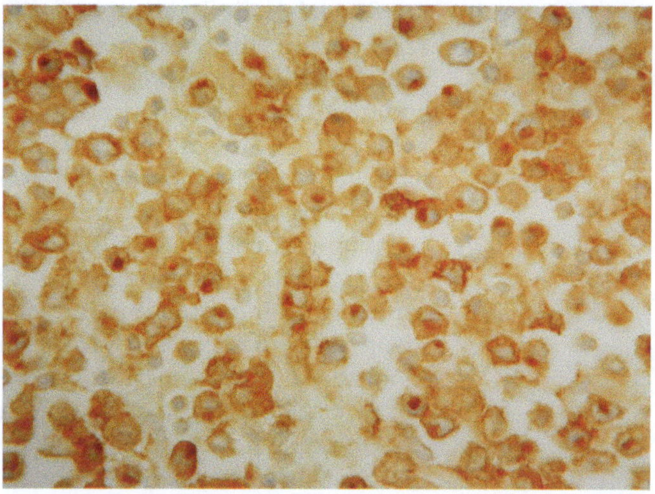

Fig. 6.113. ALCL with variant translocation showing characteristic pattern of CD30 staining of membrane and cytoplasm with Golgi enhancement.

Table 6.27
Anaplastic large cell lymphoma, ALK-positive – immunohistology

T cell or "null" cell lineage
CD30+ (membrane and Golgi staining)
ALK+ (commonly nuclear, nucleolar, and cytoplasmic staining) in t(2;5)
Variant translocations produce different staining patterns including diffuse cytoplasmic, granular cytoplasmic, membrane, and nuclear or cytoplasmic staining alone
CD3+, CD68+, cytotoxic granules+
Variable EMA+; variable CD45 – with morphologic appearance need distinction from metastatic carcinoma
Often loss of pan-T-antigens including CD5 and CD7
EBV–, Bcl2– , CD15–

Table 6.28
Anaplastic large cell lymphoma, ALK+ – genetics

t(2;5)(p23;q35)/*ALK-NPM* is most common (80%)
Variant translocations involve *ALK* and partner genes on chromosomes 1, 2, 3, 17, 19, and 22
t(2;5) translocation detected by RT-PCR but variant translocations cannot be detected when primers specific to *ALK* and *NPM* are employed
About 90% show clonal rearrangement of TCR genes

Several clinical variants of ATLL have been described. An acute variant, the most common, is characterized by a leukemic phase, often with markedly elevated white cell counts, skin rash, and generalized lymphadenopathy. There may be hypercalcemia with or without lytic bone lesions. Patients with acute variant have hepatosplenomegaly with constitutional symptoms, leucocytosis, and eosinophilia being common. Many patients exhibit T cell immunodeficiency and suffer opportunistic infections.

In the lymphomatous variant, prominent lymphadenopathy is the presenting symptom but without peripheral blood involvement. As with the acute variant, skin involvement is also common and can be clinically diverse, presenting as erythematous rashes, papules, and nodules that may ulcerate. Hypercalcemia is uncommon.

The chronic variant is often associated with an exfoliative skin rash and lymphocytosis, although atypical lymphocytes in the peripheral blood are not numerous. Hypercalcemia is absent.

The smothering variant is accompanied by skin or pulmonary lesions but not by hypercalcemia. White blood cell counts are within the normal range with >5% circulating neoplastic lymphocytes. Both chronic and smothering variants may progress to the acute variant in about 25% of cases but over a long period of time.

Prognosis is variable. In the acute and lymphomatous variants, survival ranges from 2 weeks to over a year, death occurring from infectious complications. The chronic and smothering variants show a more protracted course but can transform to an aggressive phase (**Table 6.29**).

Morphology

ATLL shows a wide cytomorphological spectrum. The atypical cells range from small to large and are characterized by marked atypia with pronounced nuclear pleomorphism. Chromatin is coarsely clumped and nucleoli are distinct, sometimes prominent. A striking feature of the neoplastic cells is the nuclear convolutions which can be seen in both large and small cells. Giant cells are occasionally present and blast-like cells may be seen, sometimes with an inflammatory background that contains eosinophils.

The pattern of infiltration is diffuse with paracortical expansion. Some cases display a leukemic pattern of infiltration with atypical cells distending and percolating through lymph node sinuses. Epstein–Barr-virus-positive B cells with Hodgkin-like features may be interspersed among the infiltrating neoplastic cells. This population of EBV+ B cells are thought to be secondary to the associated underlying immunodeficiency.

Atypical cells found in the peripheral blood in all variants of ATLL display nuclear convolutions characteristic of this disease. They have deeply basophilic cytoplasm and polylobated nuclei and are called "flower cells."

Table 6.29
Adult T Cell leukemia/lymphoma – clinical

Associated with endemic HTLV-1 in Southwestern Japan, Caribbean basin, and central Africa
Long latency period, other genetic alterations required to develop ATLL
Presents only in adults, mean age 58 years
Widespread lymphadenopathy, involvement of peripheral blood, skin, spleen, liver, gastrointestinal tract, and CNS
Acute variant: Leukemia, generalized lymphadenopathy, skin rash, hypercalcemia, and lytic bone lesions
Lymphomatous variant: Prominent lymphadenopathy, skin rash, peripheral blood not involved, hypercalcemia uncommon
Chronic variant: Exfoliative skin rash and lymphocytosis. Hypercalcemia absent
Smothering variant: Skin and pulmonary involvement; atypical cells in peripheral blood but WBC count normal, no hypercalcemia
Survival ranges from 2 weeks to >1 year in acute and lymphomatous variants; more protracted clinical course in chronic and smothering variants.
Both chronic and smothering variants can transform to acute variant in about 25% of cases, after long durations

The skin lesions that are seen in more than 50% of cases show epidermotropism with Pautrier-like microabscesses. Dermal infiltration is largely perivascular. Osteoclastic activity accounts for hypercalcemia and lytic bone lesions, and can be seen even in the absence of infiltration by ATLL (**Figs. 6.114, 6.115, 6.116, 6.117, 6.118, 6.119, 6.120, 6.121, 6.122, 6.123, 6.124, 6.125; Table 6.30**).

Immunohistology and Genetics

ATLL expresses T cell-associated antigens, namely CD3, CD5, and CD2 but often show aberrant loss of CD7. Most tumors are CD4+ CD8– but few may be CD4– CD8+ or CD4+ CD8+. The large transformed cells may express CD30 but are negative for ALK protein and cytotoxic molecules. In addition, there is frequent expression of the regulatory T cell antigens CCR4 and FOXP3 (**Table 6.31**).

T cell receptor genes are clonally rearranged.

Nodal Involvement by the Cutaneous T Cell Lymphomas

The term cutaneous T cell lymphoma (CTCL) has been replaced by five separate entities, namely, mycosis fungoides (MF) and its variants, Sezary syndrome (SS), primary cutaneous CD30+ T cell lymphoproliferative disorders, subcutaneous panniculitis-like T cell lymphoma, and primary cutaneous peripheral T cell lymphoma, rare subtypes. All these conditions can involve the lymph node secondarily and it is often necessary to exclude nodal

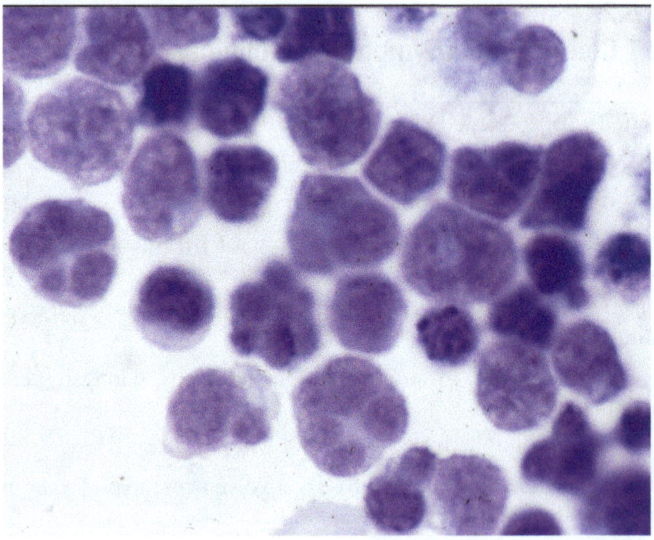

Fig. 6.114. ATLL. Buffy coat smear of peripheral blood showing medium-sized and large atypical cells with markedly convoluted nuclei and small quantities of basophilic cytoplasm, so-called "flower cells" (Giemsa stain).

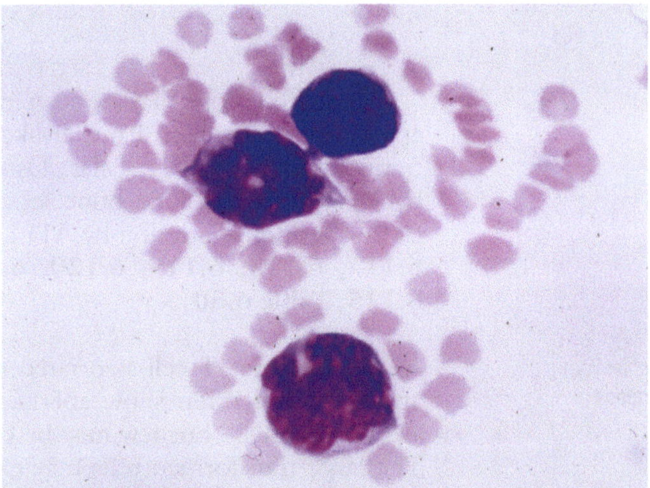

Fig. 6.115. ATLL. Peripheral blood shows spontaneous rosettes with sheep red blood cells, a property of T cells, around atypical cells with marked nuclear convolutions.

involvement as requirement of prognostication and treatment especially in MF and SS, and it is for this reason that these two entities will be discussed.

Morphology

The identification of nodal involvement by cutaneous T cell lymphoproliferative disorders is complicated by the presence of dermatopathic lymphadenopathy (DL) in draining lymph nodes,

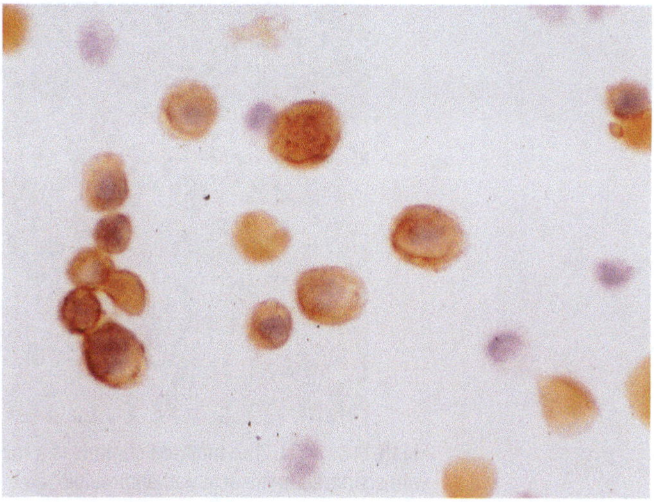

Fig. 6.116. The atypical cells in the peripheral blood buffy coat stain for CD3.

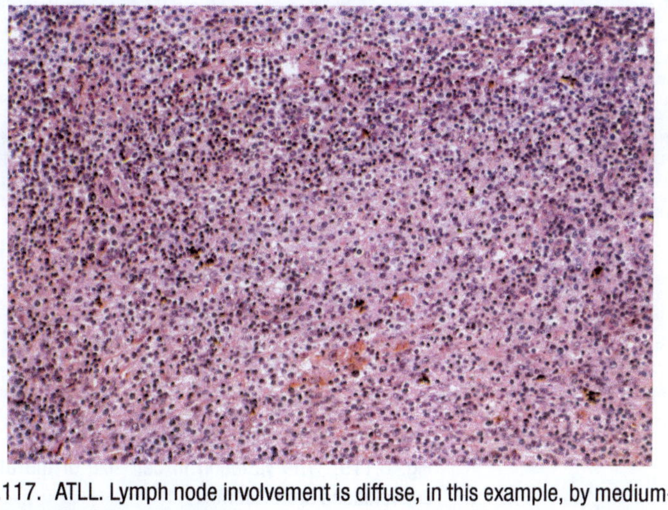

Fig. 6.117. ATLL. Lymph node involvement is diffuse, in this example, by medium-sized cells that expand the paracortex.

especially in MF and its variants, namely, folliculotropic MF, pagetoid reticulosis, and granulomatous slack skin.

The negative impact of palpable lymphadenopathy on survival in MF is well recognized but the correlation of histologic detection of nodal involvement with prognosis is less established suggesting that morphological examination may miss low-level disease present in a proportion of cases. The presence of atypical cells, when identified, has given rise to at least two staging systems for MF and SS, ranging from DL only to complete effacement of nodal architecture, with intermediate stages depending on the number or quantity of atypical cells.

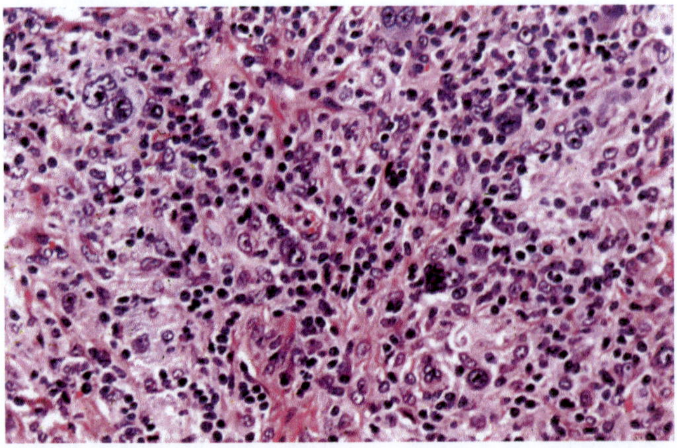

Fig. 6.118. ATLL. The infiltrate comprises a mixture of medium and large atypical cells with scattered multinucleated and multilobated cells.

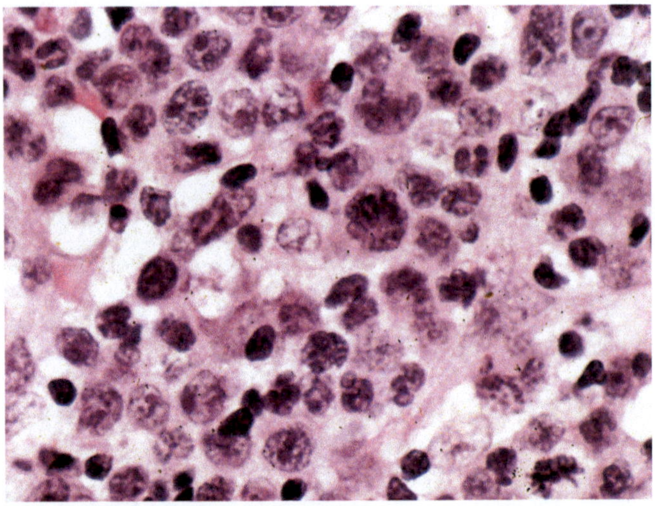

Fig. 6.119. The variation in cell size of the atypical cells and their marked nuclear convolutions are evident.

Mycosis cells initially infiltrate the subcapsular and paracortical regions and occur singly and in clusters in the early stages so that a careful search for these cells must be made. It is generally easier to evaluate nodes from patients with SS in that pronounced DL changes are uncommon in SS and the nodes are partially replaced by sheets of a monotonous population of atypical cells. The atypical cells in both MF and SS display varying degrees of nuclear size and irregularity, ranging from slight nuclear indentations to prominent cerebriform convolutions and serpentine shapes. These cells can be found in the peripheral blood in SS. Focal necrosis may be present but fibrosis generally does not occur. Plasma cells, lymphocytes, eosinophils,

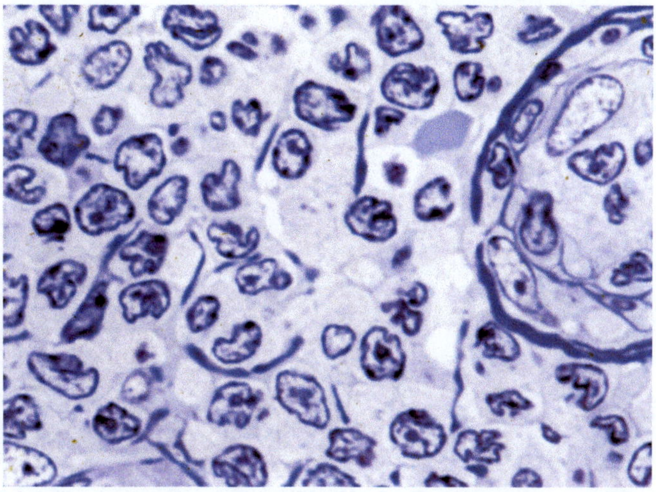

Fig. 6.120. Epon-embedded section of lymph node showing the prominent nuclear indentations and lobation.

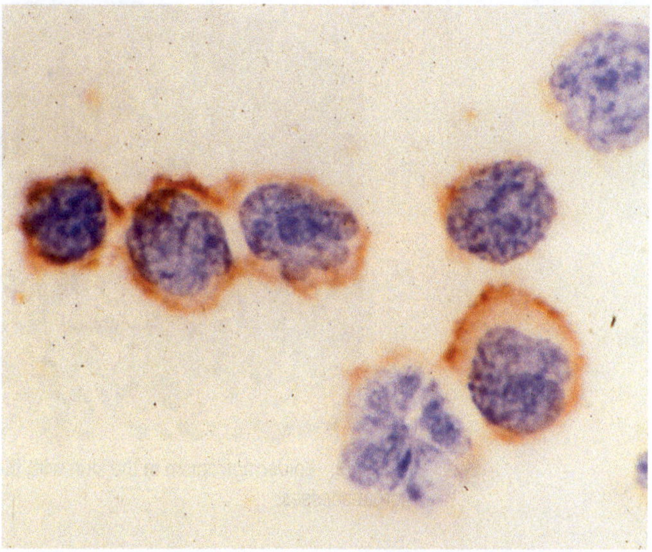

Fig. 6.121. Imprint of lymph node showing expression of CD4 in cells with prominent nuclear convolutions.

interdigitating reticulum cells (IDC), and Langerhans cells are mixed with the atypical cells (**Figs. 6.126**, **6.127**, **6.128**, **6.129**, **6.130**, **6.131**, and **6.132**; **Table 6.32**).

Immunohistology and Genetics

The normal counterpart of MF and SS is thought to be the central memory T cell. The cells of MF and SS display a mature T cell immunophenotype and invariably show CD4+/CD8− phenotype with CD3+, CD5+, CD2+, CD45RO+, and usually the TCR for α/β receptor. CD7 may be aberrantly lost. They may also express

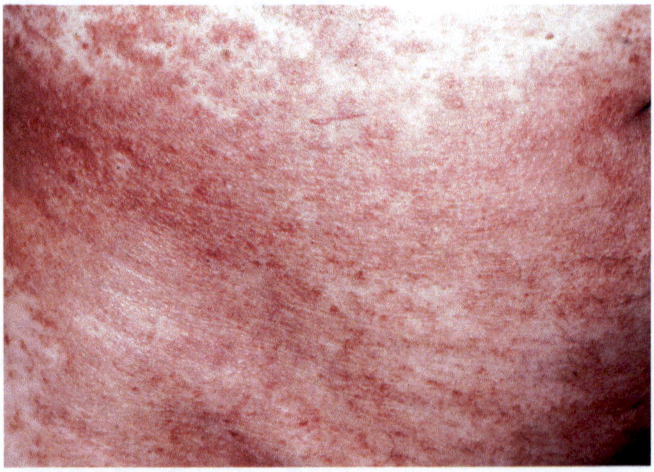

Fig. 6.122. ATLL, smothering variant, with exfoliative skin rash over the abdominal wall. Enlarged right inguinal nodes are also evident (*arrows*).

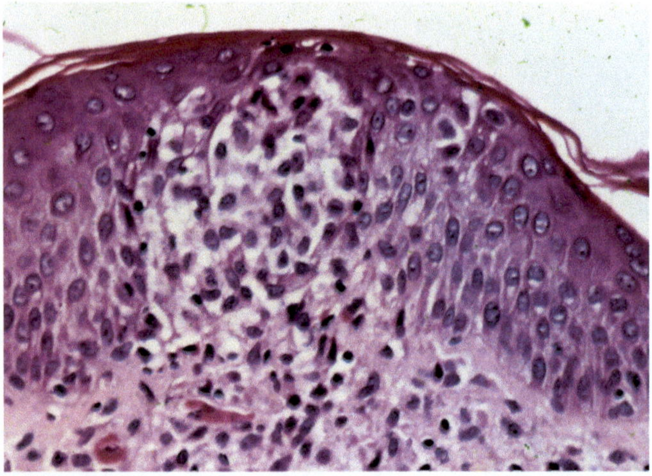

Fig. 6.123. Epidermotropism in the skin with the neoplastic cells producing Pautrier-like microabscesses.

Bcl2, and in rare cases, typical in all other ways, can be CD8+. The neoplastic cells of these two conditions are CD1a–, TdT–, NK cell-associated antigens negative and myeloid-associated antigens negative (**Table 6.33**).

Histiocytic and Dendritic Neoplasms

These neoplasms originate from mononuclear phagocytes (macrophages and dendritic cells) or histiocytes that are bone

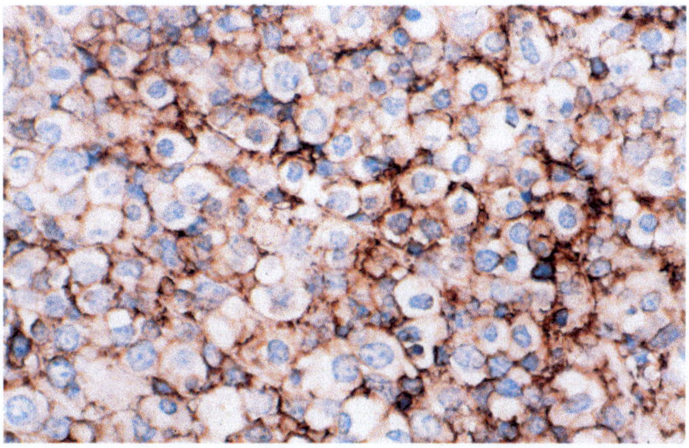

Fig. 6.124. The atypical cells in the lymph node stain for CD3 and often show clear cytoplasm.

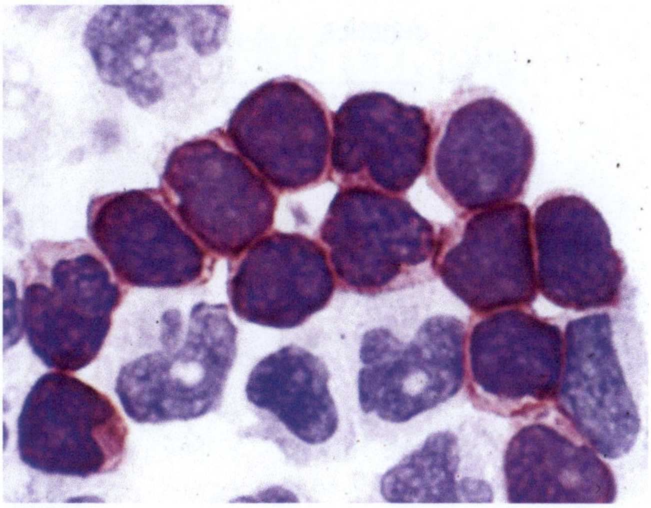

Fig. 6.125. Imprint of lymph node showing CD4 expression in the atypical cells.

marrow-derived. The dendritic cells have a role in phagocytosis, processing and presenting the antigen to lymphoid cells and are divided into several different lineages of accessory antigen-presenting cells. There are three main groups of neoplasms in this category, viz, those of myeloid-derived macrophages, myeloid-derived dendritic cells, and stromal-derived dendritic cells. While the myeloid-derived macrophages and myeloid-derived dendritic cells represent divergent lines of differentiation, hybrids can occur. Macrophage activation or hemophagocytic syndromes can have large numbers of histiocytes but these are not neoplastic and needed to be differentiated from the histiocytic neoplasms. The Rosai–Dorfman disease is probably non-neoplastic and has been previously discussed.

Table 6.30
Adult T cell leukemia/lymphoma – morphology

Broad spectrum of cytomorphology
Diffuse or partial effacement of nodal architecture with leukemic infiltration of sinuses
Range of cell types and mixtures of medium and large cells
Striking feature is the presence of multilobated cells, often with marked nuclear convolutions
Giant tumor cells and inflammatory background may mimic Hodgkin lymphoma
Expansion of EBV+ B cell population due to underlying immunodeficiency in ATLL
Atypical "flower cells" circulate in peripheral blood
Skin involvement by epidermotropic atypical T cells to produce Pautrier-like microabscesses

Table 6.31
Adult T cell leukemia/lymphoma – immunohistology and genetics

CD3+, CD5+, CD2+
Often aberrant loss of CD7
CD4+CD8– , uncommonly CD4-CD8+ or CD4+CD8+
Frequently express antigens of the peripheral regulatory T cell CCR4 and FOXP3
Clonal rearrangement of T cell receptor genes

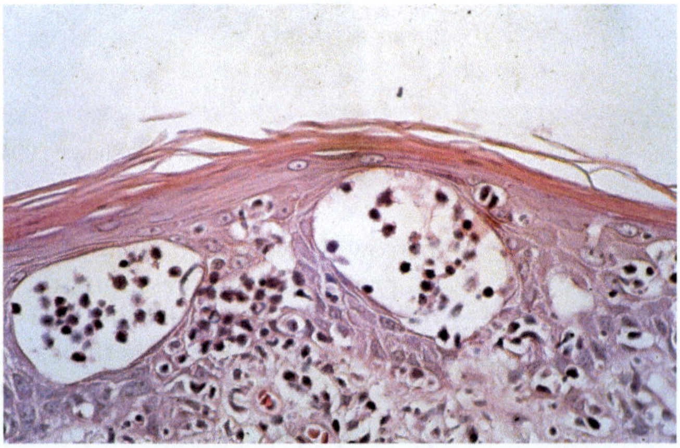

Fig. 6.126. MF, plaque stage, with a band-like polymorphous infiltrate in the papillary dermis, Pautrier microabscesses, and epidermotropism.

Histiocytic Sarcoma

Histiocytic sarcoma is defined by the WHO classification as a malignant neoplasm composed of cells with morphologic and immunophenotypic features of mature, myeloid-derived,

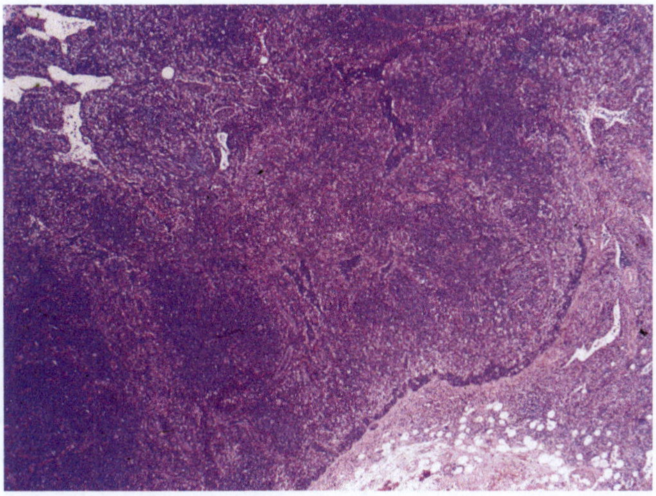

Fig. 6.127. MF showing preservation of nodal architecture and infiltration of the subcapsular sinus. The pale areas in the paracortex represent DL and contain clusters of mycosis cells.

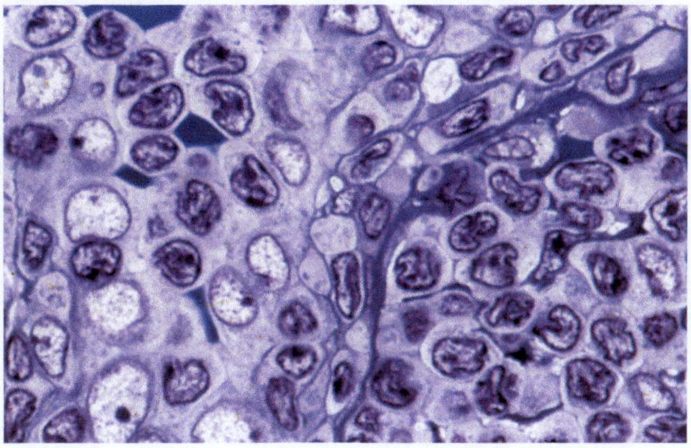

Fig. 6.128. Mycosis cells with pronounced nuclear indentations are seen in a plastic-embedded section of lymph node.

phagocytic histiocytes. However, phagocytosis is seen only in a minority of cases, contributing to the considerable morphologic overlap between this entity and large cell lymphomas of B or T cell origin, as well as metastatic tumors such as melanoma or carcinoma.

Clinical

These rare tumors are most commonly encountered in adults (median age around 50), although examples have been reported in infants and the elderly. While some patients present with lymphadenopathy, extranodal disease is seen more frequently, particularly involving the gastrointestinal tract. Even among cases in

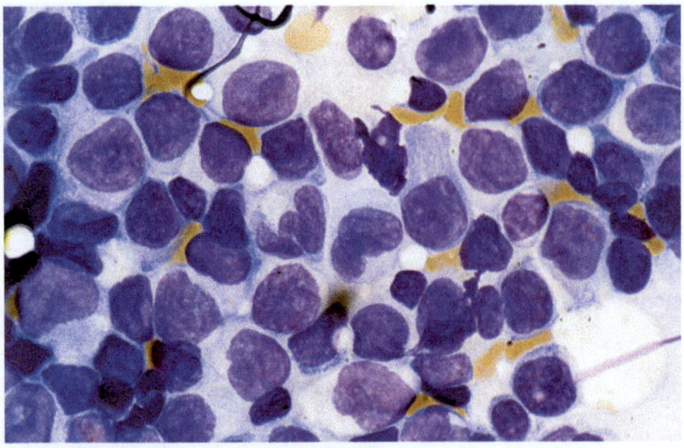

Fig. 6.129. Cytospin preparation of lymph node in MF-containing cells with convoluted nuclei (Giemsa stain).

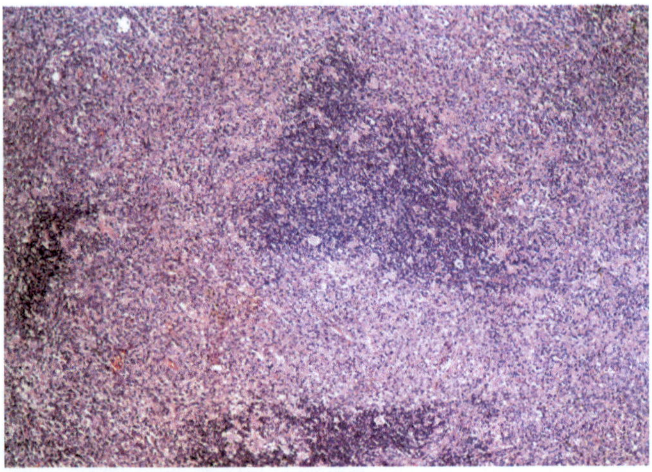

Fig. 6.130. SS with almost complete effacement of nodal architecture by pale Sezary cells.

which neoplastic involvement is localized, constitutional symptoms are sometimes observed (**Table 6.34**).

Morphology

Involved lymph nodes typically show diffuse infiltration, ranging from predominantly paracortical to near-total effacement, by a population of intermediate to large cells with abundant eosinophilic cytoplasm and pleomorphic nuclei that range from round to oval to irregular. Multinucleated cells may be seen, as can vacuolated cells and areas exhibiting spindle cell morphology. Hemophagocytosis, while sometimes present, is generally inconspicuous. The neoplastic cells are accompanied by a mixed leucocytic infiltrate that may include lymphocytes, plasma cells,

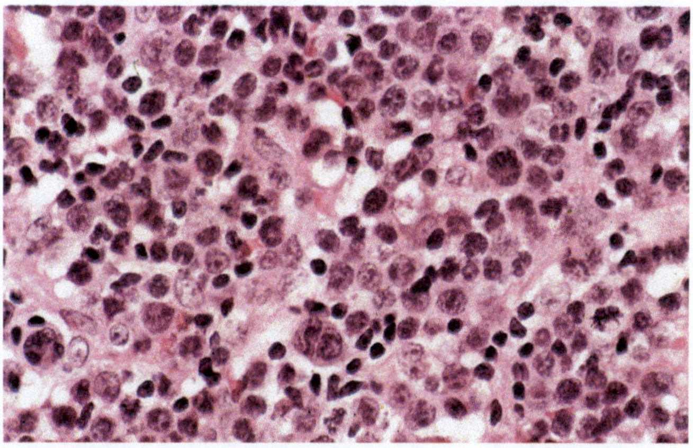

Fig. 6.131. There is marked nuclear atypia of both medium-sized and large Sezary cells, several with cerebriform nuclei.

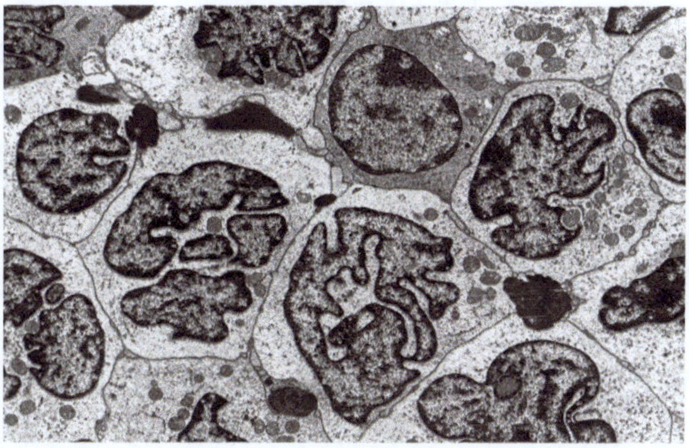

Fig. 6.132. The distinctive cerebriform nuclei of SS are seen in this electron micrograph of a lymph node.

eosinophils, and neutrophils (**Figs. 6.133, 6.134, 6.135, 6.136; Table 6.35**).

Immunohistology

Tumor cells show evidence of histiocytic differentiation through the expression of CD68 (KP1, PG-M1, and HAM56), CD163, and lysozyme, as well as occasional weak expression of CD4. Immunoreactivity for S100 is variable, but FDC markers such as CD21 are generally negative, as CD1a and other Langerhans cell markers. Markers associated with B and T cell lineage are consistently negative, as markers specific to the myeloid lineage, such as myeloperoxidase and CD33. Consistent positivity for CD45 and/or CD45RO facilitates recognition of this lesion as leucocytic in origin when the differential diagnosis includes non-hematopoietic neoplasms; histiocytic sarcomas is negative for cytokeratins, EMA, and for more specific melanoma markers such

Table 6.32
Nodal involvement by mycosis fungoides and Sezary syndrome

Palpable lymphadenopathy poor prognostic sign
Staging depends on extent of nodal involvement
Pronounced DL frequent in mycosis fungoides and variants
Mycosis cells infiltrate subcapsular and paracortical areas mixed with areas of DL
Sezary cells present in peripheral blood
Atypical cells may be mixtures of large and small
Nuclei range from mild indentations to marked convolutions
Necrosis may be present, fibrosis absent
Eosinophils, lymphocytes, plasma cells, IDC, Langerhans cells, melanophages are present

Table 6.33
Mycosis fungoides and Sezary syndrome – immunohistology and genetics

Express mature T cell antigens CD3, CD5, CD2, and CD45RO
Almost always CD4+/CD8–
May be CD7–
Bcl2+
CD1a–, TdT–
NK-associated and myeloid-associated antigens negative
Monoclonal TCR gene rearrangement

Table 6.34
Histiocytic sarcoma – clinical

Affects middle aged and older adults most frequently, though age range is wide
Extranodal disease more common than nodal involvement (especially in skin, gastrointestinal)
Constitutional symptoms common
Subsets associated with germ cell tumors and with other hematopoietic disorders

as HMB45 and Melan A. The proliferative rate as assessed by Ki67 staining is highly variable (**Figs. 6.137**, **6.138**, **6.139**, and **6.140**).

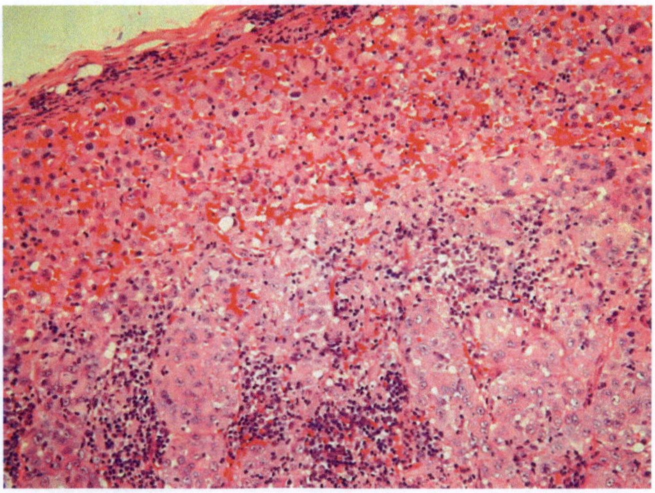

Fig. 6.133. Histiocytic sarcoma showing lymph node infiltration by epithelioid cells that are somewhat cohesive.

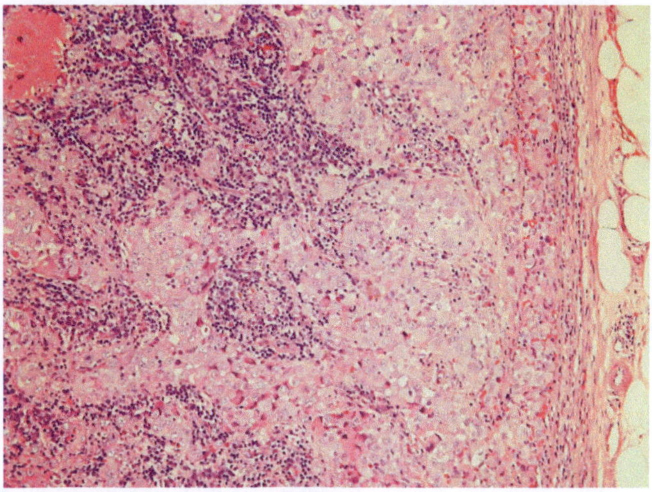

Fig. 6.134. A focus of prominent subcapsular involvement by histiocytic sarcoma.

Genetics

Clonal gene rearrangement of TCR or IGH may be encountered in a subset of cases; negativity of the neoplastic cells for immunophenotypic markers of the corresponding lineage will avert misclassification.

Other large cell neoplasms included in the differential diagnosis include non-Hodgkin lymphomas, poorly differentiated carcinoma, and melanoma. DLBCL and T cell lymphomas such as ALCL both differ immunophenotypically from histiocytic sarcoma, and the latter contains hallmark cells. Carcinoma and melanoma may likewise be excluded on the basis of immunophenotypic data. In contrast, such data may be less useful in

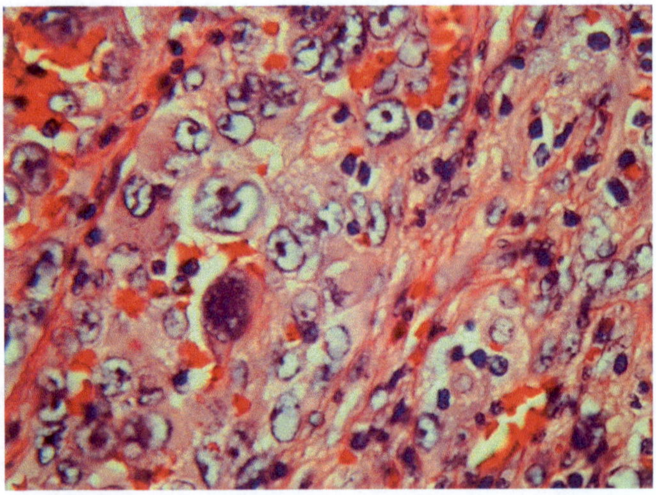

Fig. 6.135. Histiocytic sarcoma. Large cells with vesicular nuclei and eosinophilic cytoplasm are accompanied by large multinucleated cells.

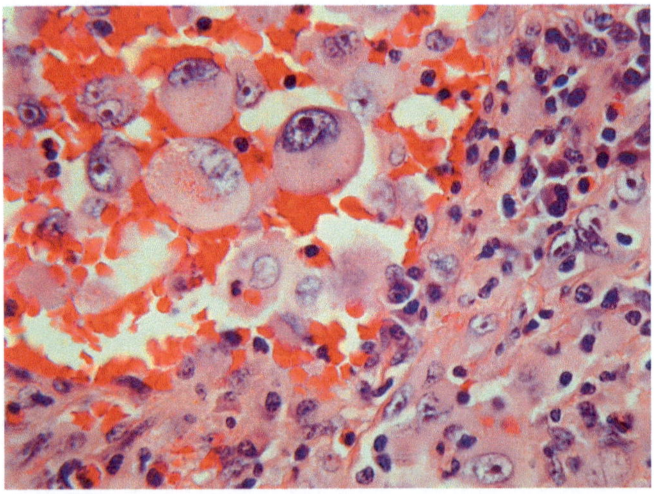

Fig. 6.136. The neoplastic cells have abundant eosinophilic cytoplasm and nuclei that range from oval to irregular with variably prominent nucleoli. Pleomorphism is typical of histiocytic sarcoma.

distinguishing histiocytic sarcoma from extramedullary involvement by acute monoblastic leukemia (i.e., monoblastic sarcoma) (**Table 6.36**).

Langerhans Cell Histiocytosis

Clonal proliferations of cells with the morphologic, immunophenotypic, and ultrastructural features of Langerhans cells are designated Langerhans cell histiocytosis (LCH), unless overtly malignant cytologic features warrant classification as Langerhans cell sarcoma.

Table 6.35
Histiocytic sarcoma – morphology

Intermediate to large cells with eosinophilic cytoplasm
Pleomorphic nuclei ranging from round to oval to irregular
May see multinucleated cells, vacuolated cells, spindle cells
Hemophagocytosis generally inconspicuous
Mixed leucocytic infiltrate in background
May resemble large cell lymphomas or non-hematopoietic neoplasms

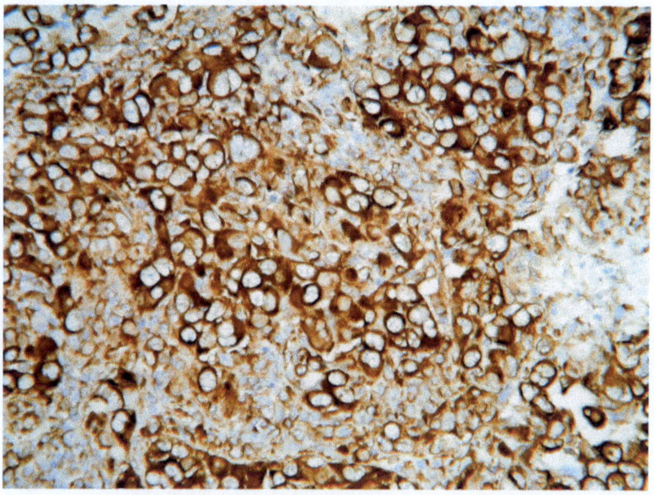

Fig. 6.137. Diffuse positivity of tumor cells for CD163 is indicative of monocytic differentiation.

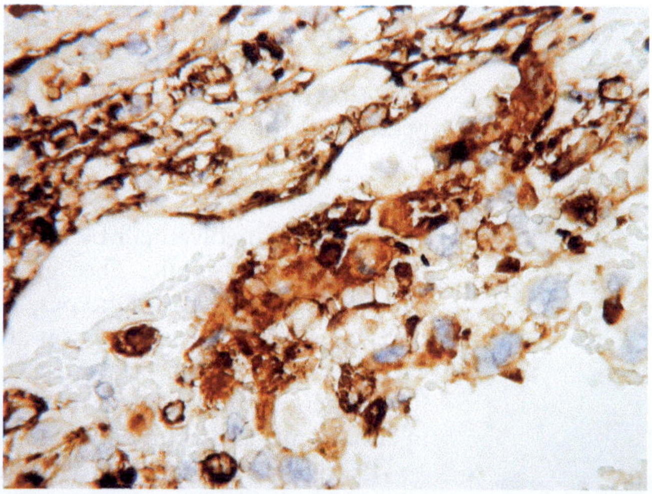

Fig. 6.138. Staining for CD68 likewise fits with histiocytic differentiation of the neoplastic cells.

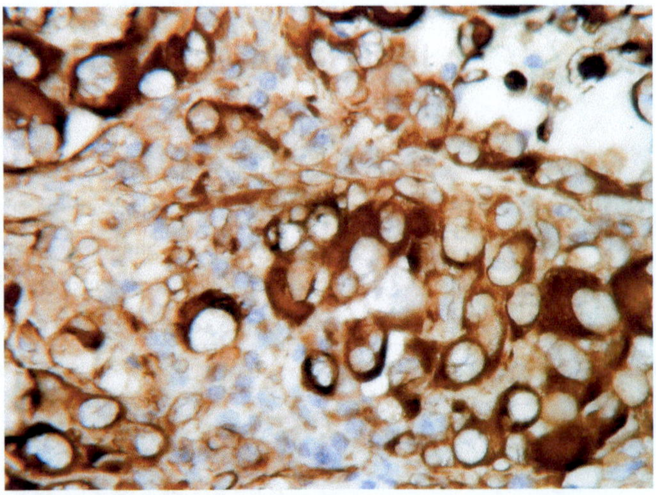

Fig. 6.139. Cytoplasmic immunoreactivity for lysozyme is characteristic of histiocytic sarcoma.

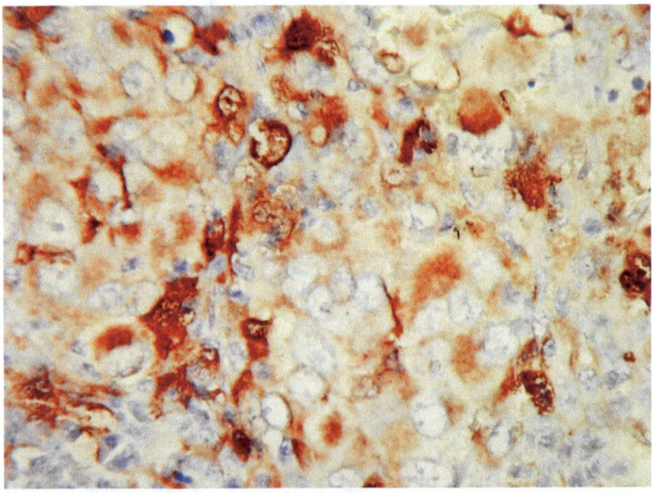

Fig. 6.140. The variation in positivity and staining intensity for S100 in this field is typical of histiocytic sarcoma.

Clinical

The extent of involvement by LCH ranges from localized to multifocal to multisystemic. The age range of those affected is similarly broad, but across subtypes, young children have been recognized as the most frequently affected age group. A possible exception may be the rare subset of cases presenting as isolated lymphadenopathy, which, in one series, more such cases were seen in adolescents and young adults than in infants and toddlers.

LCH affects bone more frequently than any other tissue; while a small fraction of cases may present with nodal disease as the sole or primary finding. Lymph node involvement is more

Table 6.36
Histiocytic sarcoma – immunohistology and genetics

Positive for markers of histiocytic differentiation: CD68, CD163, lysozyme
Variable positivity for S100, CD4
CD45 and CD45RO are expressed
Negative for FDC markers (CD21, CD35) and Langerhans cell markers (CD1a, CD207 (langerin))
Negative for myeloid and lymphoid markers
Clonal rearrangement of *TCR* or *IGH* may be seen

frequently encountered in children with multifocal, multisystem disease. Such patients, typically infants, often present not only with lesions of bone and soft tissue but also with fever and cytopenias.

Morphology

Lymph node involvement by LCH ranges from focal disease, limited to sinuses, to subtotal or total effacement of nodal architecture by a diffuse infiltration in a sinus and paracortical pattern. Cytologically, the LCH cells are generally intermediate to large and feature nuclei that are irregular or folded in appearance with linear grooves. Nucleoli are generally small, and variable quantities of eosinophilic cytoplasm are present. Eosinophils are present in variable numbers, and multinucleated cells and neutrophils may be seen; plasma cells are uncommonly noted.

Electron microscopy reveals the presence of characteristic Birbeck granules, which are structures shaped like tennis racquets with a "zipper-like" appearance in the "handle," and range from 200 to 400 nm in length. These structures are thought to represent internalized cell membrane receptors (**Figs. 6.141**, **6.142**, **6.143**).

Immunohistology

LCH cells, like normal LCs, express CD1a, S100, and CD207 (langerin). Positivity for CD68 is variable, as is that for CD45, while staining for markers of B cell and T cell lineage, epithelial markers, and FDC markers are negative (**Figs. 6.144, 6.145, 6.146**).

Genetics

Clonality of LCH cells has been demonstrated in female patients using the HUMARA assay. TCR and IGH rearrangements are absent with only rare exceptions.

Recognition of the characteristic nuclear features and immunophenotypic profile permits discrimination between LCH and other histiocytic lesions.

Langerhans cell sarcoma is a high-grade neoplasm which shares immunophenotypic features with LCH but displays overtly malignant cytology that is incompatible with a diagnosis of LCH.

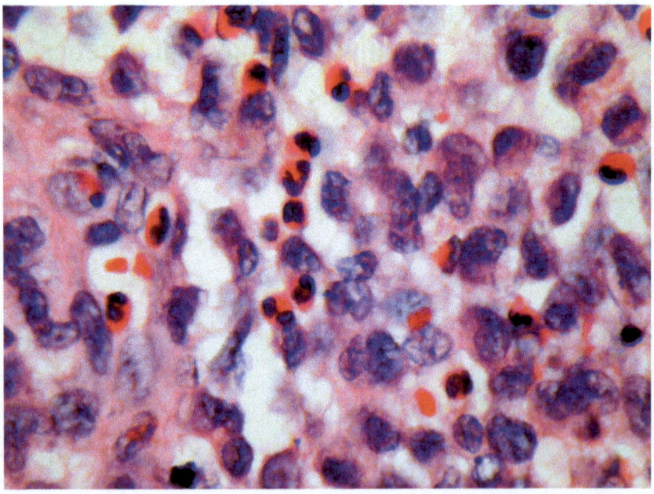

Fig. 6.141. LCH. The neoplastic cells have vesicular nuclei with prominent nuclear grooves and folds, and inconspicuous nucleoli. The cells display moderate quantities of cytoplasm and the presence of interspersed eosinophils is typical.

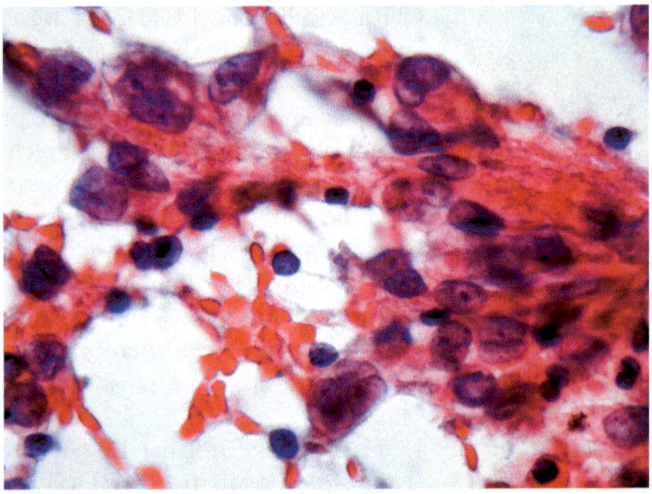

Fig. 6.142. Imprint of LCH involving a lymph node showing the cytologic appearance of the neoplastic cells with their prominent nuclear grooves that lie along the long axis of the nucleus.

Interdigitating Dendritic Cell (IDC) Sarcoma

Clinical

This extremely rare neoplasm may present as a solitary nodal or extranodal mass, or as diffuse lymphadenopathy, splenomegaly or hepatomegaly. While many of the reported cases have occurred in adults, pediatric cases have also been encountered. Constitutional

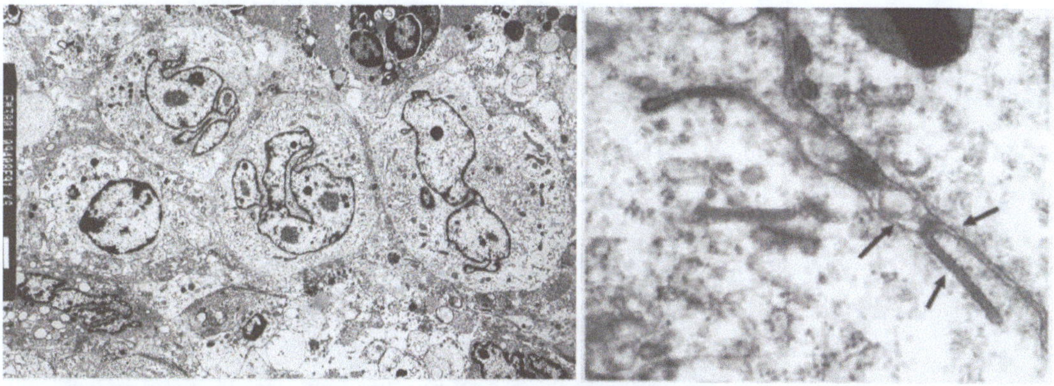

Fig. 6.143. Electronmicrograph of LCH cells. The large cells display deep nuclear indentations and small nucleoli. The moderate to abundant cytoplasm contains numerous organelles that include smooth endoplasmic reticulum, lysosomal bodies, and Birbeck granules. The latter shown in the *inset* are tri-lamella zipper-like structures that appear to be internalized from the cell membrane which is indicated by *arrows*.

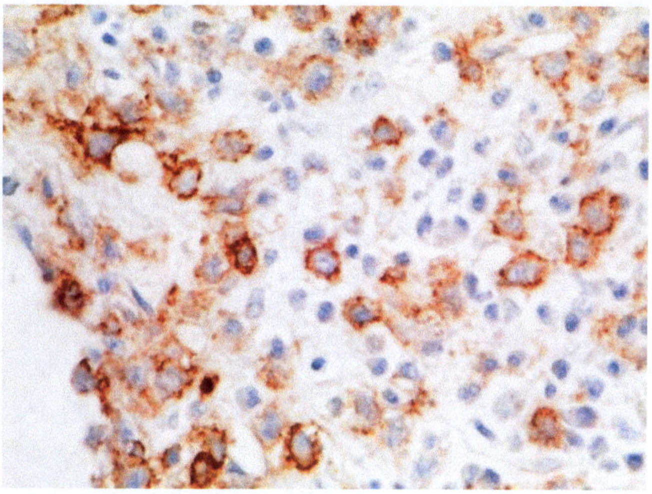

Fig. 6.144. Staining of LCH cells for CD1a shows membranous positivity.

symptoms have been variably reported. Rarely, there has been associated low-grade B or T cell lymphoma.

Morphology

Diffuse paracortical infiltration by medium to large spindled cells with vesicular chromatin and prominent nucleoli is typical. Oval or indented nuclei may also be seen. Storiform arrangement of the cells is common, while multinucleated forms and necrosis are not. The mitotic rate is usually low. Small lymphocytes are present amidst the neoplastic infiltrate and are in some instances accompanied by plasma cells.

While FDC sarcoma exhibits similar histologic features, electron microscopy reveals interdigitating cell junctions in IDC

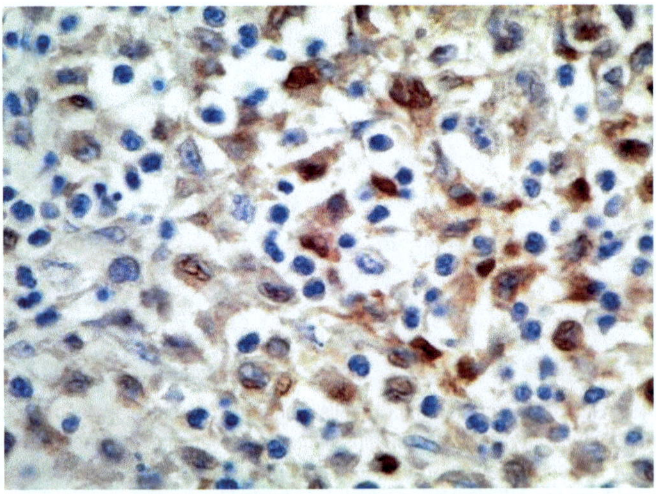

Fig. 6.145. S100 positivity is uniformly seen in cases of LCH.

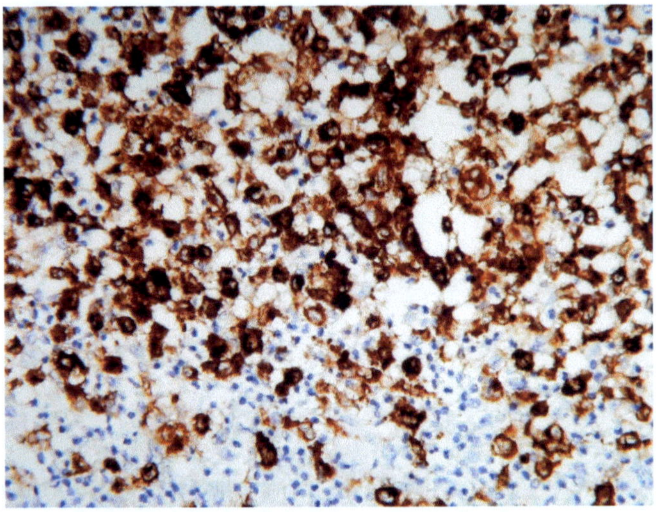

Fig. 6.146. LCH cells are diffusely positive for CD207 (langerin).

sarcoma, in contrast to the long cytoplasmic processes and desmosomes observed in FDC sarcoma (**Figs. 6.147**, **6.148**, and **6.149**).

Immunohistology

Positivity for S100 and vimentin is characteristic of this lesion, as is negativity for lymphoid and FDC markers (CD21, CD35). Expression of CD68 and lysozyme is variable, while the neoplastic cells are generally negative for CD1a and langerin. There is often staining for fascin and p53. Negativity for HMB-45 permits distinction from melanoma (**Figs. 6.150**, **6.151**, **6.152**).

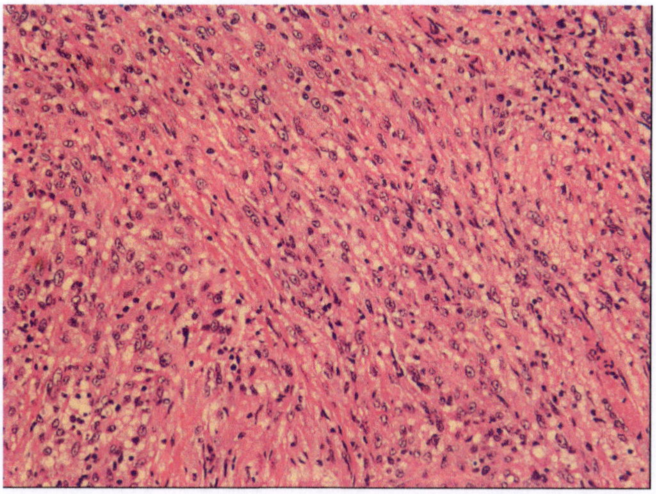

Fig. 6.147. IDC sarcoma in an axillary lymph node showing diffuse infiltration by spindled to oval cells.

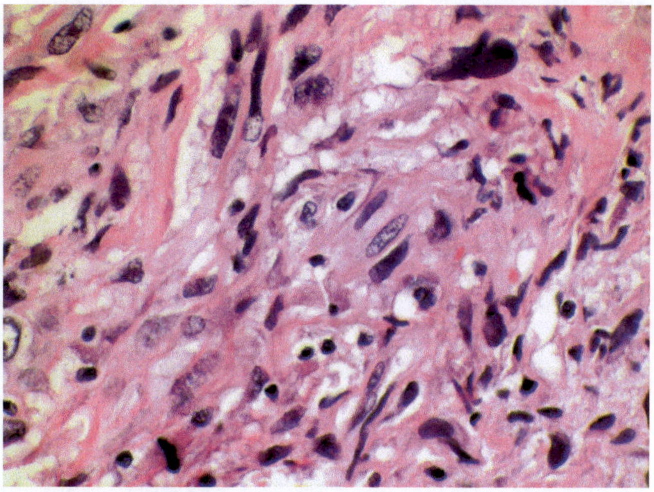

Fig. 6.148. The neoplastic cells display vesicular nuclei with prominent nucleoli. Folds and indentations in the nuclear membrane are common.

Genetics

Karyotypic data are extremely scarce. Clonal rearrangement of TCR or IGH is not seen.

Follicular Dendritic Cell (FDC) Sarcoma

Clinical

Follicular dendritic cell (FDC) sarcoma is a rare lesion often presenting as a painless mass of considerable size, occurring most commonly in cervical lymph nodes, mediastinum, and abdomen. Characterized by a wide age range, FDC sarcoma typically

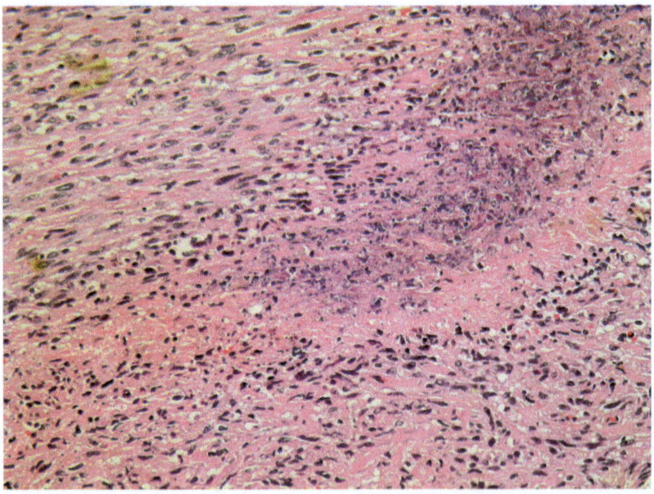

Fig. 6.149. There is focal necrosis in this tumor, an uncommon feature of IDC sarcoma.

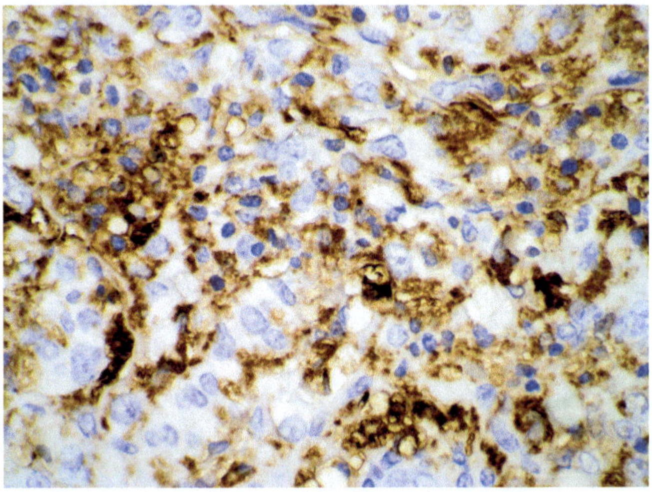

Fig. 6.150. Diffuse positivity for S100 is typical in IDC sarcoma.

presents without constitutional symptoms. A minority of cases arise in association with Castleman disease (hyaline–vascular). While an indolent course is frequently seen, in contrast to the generally more aggressive course typical of IDC sarcoma, late recurrence and metastasis occur in a subset of patients.

Morphology

Spindled cells with oval nuclei, vesicular chromatin, and small nucleoli are typically arranged in a storiform or whorled pattern. Cytologic atypia is generally mild, and mitoses are usually few. Small lymphocytes are admixed with the neoplastic cells. As noted above, ultrastructural differences between FDC sarcoma and IDC

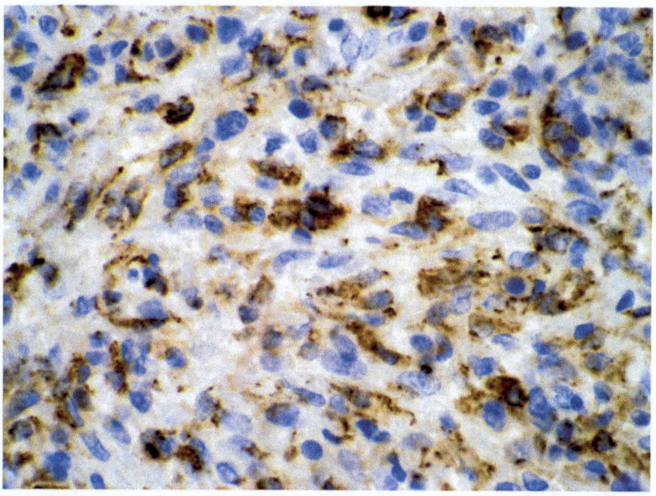

Fig. 6.151. Strong immunoreactivity for CD68 is present, although this is generally variable in IDC sarcoma.

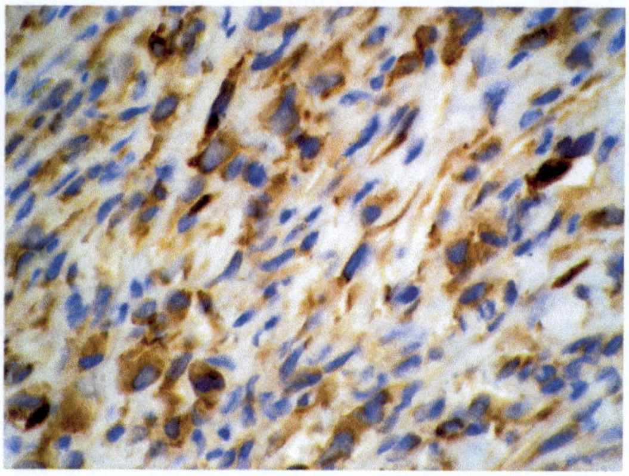

Fig. 6.152. There is also strong staining for fascin in the tumor cells.

sarcoma may be of assistance in distinguishing these lesions (**Figs. 6.153, 6.154, 6.155, 6.156**).

Immunohistology

Expression of at least one of the standard markers of FDC differentiation (CD21, CD23, and CD35) is necessary to establish the diagnosis. Positivity for podoplanin (D2-40) and clusterin is also seen. Expression of CD68 and S100 is variable, while stains for CD1a and lysozyme are negative, as are those for lymphoid and epithelial differentiation. Negativity for HMB45 rules out melanoma.

Genetics

Karyotypic data are extremely scarce. Clonal rearrangement of TCR or IGH is not seen.

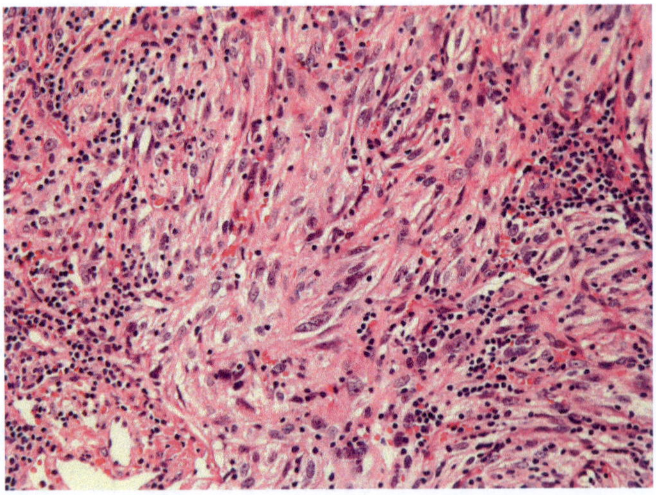

Fig. 6.153. FDC sarcoma in a cervical node showing diffuse replacement of the node by a spindled tumor with interspersed small lymphocytes.

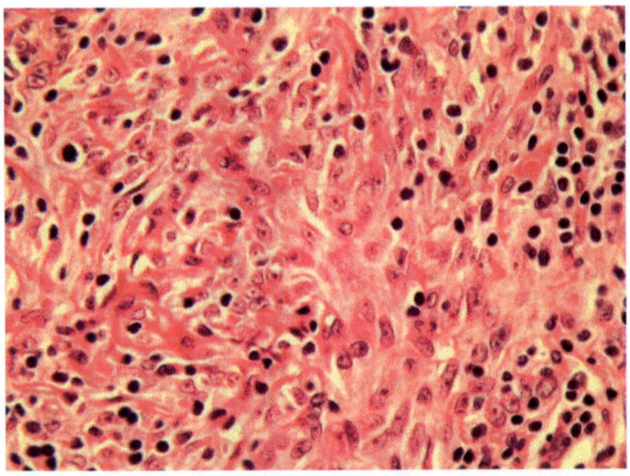

Fig. 6.154. The spindled tumor cells have vesicular nuclei with distinct nucleoli and abundant bipolar eosinophilic cytoplasm. Nuclear pleomorphism is moderate. Mitosis is infrequent.

Immunophenotypic data may be of considerable assistance in distinguishing among the tumors of histiocytic and dendritic cell origin (**Table 6.37**).

Hodgkin Lymphoma

As described in detail in Chapter 5, mixed cellularity classical Hodgkin lymphoma, while sometimes vaguely nodular, is often diffusely infiltrative. Lymphocyte-depleted CHL, while diffuse, is rare; lymphocyte-rich CHL, on the other hand, only rarely exhibits a diffuse pattern, and the same is true of nodular lymphocyte-predominant Hodgkin lymphoma. Nodular sclerosis CHL by definition lacks a diffuse pattern of infiltration.

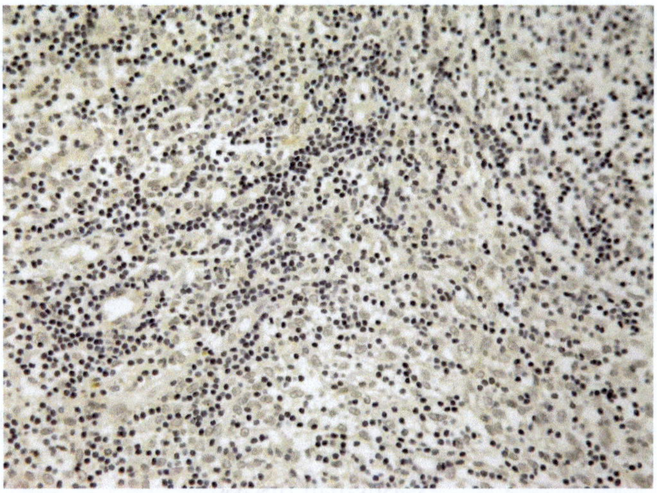

Fig. 6.155. Reticulin stain fails to demonstrate reticulin around the tumor cells, a feature which contrasts with most mesenchymal neoplasms whose cells are invested by reticulin.

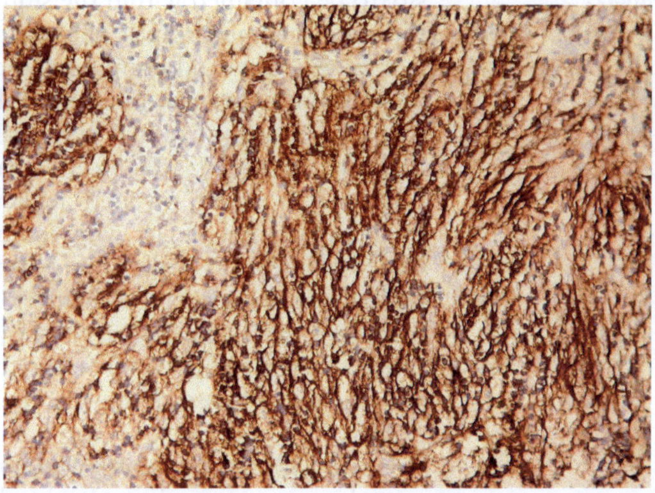

Fig. 6.156. The cells of FDC sarcoma show distinct membrane staining for CD21. CD23 and CD35 were also expressed by this tumor (not shown). Other markers for FDC cells include D2-40 and clusterin.

Diagnostic Approach to Diffuse Infiltrates in lymph Nodes

As with follicular and nodular infiltrates, it is helpful to formulate an approach to diffuse infiltrates through a series of questions.

Is the Infiltrate Truly Diffuse?

Stain for FDC meshworks with CD21, CD35, D2-40, or CD23. This helps to display the lymph node architecture and may reveal

Table 6.37
Immunophenotypic profiles of histiocytic and dendritic cell neoplasms

	CD68	Lysozyme	CD1a	S100	CD21/CD35
HS	+	+	–	–/+	–
LCH	+	–/+	+	+	–
IDC sarcoma	+/–	–/+	–	+	–
FDC sarcoma	+/–	–	–	–/+	+

residual follicles, colonization of follicles by DLBCL, confluence of FL, constricted follicles in MCL, and proliferation of FDC in Castleman disease.

Does the Diffuse Infiltrate Involve the Node Partially or Completely?

Often the extent of involvement is a reflection of severity and not specific to the entity, i.e., the same entity can produce a partial or complete involvement of the node. The leukemias have a propensity to be contained within the sinuses and medulla, and produce localized accumulations in the paracortex, each with their specific cytomorphology and immunophenotypic profile.

Myeloid sarcoma infiltrates the sinuses, paracortex and medullar, sparing residual germinal centers, alternatively, it can infiltrate as sheets. The cells may reflect the full spectrum observed in acute myeloid leukemia, comprising blasts with medium to large nuclei with multilobated, round, reniform or folded contours, small to inconspicuous nucleoli and a high nuclear/cytoplasmic ratio. Mitosis is brisk. The identification of myelocytes and promyelocytes showing evidence of granulocytic differentiation help confirm the diagnosis, and immunostains for myeloperoxidase, lysozyme, CD43, CD117, and CD68 are positive.

Lymphoblastic leukemia/lymphoma produces a diffuse infiltrate but may sometimes be localized to the sinuses producing pseudonodules encircled by thin fibrous strands. Sometimes residual lymphoid follicles, so-called naked germinal centers, and areas of residual paracortical tissue and patient sinuses may be present. A helpful clue is the single file infiltration of the lymph node capsule, fibrocollagenous tissue within the node, and perinodal tissue. A focal starry sky pattern may be present. The small- to intermediate-sized neoplastic cells show highly irregular and indented nuclei that display fine dusty chromatin and inconspicuous nucleoli. Cytoplasm is negligible and mitotic figures are frequent. The lymphoblasts are acid-phosphatase positive and Tdt+/CD7+/CD2+/CD5+/CD3+/CD43+/CD99+, and may be CD4+/CD8+ or CD4-/CD8– or CD4–/CD8+ or CD4+/CD8–.

Hairy cell leukemia, B-pro-lymphocytic leukemia, aggressive NK cell leukemia, enteropathy-associated T cell lymphoma, extranodal NK/T cell lymphoma, nasal type, hepatosplenic T cell lymphoma, cutaneous T cell lymphoma, and T-prolymphocytic leukemia can produce focal nodal infiltrates (discussed in Chapter 8).

Is the Infiltrate Monomorphous or Polymorphous? Are the Cells Small or Large?

Diffuse monomorphous, small to intermediate cell infiltrates include CLL/SLL, Burkitt lymphoma (BL), and lymphoblastic lymphoma.

CLL/SLL produces a "wall-to-wall" infiltrate of densely packed "blue" cells which may contain proliferation or growth centers of pallor occupied by variable numbers of prolymphocytes and paraimmunoblasts, which are larger and less densely packed. There may be areas of transformation to DLBCL or classical HD in the same node. The neoplastic cells are CD23+/CD20+/CD79a+/CD3–/CD10– with variable staining for CD5 and CD43. CD38 and ZAP70 expression correlate with unmutated cases and a poorer prognosis.

Burkitt lymphoma (BL) is composed of monotonous medium-sized cells that diffusely replace the lymph node. Chromatin is finely clumped and dispersed and there are multiple basophilic paracentral nucleoli present with moderate amounts of deeply basophilic, occasionally vacuolated cytoplasm. A starry sky pattern is evident, and cell moulding with retracted squared-off cell shapes may be seen. Plasmacytoid differentiation and a granulomatous response may be present. BL cells are CD20+/CD79a+/CD10+/Bcl6+/CD43+/CD38+. The proliferative index approaches 95%.

Lymphoblastic lymphoma can sometimes produce a complete effacement of nodal architecture as described above.

Diffuse monomorphous, large cell infiltrates include lymphoplasmacytoid lymphoma (LPL) and DLBCL.

Lymphoplasmacytic lymphoma (LP) shows a monotonous population of small lymphocytes, plasma cells, and intermediate plasmacytoid forms alongside distended sinusoids and vessels filled with PAS+ material. Dutcher bodies may be present. The cells are CD79a+/CD38+/CD138+/MUM1+ and are CD5–/CD23–/CD10–/Bcl6+/–.

DLBCL produces diffuse infiltrates that may partially or completely replace the lymph node architecture. A variety of cell types may be seen. The *centroblastic variant* is most common and comprises medium to large cells with oval vesicular nuclei containing two to four nucleoli that often appear attached to the nuclear membrane. Cytoplasm is scanty and amphophilic to basophilic. A mixture of centroblasts and immunoblasts may be present, the latter showing a single central nucleolus and moderate quantities of basophilic cytoplasm. The *immunoblastic variant* contains >90% of immunoblasts. The *anaplastic variant* shows large bizarre cells that resemble RSC and cells of ALCL. They may have a sinusoidal and cohesive growth pattern. DLBCL is CD20+/CD79a+/CD10+/Bcl6+ and may show immunoglobulin light-chain restriction. There is variable expression of MUM1, and a smaller percentage express CD5 and Bcl2.

Monomorphous infiltrate of bizarre large cells can represent anaplastic large cell lymphoma or a true histiocytic sarcoma.

Anaplastic large cell lymphoma (ALCL) can be mistaken for carcinoma because of its propensity to infiltrate subcapsular and nodal sinuses, and sometimes poor cohesiveness. The large pleomorphic cells have bizarre nuclei that contain prominent nucleoli. Wreath-like, horse-shoe shaped and kidney-shaped nuclei with paranuclear hopf may be seen and hallmark cells are often present. Mitosis is brisk. Variants include small cell, lymphohistiocytic, hypocellular, and sarcomatoid types. The neoplastic cells express T cell antigens or are of "null" cell type. They are CD30+/ALK+/CD3+/CD68+ and often express cytotoxic proteins. There is also often aberrant loss of CD5 and/or CD7. Variable EMA positivity and often negative CD45 further mimic carcinoma. ALCL, ALK–negative is not morphologically distinguishable from the ALK-positive counterpart and is also CD30+.

Histiocytic sarcoma is very rare. It shows marked cellular pleomorphism with large atypical cells displaying irregular vesicular nuclei and abundant eosinophilic cytoplasm, occasionally with phagocytic activity. Mitosis is frequent and the neoplastic cells are CD163+/CD68+/CD45+/CD4+, and express lysozyme, acid phosphatase, and non-specific esterase.

Polymorphous infiltrates include T cell/histiocyte-rich large B cell lymphoma (THRLBCL) and T cell and NK cell neoplasms.

THRLBCL is a polymorphous infiltrate of scattered large neoplastic B cells in a background of abundant small T cells and variable numbers of histiocytes. While mostly diffuse, it can sometimes produce a vague nodularity so that Hodgkin disease needs to be excluded. In this regard, eosinophils and plasma cells are often not found in THRLBCL. The large atypical cells have vesicular nuclei that may be oval or multilobated and contain prominent nucleoli. They are CD20+/CD79a+/Bcl6+. Staining for CD15, CD30, and CD38 is negative.

T cell and NK cell lymphomas are typically characterized by a polymorphous infiltrate that commences in the paracortex and may replace the entire node. Response to chemokines and cytokines secreted by the neoplastic population produces a background of small lymphocytes, eosinophils, plasma cells, and histiocytes. High-endothelial vessels are frequently prominent and the neoplastic cells are large with vesicular nuclei that are irregular, multilobated, and even convoluted. Nucleoli are prominent and may be multiple. Cytoplasm is variable in quantity and may be eosinophilic, basophilic, or clear. Mitosis is brisk. The *lymphoepithelial variant (Lennert lymphoma)* shows confluent clusters of epithelioid histiocytes, often in such abundance that the neoplastic population of small and large convoluted cells can be hidden. In the *T-zone variant,* the neoplastic cells occupy perifollicular areas to produce a pattern that may be mistaken for benign paracortical hyperplasia and a rarer *follicular variant* presents as perifollicular and intrafollicular nodules of atypical clear cells in a background of progressively transformed germinal centers. CD2+/CD4+/CD8- phenotype predominates in nodal T cell lymphoma and an aberrant loss of CD5 and CD7 may be seen. There may be expression of cytotoxic proteins whereas CD57 and CD56 expression are uncommon.

Angioimmunoblastic T cell lymphoma (AITL) comprises a polymorphous infiltrate associated with a striking proliferation of arborizing high-endothelial venules. The neoplastic cells are both large and small, and mixed with reactive cells that include plasma cells, eosinophils, histiocytes, small lymphocytes, and follicular dendritic cells (FDC). In the early phase, the infiltrate may be more monotonous and the atypical cells may show clear cytoplasm. Germinal centers may be preserved but these progressively regress and are replaced by a pronounced proliferation of FDC which extend to encompass surrounding proliferating vessels. As with other peripheral T cell lymphomas, AITL is commonly CD4+/CD8– and expresses other T cell antigens such as CD2, CD3, CD5, CD45RO, and CD43, sometimes with aberrant loss of CD7. In addition, AITL expresses antigens of follicular helper T cells including CD10, Bcl6, CXCL13, and PD-1. FDC meshworks around the vessels are CD21+/CD35+/D2-40+.

Other T cell neoplasms that involve the lymph node include adult T cell leukemia/lymphoma and cutaneous T cell lymphoma, both showing partial node involvement by cells with marked nuclear convolutions and typical immuno-phenotype.

When the infiltrate comprises somewhat bland large cells mixed with epithelioid histiocytes and inflammatory cells including eosinophils, the diagnosis of *Langerhans cell histiocytosis (LCH)* should be considered. The neoplastic cells can sometimes be localized within sinuses without significant expansion or disruption of nodal architecture. They have characteristic nuclei that have folded or convoluted nuclear membranes and linear grooves. Nucleoli are inconspicuous and their moderate quantities of cytoplasm are eosinophilic. Multinucleated giant cells may be present. The neoplastic cells are CD1a+/langerin+/S100+/HLA-DR+.

Classical Hodgkin disease, mixed cellularity type can present as a diffuse polymorphous infiltrate. The RSC and HS are CD15+/CD30+/CD20+/– and are frequently EBER+ and LMP-1+. They do not express CD45, Oct-2, or Bob.1.

Background cells include epithelioid histiocytes, eosinophils, small lymphocytes, and plasma cells.

Diffuse or localized infiltration by spindled cells should raise the possibility of *FDC sarcoma* or *IDC sarcoma*. Both conditions are rare (**Table 6.38**).

Table 6.38
A diagnostic approach to diffuse infitrates

Is the infiltrate truly diffuse?
Stain for FDC meshworks with CD21, CD35, or D2-40
Is the diffuse infiltrate involving the node partially or completely?
Extent of infiltration is largely a function of severity, not specificity
Leukemic infiltrates tend to be confined to sinuses
T cell lymphoma may be localized to the paracortex
ALCL infiltrates subcapsular and nodal sinuses mimicking carcinoma
Is the infiltrate monomorphous or polymorphous?
If monomorphous, are the cells large or small?
Small to intermediate cells
CLL/SLL
• Small dark cells packed wall-to-wall
• Proliferation centers may be present
• CD20+/CD79a+/CD23+/CD5+/CD43+/Bcl2–/Bcl6–/cyclinD1–
• Exclude synchronous DLBCL and HD
Burkitt lymphoma
• Intermediate-sized cells with high N/C ratio
• Starry sky pattern
• Proliferation index >90% (use Ki67)
• C10+/Bcl6+/CD38+/CD138+/CD43+/Bcl2–/Tdt–
• Eber+/LMP-1+
LPL
• May often show IgM paraprotein
• Diffuse or partial effacement, sinuses paten filled with PAS+ protein
• Small lymphocytes, plasma cells, and intermediate forms; also variable eosinophils, mast cells and epithelioid histiocytes
• Dutcher bodies, may show amyloid deposition
• CD38+/CD138+/CD79a+/MUM1+ with variable CD43 and Bcl6 staining; light-chain restriction
LBL
• Generally diffuse, sometimes with pseudonodular pattern, focal starry sky
• Small- to intermediate-sized blasts with fine dusty nuclei with thin nuclear membranes and inconspicuous nucleoli; scanty cytoplasm, mitosis brisk
• Tdt+/CD2+/cCD3+/CD7+/CD5+; variable expression of CD4 and CD8

Table 6.38 (continued)

Large cells
DLBCL
• Variants: centroblastic, immunoblastic, anaplastic, signet ring, microvillous
• CD20+/CD79a+/Bcl6+/CD10+/cyclinD1–/CD23–; MUM1 variable
• Ig light-chain restriction; Ki67 >40%
ALCL
• Sinus infiltration; large poorly cohesive cells, bizarre nuclei, wreath-, horse-shoe-, kidney- shaped nuclei; hallmark cells
• Mostly T or "Null" cell type; CD3+/CD2+/CD4+/CD30+/ALK+, cytotoxic proteins+
• Many CD45–, EMA+ hence mistaken for carcinoma; Bcl2– and EBV–
• Typical t(2;5)
Histiocytic sarcoma
• Large pleomorphic cells, diffuse infiltrate
• CD163+/CD68+/S100+/Lys+, variable staining with Mac387, HAM56
• Exclude metastatic carcinoma and melanoma with broad spectrum CK, HMB45, Melan A, MiTF1
FDC tumor
• Spindle cell proliferation, localized or diffuse; associated with Castleman disease
• CD21+/CD23+/CD35+/D2-40+/clusterin+/fascin+
• Also stains for vimentin, HLA-DR with variable staining for S100, CD68, and, CD45
IDC tumor
• Localized or disseminated; spindled or epithelioid; nuclear atypia and frequent mitosis
• S100+/HLA-DR+/fascin+/CD1a–/Clusterin–
Polymorphous diffuse infiltrates
THRLBCL
• Variant of DLBCL accounting for 10%
• Scattered atypical large B cells in background of small T cells and histiocytes; mimics HD especially NLPHD
• Typical B cell phenotype; small T cells are CD3+/CD2+/CD5+
T cell lymphoma
• Large and small atypical cells, often with highly irregular nuclei and large nucleoli; clear cells
• High-endothelial vessels in background
• Polymorphous cell response to cytokines from neoplastic cells – plasma cells, eosinophils, histiocytes, small lymphocytes
• Variants: Lennert lymphoma – prominent confluent epithelioid cell infiltrate; T-zone – small atypical cells in perifollicular; follicular – atypical clear cells as perifollicular nodules
• CD2+/CD3+/CD4+/CD8 – phenotype predominates; aberrant loss of CD5 and/or CD7

Table 6.38 (continued)

AITL
• Variable, initially partial effacement by largely monomorphous atypical clear cells; later diffuse effacement with regressed germinal center, perinodal involvement, pericortical sinuses spared
• Striking high endothelial vascular proliferation
• Highly polymorphous, small and large atypical cells mixed with reactive plasma cells, eosinophils, histiocytes, small lymphocytes, and FDC in regressed follicles extending around proliferating vessels; PAS+ sludge
• Characteristic follicular helper T cell phenotype – CD10+/Bcl6+/CXCL13+/PD-1+
LCH
• Distinctive histiocytes with bland appearing nuclei showing prominent folds and longitudinal grooves, small nucleoli, moderate amounts of pale cytoplasm
• Epithelioid histiocytes and variable numbers of eosinophils present • Langerhans cells stains for langerin (CD207), CD1a, S100, CD68

Chapter 7

Defining Microscopic Features

Key words: Granulomas, starry sky/mottling, necrosis/apoptosis, sinus pattern, vascular prominent, spindle cells, fibrosis/hyalinization, signet ring cells, clear cells, bizarre multinucleated cells, eosinophils, neutrophils, plasma cells, pericapsular fat infiltration, extraneous cells, pigmented cells, epithelial cells, hemosiderin, foreign material.

While the primary patterns of lymph node infiltration can be broadly divided into nodular and diffuse, morphologically distinctive changes that form defining features of a disease are important to recognize. Such defining microscopic features are identifiable at low magnification because the tinctorial and morphological properties set them apart from the background architecture and cells. Furthermore, such defining features are often localized, although the surrounding lymph node tissue may display reactive hyperplasia (**Table 7.1**).

Granulomas and Foam Cells

Granulomatous inflammation is characterized by the presence of a histiocytic response composed of mixtures of macrophages and epithelioid cells that can be diffuse or that can occur as small clusters, loose aggregates or more discrete nests, or granulomas. The presence of sheets or accumulations of foam cells or phagocytic histiocytes filled with lipid also represents a granulomatous reaction.

Infective Granulomatous Lymphadenitis

A granulomatous response is characteristic of a number of infective agents that include bacteria, fungi, and parasites. Such granulomas may be necrotizing or non-necrotizing. There is

A.S.-Y. Leong, *A Pattern Approach to Lymph Node Diagnosis*,
DOI 10.1007/978-1-4419-7176-0_7, © Springer Science+Business Media, LLC 2011

Table 7.1
Defining microscopic features as diagnostic discriminators

Granulomas and foam cells
Sinus pattern
Necrosis, apoptosis, and infarction
Clear cells
Spindled cells
Vascular prominence
Hemorrhage
Mottling
Starry sky pattern
Fibrosis/hyalinization
Signet ring cells
Mast cells
Bizarre or multinucleated cells
Extramedullary hematopoiesis
Eosinophils prominent
Neutrophils prominent
Plasma cells prominent
Infiltration of pericapsular fat
Extraneous cells – pigmented cells, epithelial cells, foreign material, dermatopathic lymphadenitis, hemosiderin

accumulating evidence that apoptosis may have a major role in producing the so-called "necrosis" in some granulomas.

Mycobacterium tuberculosis, atypical mycobacteria, *Bartonella henselae* (in cat-scratch disease), *Chlamydia trachomatis*, and *Yersinia* infections produce a granulomatous lymphadenitis that shows central necrosis. The necrotizing areas are associated with the presence of variable numbers of neutrophils, sometimes accumulating as microabscesses, resulting in the term "suppurative granulomatous lymphadenitis" (care should be taken not to mistake apoptotic bodies for neutrophils). These granulomas are found mostly in the cortex and paracortex. They are distinctive and, like most infective processes, may be associated with varying degrees of follicular and paracortical hyperplasia, the relative prominence of the microscopic features varying with time. The discrete collections of epithelioid histiocytes often occur beneath the subcapsular sinus and are surrounded by lymphocytes, plasma cells, and variable amounts of fibrosis. There are no specific features of distinction except that the necrosis in cat-scratch disease is described as stellate in shape, but other infective diseases including *M. tuberculosis* and *Yersinia* lymphadenitis can also produce stellate necrosis. Specific diagnosis is dependent on identification of the infecting organism with special stains, by immunohistochemistry, or by polymerase chain reaction.

Mycobacterial Lymphadenitis

Mycobacterial infections with *M. tuberculosis, M. avium-intracellulare* (MAIC), *and M. leprae* produce similar appearing necrotizing granulomas, but the latter two organisms are associated with a greater range of histological changes including an infiltrate of foam cells (lepra reaction), non-specific follicular hyperplasia, sarcoid-like granulomatous reaction, and, especially in the case of *M. avium-intracellulare*, a spindle cell proliferation akin to inflammatory pseudotumor (inflammatory myofibroblastic tumor). Acid-fast stains help identify the mycobacteria. Antibodies directed to mycobacteria are not sensitive (**Figs. 7.1**, **7.2**, **7.3**, **7.4**, **7.5**, and **7.6**).

Cat-Scratch Disease

Cat-scratch disease is caused by a small, pleomorphic, gram-negative bacterium, *Bartonella henselae* (previously *Rochalimaea* sp.) that is stained by the Warthin–Starry stain. The infected nodes are tender, and axillary or cervical nodes that drain the inoculation site in the hands and arms are commonly involved. There is often a recent history of contact with a cat or kitten. The lymphadenitis is characterized by sheets of histiocytes/macrophages, often arranged as discrete granulomas with central necrosis. Plasma cells and immunoblasts may be found in the sinuses (**Figs. 7.7**, **7.8**, **7.9**, and **7.10**).

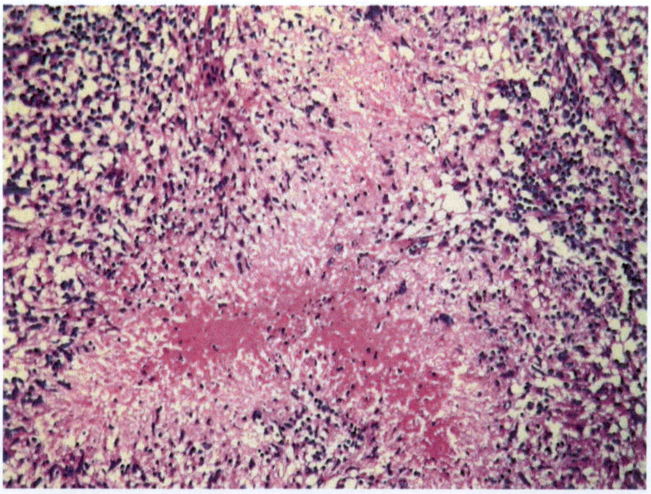

Fig. 7.1. Typical caseating/necrotizing granuloma seen in *M. tuberculosis*. In this example, the necrotic area is stellate in shape.

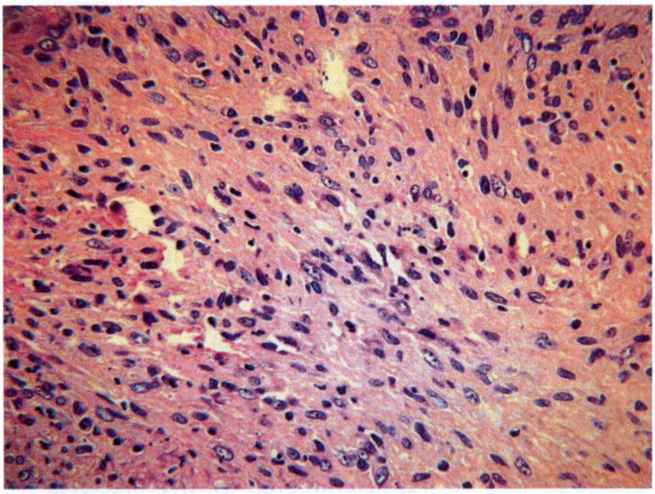

Fig. 7.2. A spindle cell proliferation akin to inflammatory pseudo-tumor (inflammatory myofibroblastic tumor) is uncommonly seen in *M. avium-intracellulare* infection.

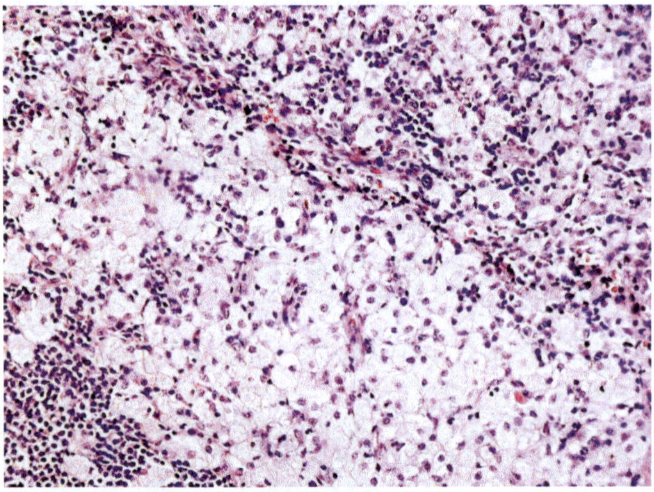

Fig. 7.3. A granulomatous infiltrate of foamy macrophages in MAIC lymphadenitis.

Lymphogranuloma Venereum

Lymphogranuloma venereum, which is caused by *Chlamydia trachomatis,* most often involves inguinal nodes and is preceded by a papule on the mucosa or on skin of the genitalia or rectum. The necrotizing granulomas commence as small necrotic foci with collections of neutrophils followed by plasma cells and lymphocytes accumulating around the necrosis. Coalescing of these foci produces a stellate pattern of necrosis within the granulomas. The 0.2–2.0 μ diameter, sand-like organisms that are blue in H&E-stained sections occur within vacuolated macrophages that accumulate in necrotic or suppurative foci. They can be stained with the Warthin–Starry stain and confirmed by the polymerase chain

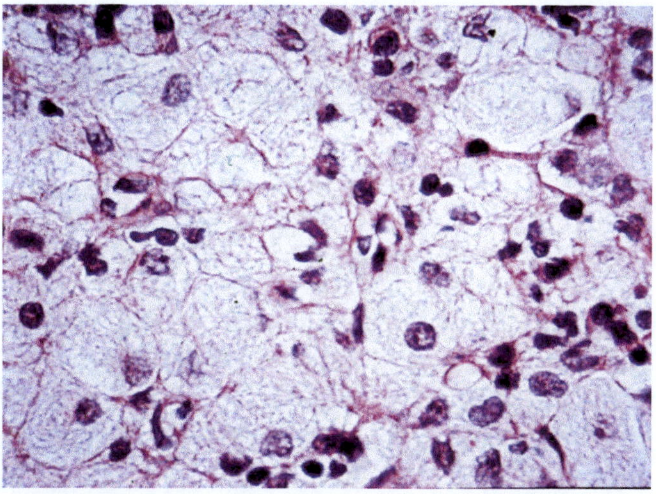

Fig. 7.4. The foamy cells contain filamentous-like organisms which are just visible in H&E sections imparting a striated appearance to the macrophages.

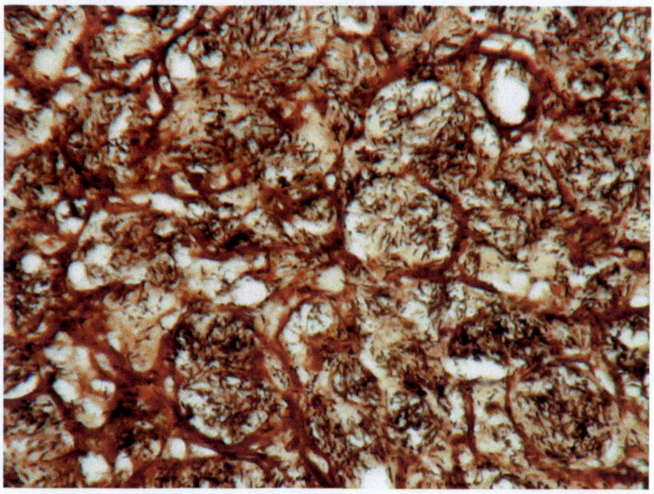

Fig. 7.5. MAIC lymphadenitis. Numerous long bacilli are contained within the foamy macrophages (methenamine silver stain).

reaction. There is a background of follicular hyperplasia with clusters of monocytoid B cells in the cortex. Vascular endothelial cells may be prominent; there is capsular fibrosis and capsular vessels may show vasculitis.

Yersinia Lymphadenitis

Yersinia pseudotuberculosis and *Y. enterocolitica* produce a self-limiting mesenteric lymphadenitis with capsular thickening, an immunoblastic proliferation in the cortical and paracortical areas, follicular hyperplasia, dilated sinuses engorged with lymphocytes, and, in the case of *Y. pseudotuberculosis,* small tuberculoid

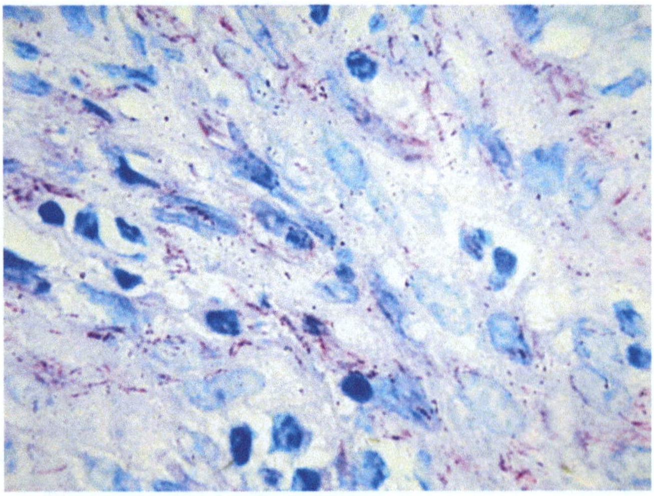

Fig. 7.6. MAIC lymphadenitis with inflammatory pseudotumor-like response showing numerous acid-fast organisms in the spindle cells.

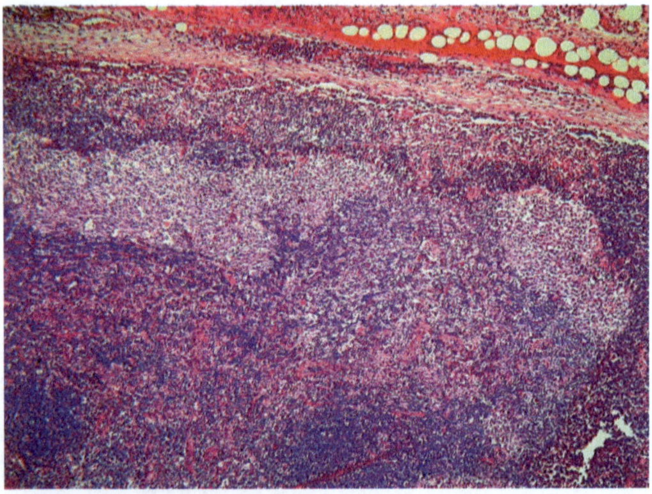

Fig. 7.7. *B. henselae* axillary lymphadenitis showing congestion and edema with distinct collections of macrophages in the cortex. The capsule is thickened and inflammatory cells spill over into the pericapsular tissue.

granulomas with microabscesses. Specific diagnosis is confirmed by culturing the organism (**Table 7.2**; **Figs. 7.11**, **7.12**, **7.13**, and **7.14**).

Whipple Disease

Whipple disease has protean clinical manifestations, most commonly fever, diarrhea, and weight loss. Infection of the small bowel results in malabsorption with prominent, edematous jejunal folds composed of villi that are pale and swollen due to engorged lymphatics, an appearance which has been likened to that of a shag rug. Besides extensive para-aortic and mesenteric

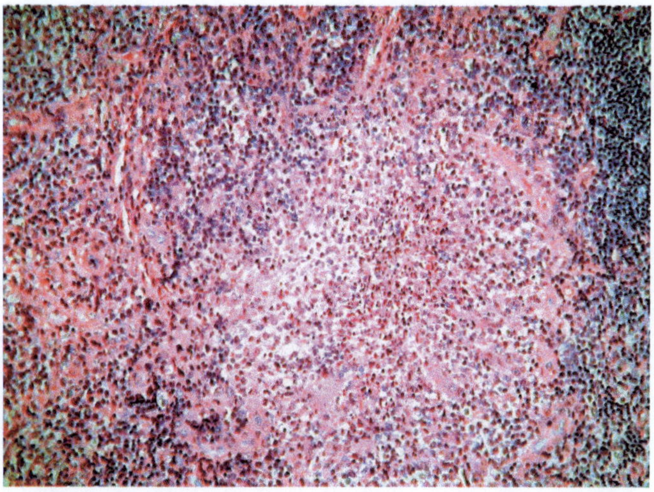

Fig. 7.8. There is early necrosis and collections of neutrophils and eosinophils are present within the granuloma.

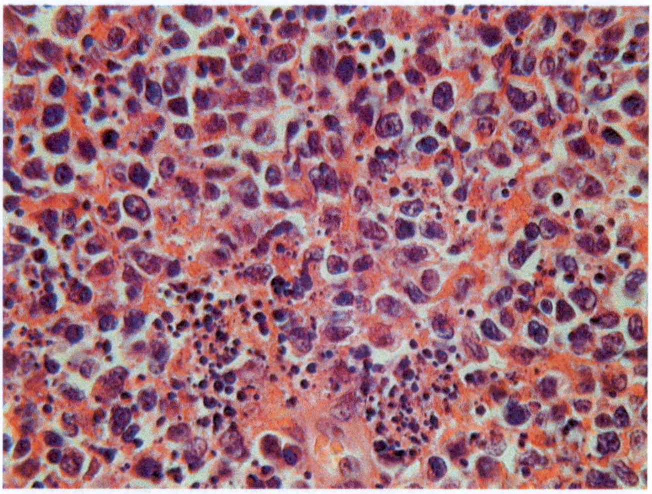

Fig. 7.9. Numerous apoptotic bodies are present among the phagocytic histiocytes.

lymphadenopathy, peripheral lymphadenopathy may be a presenting symptom, and liver, spleen, joints, heart, brain, adrenals, muscle, and eyes have been reported to be involved. The causative organism is *Tropheryma whipplei,* a rod-shaped bacillus amenable to silver staining. Affected lymph nodes are macroscopically spongy and yellow and contain large numbers of foamy macrophages as single cells and in aggregates, within sinuses as well as lymphoid areas. The foamy macrophages are filled with intracellular PAS-positive granules that represent the infecting organisms. Epithelioid cells and giant cells of foreign body type are frequent. Diagnosis is made by the demonstration of

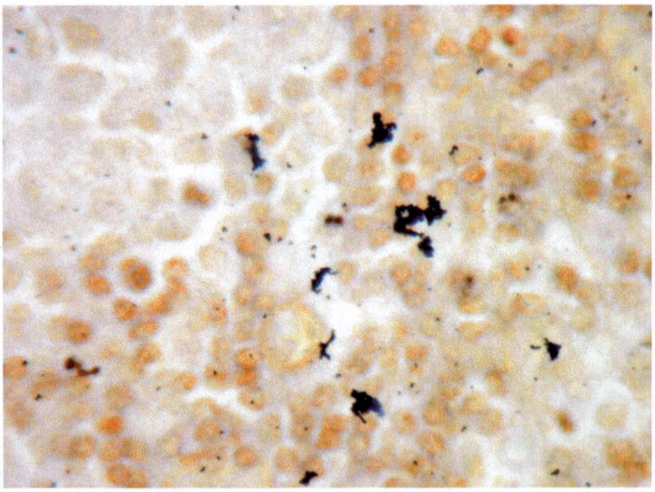

Fig. 7.10. *Bartonella henselae* stained by the Warthin–Starry stain. The bacilli are clumped, small, pleomorphic, rod- and L-shaped.

Table 7.2
Bacterial necrotizing granulomatous lymphadenitis

Mycobacterial – Typical necrotizing granulomas, acid-fast bacilli (*M. tuberculosis, M. leprae, M. avium-intracellulare*). Variant pathology – sheets of large striated macrophages with abundant MAIC; inflammatory pseudotumor-like reaction
Cat-scratch disease (B. henselae lymphadenitis) – Granulomas with stellate necrosis, pleomorphic rod-shaped bacilli demonstrated by Warthin–Starry stain
Lymphogranuloma venereum – Necrotic and suppurative granulomas with vacuolated macrophages containing sand-like organisms (*C. trachomatis*) stained with Warthin–Starry stain
Yersinia lymphadenitis – Abdominal or mesenteric nodes, small necrotizing granulomas, diagnosed by culturing organism (*Y. pseudotuberculosis*)

PAS-positive granules and specifically by staining with an anti-*T. whipplei* antibody, identification by polymerase chain reaction, or by electron microscopy in which the intact 0.2 × 1.0 μ bacilli with a distinctive trilaminar plasma membrane are found within macrophages (**Table 7.3**; **Figs. 7.15**, **7.16**, **7.17**, **7.18**, and **7.19**).

Mycotic Lymphadenitis

Fungi are generally saprophytes and become pathogenic in the debilitated, immunosuppressed or immunodeficient patient. Dissemination to the viscera and lymph nodes occurs in this setting. Fungal lymphadenitis is often granulomatous and necrotizing. Specific diagnosis is based on the identification of the fungus which can be demonstrated with the periodic acid–Schiff stain or methenamine silver stain. *Histoplasma capsulatum, Cryptococcus neoformans, Pneumocystis jiroveci* (formerly *P. carinii*), and

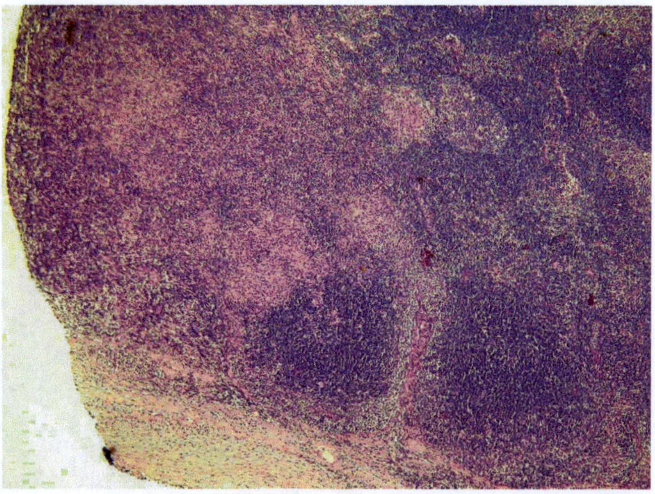

Fig. 7.11. *Y. pseudotuberculosis* mesenteric lymphadenitis. There is cortical and paracortical hyperplasia and several ill-defined granulomas are present. There is perivascular cuffing by monocytoid B cells (*arrows*).

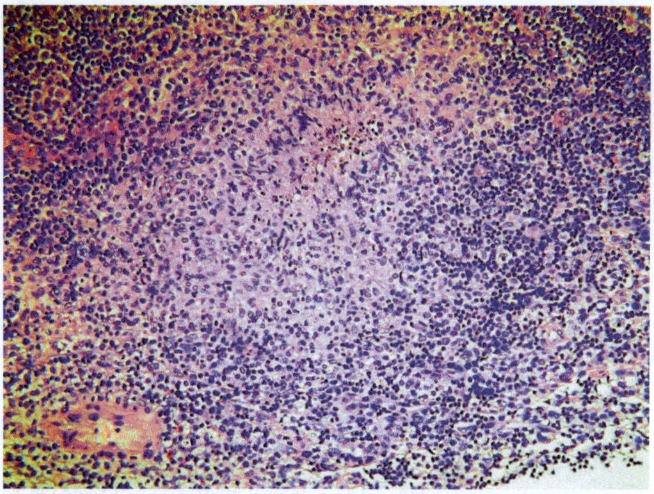

Fig. 7.12. A typical necrotizing granuloma seen in *Yersinia* mesenteric lymphadenitis.

Coccidioides immitis produce a granulomatous lymphadenitis, and the organisms have sufficiently distinctive morphology to allow identification. Except for *Coccidioides,* the other fungi occur worldwide.

Histoplasma Lymphadenitis

Histoplasma capsulatum has its natural habitat in soil especially that contaminated by excrement from birds such as chickens or pigeons, or from bats. The spores or hyphal forms are inhaled into the lungs, where the organism converts into intracellular yeast forms that, with formalin fixation, retract from their rigid

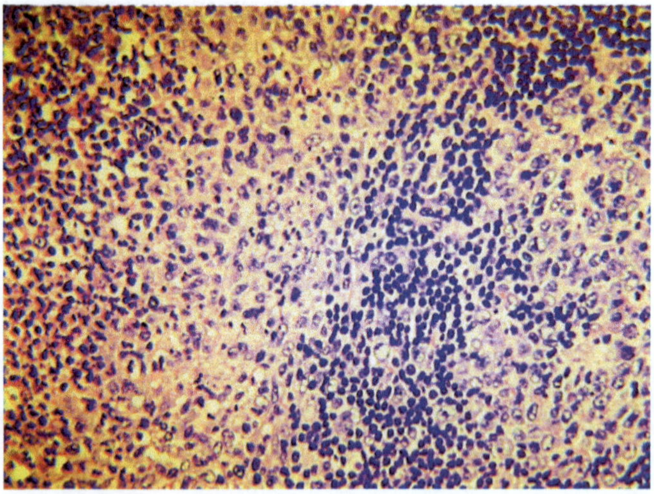

Fig. 7.13. One of the two granulomas shown is suppurative and has collections of neutrophils in its necrotic center.

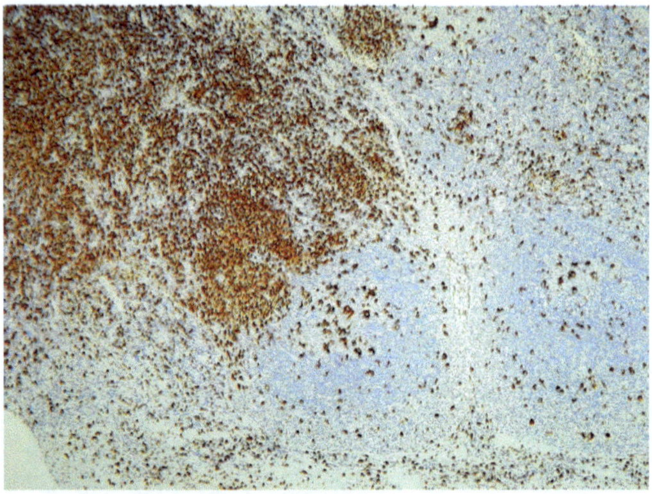

Fig. 7.14. Diffusely infiltrating histiocytes in *Yersinia* lymphadenitis should not be mistaken for immunoblasts. CD68 stain confirms their histiocyte/macrophage lineage.

cell walls to give the impression of a capsule. The granulomas comprise vast sheets of histiocytes, and epithelioid and giant cells may be present. Numerous 2–4 μ organisms are found in the macrophages. They retract from their rigid walls during fixation and become surrounded by a clear halo. Old fibrotic and calcified lesions may be indistinguishable from tuberculosis (**Figs. 7.20, 7.21**, **7.22**, and **7.23**).

Cryptococcus Lymphadenitis

Cryptococcus neoformans is found in pigeon feces, where it may remain viable for more than 2 years. Transmission is by aerosols.

Table 7.3
Whipple disease

Protean clinical manifestations
Diarrhea, fever, and weight loss as common presentation
Abdominal and mesenteric lymphadenopathy, peripheral lymphadenopathy frequent
Lymph nodes swollen and yellow
Foamy macrophages distend sinuses and lymph node parenchyma
Strong PAS+ granularity within macrophages
Epithelioid cells and multinucleated cells present, occasional eosinophils
T. whipplei is a rod-shaped, trilaminar bacillus contained within macrophage lysosomes
Organisms show various stages of degradation; after successful treatment, only capsules remain

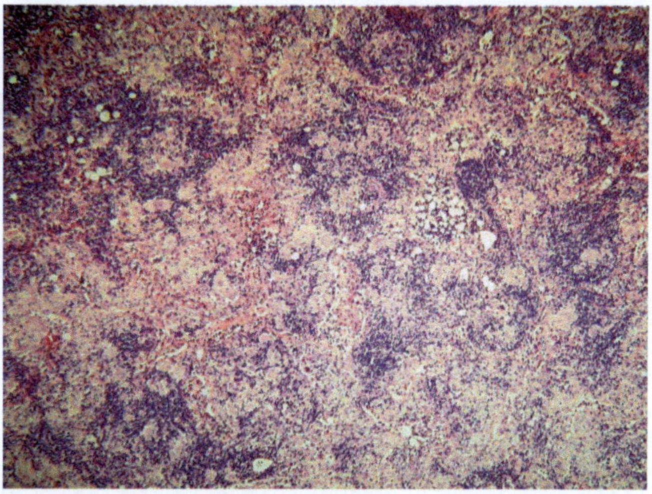

Fig. 7.15. Whipple lymphadenitis showing sinuses distended by foamy macrophages and epithelioid cells.

This monomorphic fungus forms round yeasts that are slightly larger than those of *Histoplasma*, measuring 3–6 μ and have a thick, refractile capsule. The infection generally commences as a Ghon-like complex with a primary pulmonary lesion and involved draining lymph node, both of which become fibrosed. Involved nodes contain multiple nodular and confluent, generally noncaseous granulomas composed of epithelioid histiocytes, lymphocytes, plasma cells, and multinucleated giant cells that contain phagocytosed organisms. The latter are barely visible in H&E sections but stain bright red in mucicarmine or PAS-stained sections.

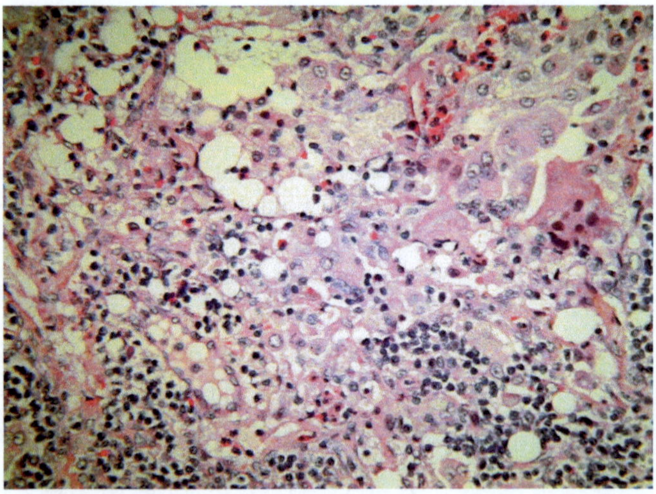

Fig. 7.16. Multinucleated giant cells are present among the epithelioid cells. Scattered eosinophils and adipocytes are also present.

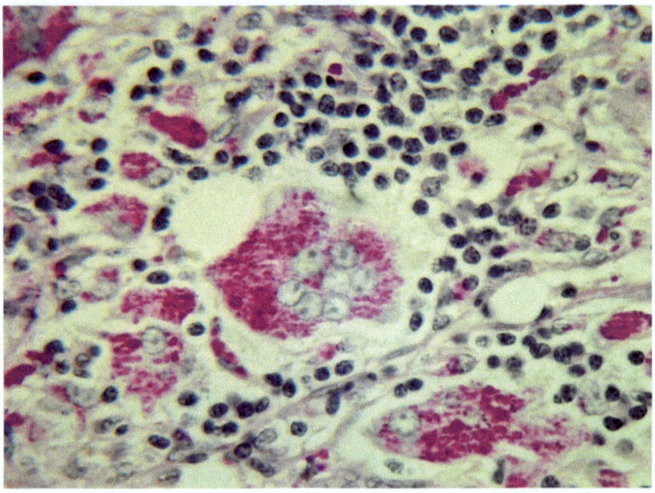

Fig. 7.17. PAS-positive granules within foam cells and a multinucleated giant cell.

The mucopolysaccharide capsules appear as clear spaces around the yeasts and forms the gelatinous material that accumulates in cystic spaces when the yeasts degenerate (**Figs. 7.24** and **7.25**).

Coccidioides Lymphadenitis

Coccidioides immitis is endemic in the southwestern United States, Mexico, and parts of Central and South America (e.g., Brazil). The fungus is airborne and highly infectious. The sporangia, 20–60 μ in diameter, are one of the largest infecting yeasts seen in man. Septate hyphae and sporangia containing multiple endospores of 2–5 μ are found mainly in necrotic cavities.

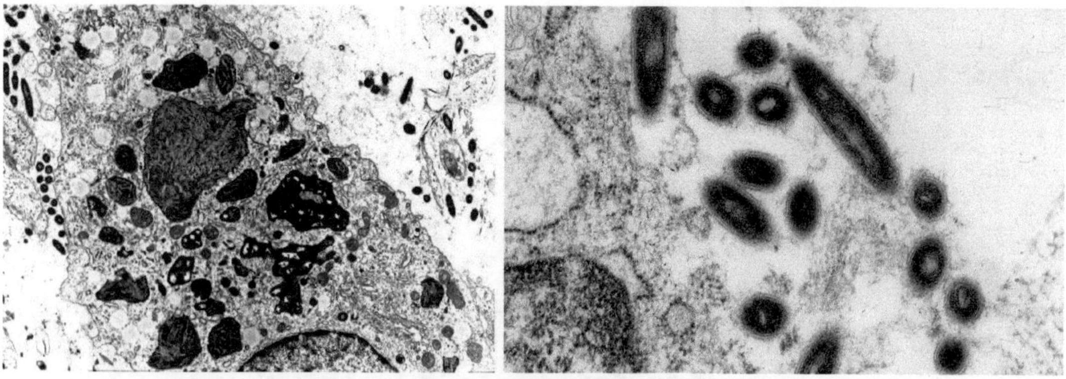

Fig. 7.18. Electron micrograph of a macrophage with numerous bacilli within lysosomes in various stages of degradation. There are intact bacilli in the intercellular spaces. *Inset* shows the trilaminar structure of the organism.

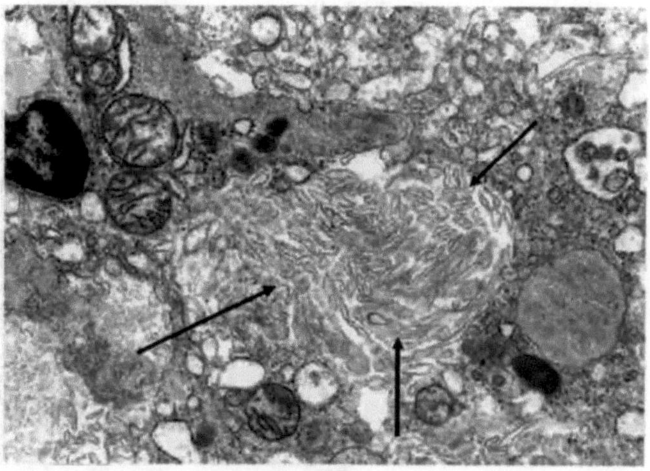

Fig. 7.19. After successful antibiotic treatment, only remnants of bacterial capsular material are present in the macrophages (*arrows*).

Pneumocystis Lymphadenitis

Pneumocystis jiroveci (formerly *P. carinii*) is the most common cause of opportunistic infections in patients with AIDS. The organism was previously classified as protozoan but has subsequently been shown to possess fungus-type ribosomal RNA and appropriately reclassified. Infection is generally limited to the lungs, though corresponding mediastinal and retroperitoneal nodes may be affected. Grossly recognizable necrotic areas are present, and histologic examination reveals the characteristic eosinophilic, PAS-positive foamy exudate within which the organisms are found. Methenamine silver stains reveal round or helmet-shaped *Pneumocystis* cysts, which can also be stained using monoclonal antibodies. In some instances, epithelioid histiocytes and multinucleated giant cells may be present adjacent to necrotic areas (**Table 7.4**).

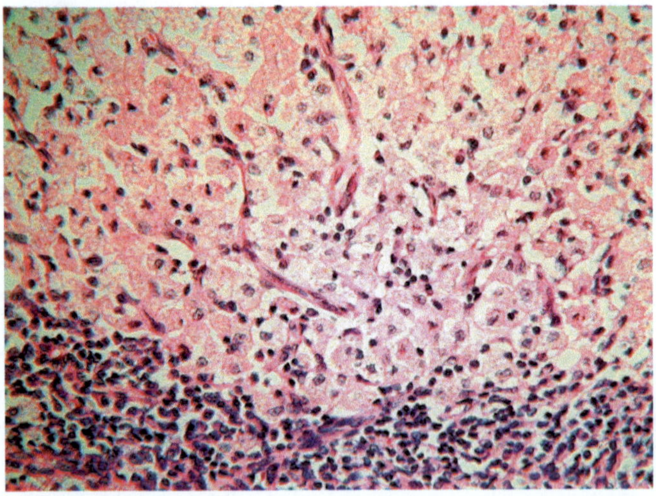

Fig. 7.20. Histoplasma lymphadenitis. Sheets of poorly circumscribed large pale histiocytes expand the paracortex with sparing of a lymphoid follicle.

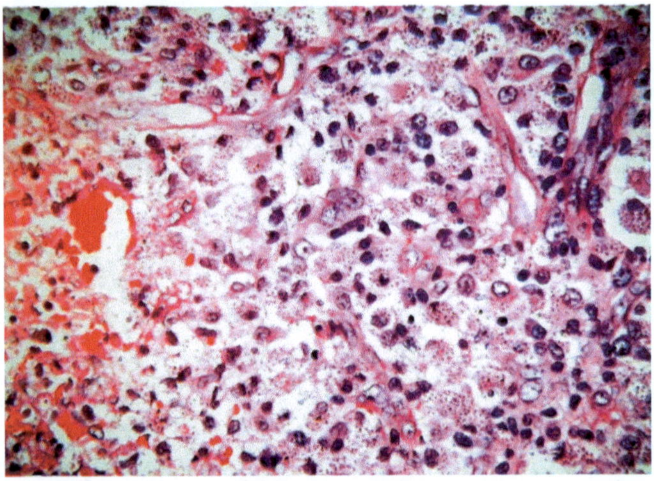

Fig. 7.21. Early necrosis is evident in the granulomatous infiltrate and the organisms impart a coarse granularity to the histiocyte cytoplasm.

Protozoan and Parasitic Lymphadenitides

In parasitic infections such as schistosomiasis, filariasis, and hookworm infestation, a granulomatous response, often accompanied by marked fibrosis, is evoked by the ova, adult worm, or larvae. Amoebae can sometimes be seen percolating through the sinuses of the draining lymph nodes in amoebic colitis. *Toxoplasma* lymphadenitis, previously discussed in **Chapter 5**, manifests as the Piringer–Kuchinka reaction with small discrete, non-necrotizing granulomas present throughout the lymph node, many impinging on or lying within hyperplastic germinal centers. There is

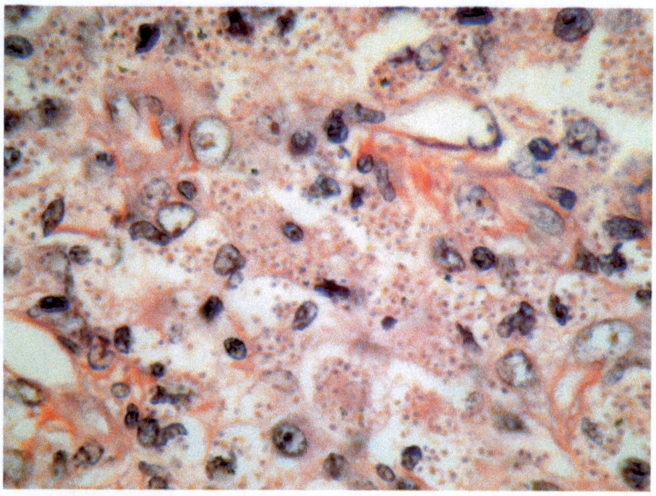

Fig. 7.22. The yeasts of *H. capsulatum* are small, round, and retract from their rigid walls to be surrounded by a halo.

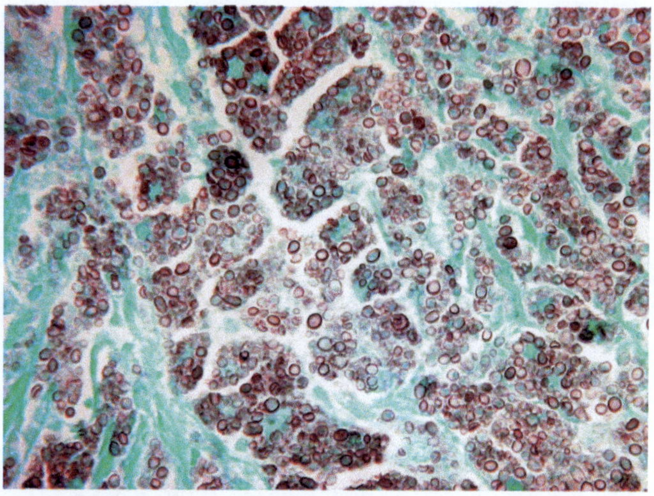

Fig. 7.23. The yeasts are 2–4 μ and multiply by narrow-based buds (Gomori methenamine silver).

accompanying expansion of the paracortex (**Table 7.5**; **Figs. 7.26** and **7.27**).

Non-infective Granulomatous Lymphadenitis

Kikuchi–Fujimoto disease and systemic lupus erythematosus produce a granulomatous lymphadenitis that is necrotizing but does not contain neutrophils. Both conditions produce very similar histological changes, the main difference being the presence of plasma cells and hematoxylin bodies within the sinuses and vessels in systemic lupus erythematosus. Both conditions have been previously discussed in detail.

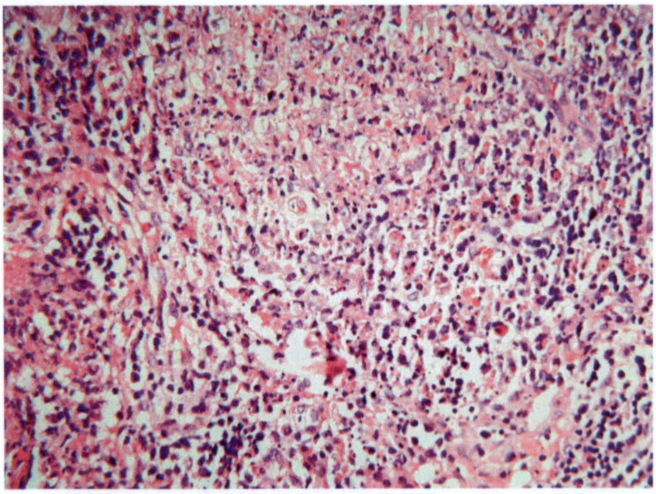

Fig. 7.24. *Cryptococcus* lymphadenitis showing a granulomatous reaction of epithelioid cells, lymphocytes and plasma cells. The "loose" nature of the granuloma is due to the mucopolysaccharide capsules of the phagocytosed organisms.

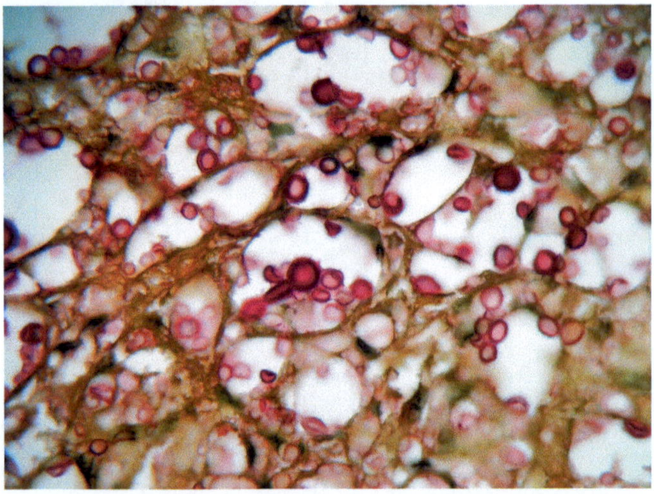

Fig. 7.25. Mucicarmine stain showing bright red 3–6 μ *Cryptococcus* yeasts. The clear spaces surrounding the organisms represent capsular mucopolysaccharide.

Kawasaki disease or the "mucocutaneous lymph node syndrome" is a self-limited, acute exanthematous disease of childhood of unknown etiology. It occurs mostly in Japan but has been reported from elsewhere. Few lymph node biopsies have been reported. The most striking findings include the presence of multiple foci of necrosis and fibrin thrombosis in small vessels, the latter resembling that seen in thrombotic thrombocytopenic purpura. The necrosis may resemble small infarcts in the initial stages, but later numerous neutrophils supervene and concentric infiltrates of transformed lymphocytes and histiocytes may occur

Table 7.4
Mycotic granulomatous lymphadenitis

Histoplasmosis – *H. capsulatum*, narrow-based budding yeast, epithelioid and giant cell necrotizing granulomas, 2–4 μ organisms retract from their rigid walls during fixation, stained by methenamine silver but not by PAS
Cryptococcal lymphadenitis – *C. neoformans*, non-caseating granulomas, 3–6 μ yeasts in histiocytes, gelatinous capsular mucopolysaccharide material released into stroma, mucicarmine and PAS-positive organisms
Coccdioidomycosis – *C. immitis*, endemic areas include southwestern United States, airborne spores, necrotizing granulomas, 20–60 μ sporangium contain endospores, stained by methenamine silver
Pneumocystosis – *P. jiroveci*, coalescent necrotic areas, granulomatous infiltrate, scanty inflammatory response, fibrinous PAS+ foamy exudate that contains helmet-shaped collapsed cysts (1–2 μ), stained by methenamine silver

Table 7.5
Protozoan and parasitic lymphadenitides

Frequently characterized by marked fibrosis with variable inflammatory response
Acute inflammation with eosinophils followed by chronic inflammation
Protozoan parts, larva, or ova present; often calcified and non-viable
Schistosoma – ova
Hookworm – larva
Filaria – adult worm and larva
Toxoplasmosis – Piringer–Kuchinka reaction; pseudocysts rare
Amoebiasis – amoeba percolating through lymph node sinuses

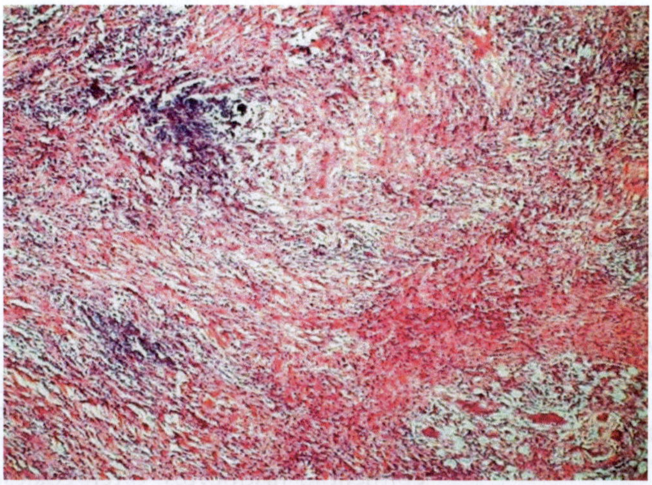

Fig. 7.26. *Brugia malayi* lymphadenitis. Enlarged inguinal node with non-necrotizing granulomatous inflammation, marked fibrosis, and focal calcification.

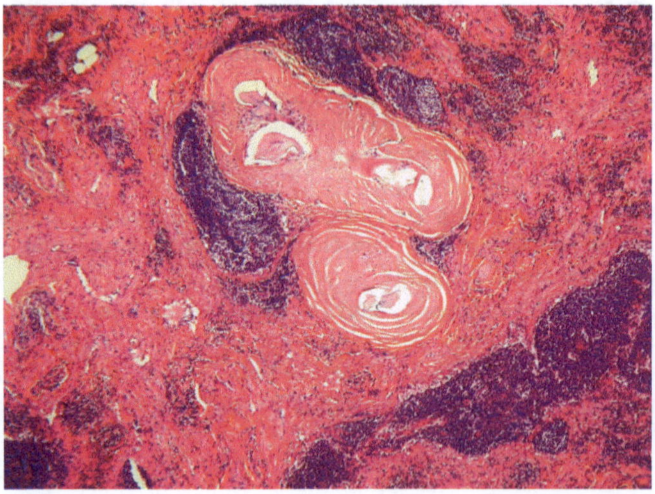

Fig. 7.27. Within the densely fibrotic areas are parts of non-viable adult worm (*arrows*).

in the vascular adventitia. The bland necrosis in the early phases can resemble systemic lupus erythematosus.

Sarcoidosis

Sarcoidosis is a multisystem disease whose etiology and pathogenesis still remain idiopathic. The lungs, lymph nodes, heart, skin, eyes, and joints are most commonly involved. It is characterized by discrete, round, non-necrotizing epithelioid granulomas in which multinucleated cells of Langhans type may be present and central fibrinoid necrosis in the granulomas is uncommon. The granulomas may partially or totally replace the lymph node and may coalesce. Asteroid bodies, Schaumann bodies, and calcium oxalate crystals may be present within the giant cells but these are not specific for sarcoidosis. Hamazaki–Wesenberg bodies may be observed. These are giant lysosomes, usually seen extracellularly at or close to the peripheral sinus and almost always away from the granulomas. Calcification is absent and there is generally no necrosis, which, if present, is only focal (**Table 7.6**; **Figs. 7.28**, **7.29**, **7.30**, and **7.31**).

Granulomas, Non-necrotizing

Peripheral T Cell Lymphoma, NOS – Lymphoepithelioid Variant (Lennert Lymphoma)

One neoplastic entity that is characterized by the presence of numerous small granulomas throughout the lymph node is the lymphoepithelioid variant (Lennert lymphoma) of peripheral T cell lymphoma (*see* **Chapter 6**). Distinctive small collections of epithelioid histiocytes, often coalescing, are found among a diffuse infiltrate of mostly small atypical T cells that are commonly CD3+ and CD8+. These cells show irregular nuclear outlines and

Table 7.6
Non-infective granulomatous lymphadenitis

Kikuchi–Fujimoto disease – Necrotizing granulomas but no neutrophils
SLE – Necrotizing granulomas very similar to Kikuchi, no neutrophils or eosinophils, plasma cells present, hematoxylin bodies may be found
Sarcoidosis – Discrete granulomas, necrosis absent or focal, Schaumann, asteroid, and Hamazaki–Wesenberg bodies, and calcium oxalate crystals
Kawasaki disease – Mucocutaneous syndrome, acute exanthematous disease of mostly Japanese children, necrosis prominent, fibrin thrombosis, numerous neutrophils

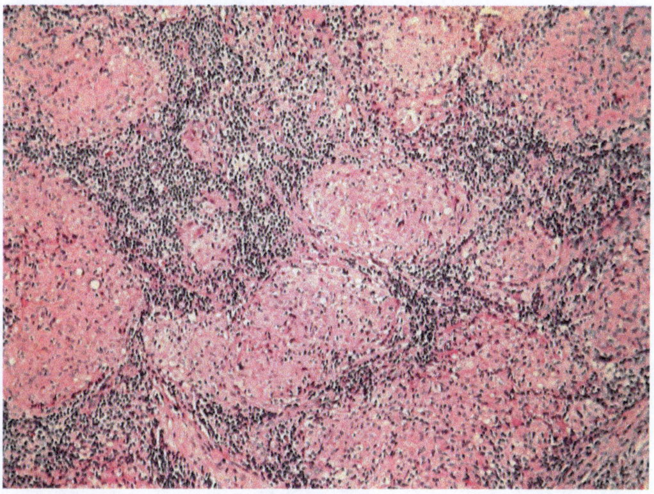

Fig. 7.28. Sarcoidosis. Discrete "hard" granulomas are closely packed in the node. Necrosis is absent.

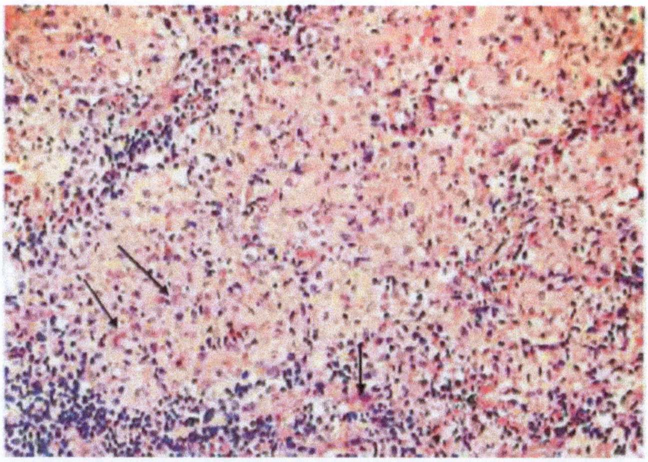

Fig. 7.29. The granulomas comprise epithelioid cells with surrounding lymphocytes and plasma cells. Multinucleated giant cells are present (*arrows*).

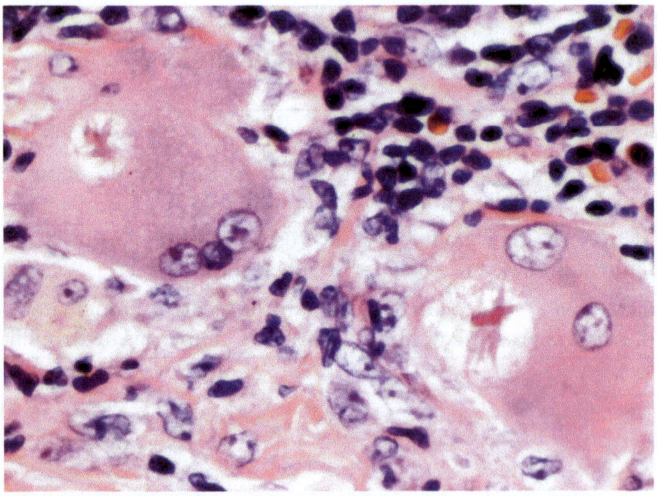

Fig. 7.30. Giant cells containing asteroid bodies which are eosinophilic stellate structures within a clear space.

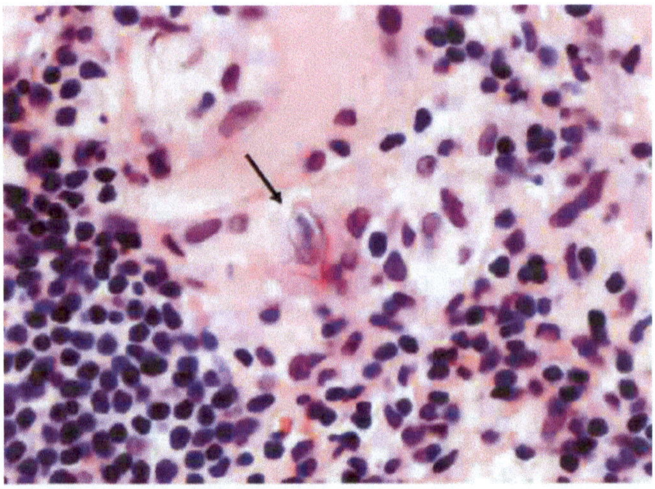

Fig. 7.31. Giant cell with Schaumann body (*arrow*). The calcified body shows concentric lamellation.

vesicular nuclei. Larger atypical proliferating blast cells are scattered throughout the infiltrate and inflammatory cells including plasma cells and eosinophils may be admixed. This pattern of reaction with numerous epithelioid histiocytes may be less commonly found in other types of T and B cell lymphomas (**Figs. 7.32, 7.33, 7.34**, and **7.35**).

Classical Hodgkin Lymphoma

Histiocytes are common among the non-neoplastic leucocytes that outnumber Hodgkin and Reed–Sternberg cells (HRS cells), and in a minority of mixed cellularity cases, epithelioid histiocytes

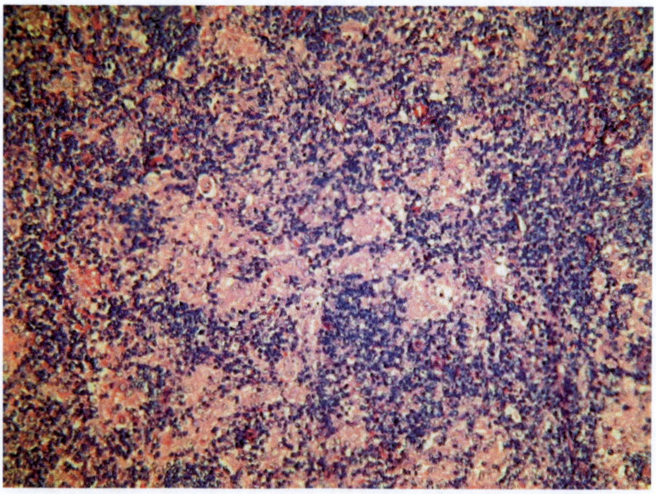

Fig. 7.32. PTCL-NOS, lymphoepithelioid variant (Lennert lymphoma). Clusters of epithelioid histiocytes infiltrate the section with intervening small- to medium-sized lymphocytes with irregular vesicular nuclei.

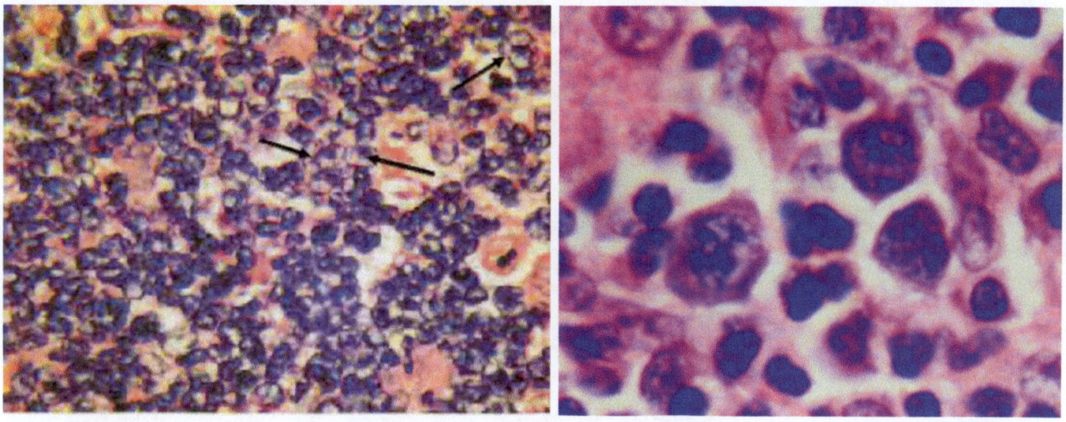

Fig. 7.33. Among the medium-sized lymphocytes and epithelioid histiocytes are large, multilobated proliferating blast cells with prominent nucleoli (*arrows*). *Inset* shows more atypical blast cells.

coalesce to form granulomas. The heterogeneity of the rest of the inflammatory cell population is striking in comparison to most other conditions associated with lymph node granulomas, with lymphocytes, plasma cells, eosinophils, and even neutrophils comprising the milieu in which diagnostic HRS cells are found.

Foreign Body and Lipid Granulomatous Lymphadenitis

The lymph node may show a prominent granulomatous response to a variety of foreign material and lipid, the latter of exogenous or endogenous origin. Foreign materials can be inhaled or implanted and include tattoo pigment and debris from prostheses. The foreign material may be pigmented, refractile, or birefringent and

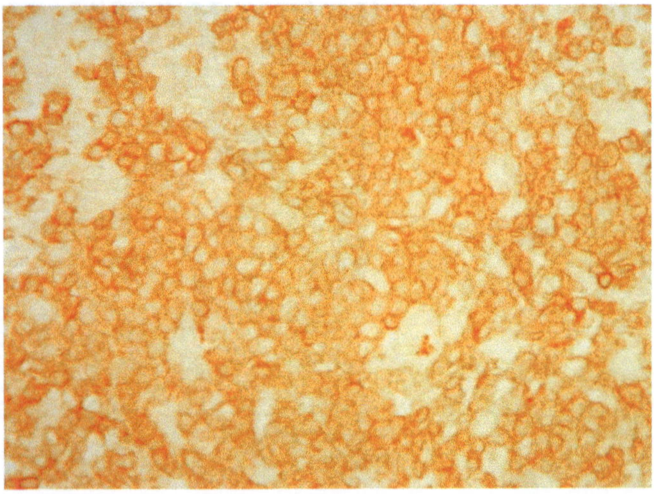

Fig. 7.34. The background medium-sized lymphocytes express CD3 and only scattered CD20+ cells are present (not shown).

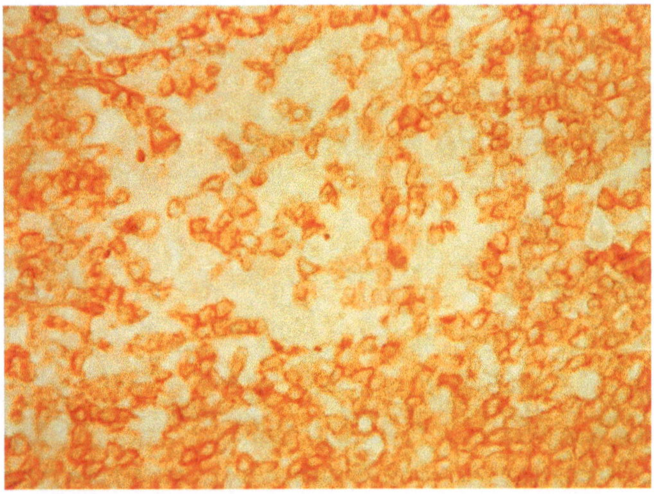

Fig. 7.35. The lymphoma cells are also CD8+. The large cells that do not label with the antibody are epithelioid histiocytes.

may evoke either no reaction or a reaction in the form of foreign body granulomas with or without necrosis.

Silicone Lymphadenopathy

Silicone, a methyl-polysiloxane, is used extensively in implantable medical devices employed in orthopedic and plastic surgery. The length of the polymer and extent of methylation and cross-linkage determine whether the polymer is in solid, gel, or liquid state, and the appearance of the embolized material varies accordingly. Silicone is not biodegradable and was thought to be relatively inert until shown to evoke a granulomatous response when embolized throughout the body as seen in patients on chronic dialysis when silicone tubing was employed in the peristaltic dialysis pump. In lymph nodes draining the site of a silicone prosthetic implant, a variable granulomatous response occurs, depending on particle size. Solid silicone produces a prominent granulomatous response with epithelioid and giant cells containing the silicone in the form of flakes and particles. Liquid silicone elicits less reaction and is seen as lipid-like vacuoles within lymph node sinuses and lymphoid parenchyma with or without a granulomatous response. A rim of oily-appearing silicone often remains at the periphery of these vacuoles. Silicone is refractile but not birefringent and is best seen when the substage diaphragm is partially closed or in Nomarski illumination. It is specifically identified by energy dispersive X-ray analysis (EDXA) or atomic absorption spectrometry (**Figs. 7.36**, **7.37**, **7.38**, **7.39**, **7.40**, **7.41**, and **7.42**).

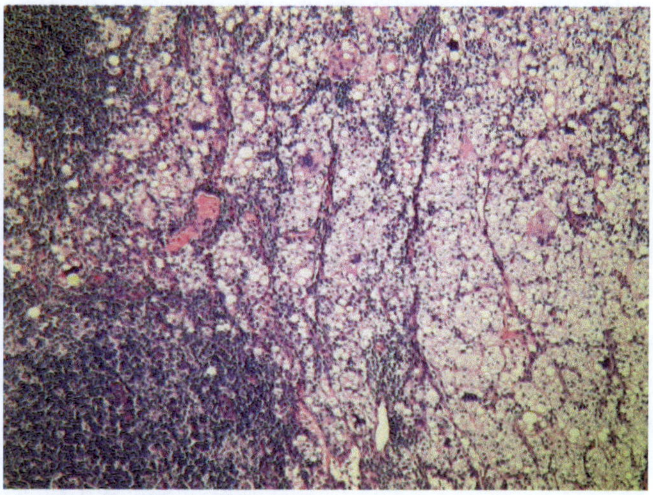

Fig. 7.36. Silicone lymphadenopathy in an axillary lymph node draining breast silicone prosthesis. There is a marked granulomatous response with sheets of foamy macrophages.

Detritic Lymphadenopathy

So-called detritic lymphadenopathy results from the histiocytic response to abraded metal and cementing material drained from the sites of joint prosthesis. Contemporary joint prostheses are made predominantly of composite metals that may include stainless steel, cobalt, chromium, and titanium; ceramics and polyethylene are often used for articular surfaces, and poly-methyl methacrylate is a common cementing material. With wear and tear, the superficial coating of the prosthesis and cementing material becomes released into the periarticular tissues. Tissue macrophages clear the wear debris and drain to regional nodes, producing a granulomatous response which can be marked and may mimic other granulomatous lymphadenitides

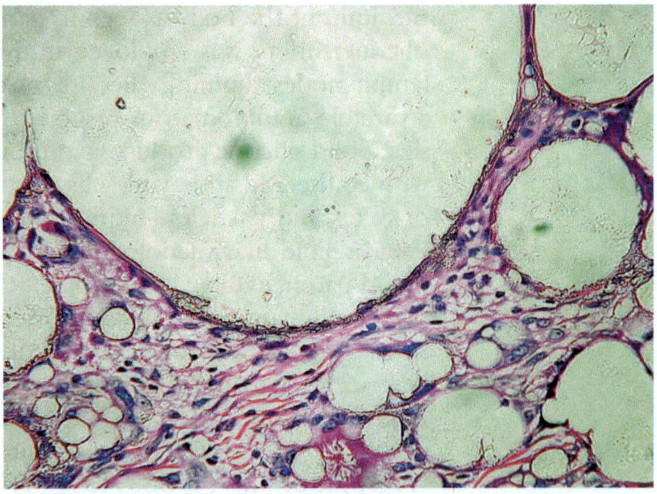

Fig. 7.37. The large vacuoles in the parenchyma and macrophages contain a transparent refractive but non-birefringent material (*arrows*) (substage diaphragm partially closed).

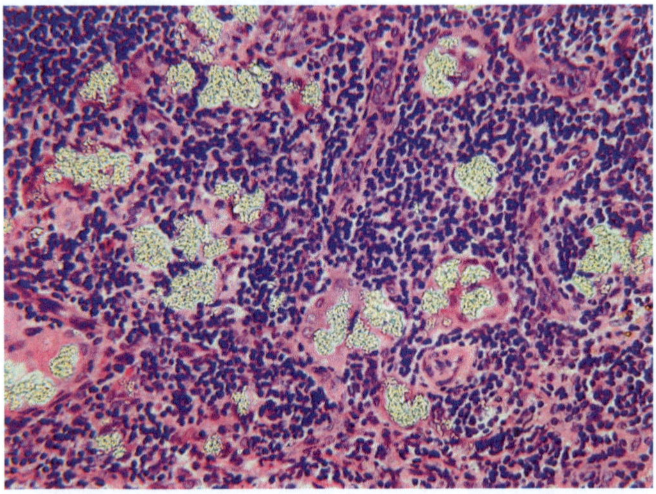

Fig. 7.38. Multinucleated giant cells contain flakes of refractile solid silicone abraded from a silicone joint prosthesis.

like Whipple disease, Rosai–Dorfman disease, and storage diseases. The abraded debris is found in the macrophages, especially polyethylene and poly-methyl–methacrylate, both of which are birefringent, together with irregular shards or flakes of titanium and cobalt which are black, refractile, and birefringent (**Figs. 7.43** and **7.44**).

Lipid Lymphadenopathy

Lipid incites a lipogranulomatous response in lymph nodes and may be exogenous or endogenous. The reactions are identical and the origin of the lipid is not identifiable other than by clinical

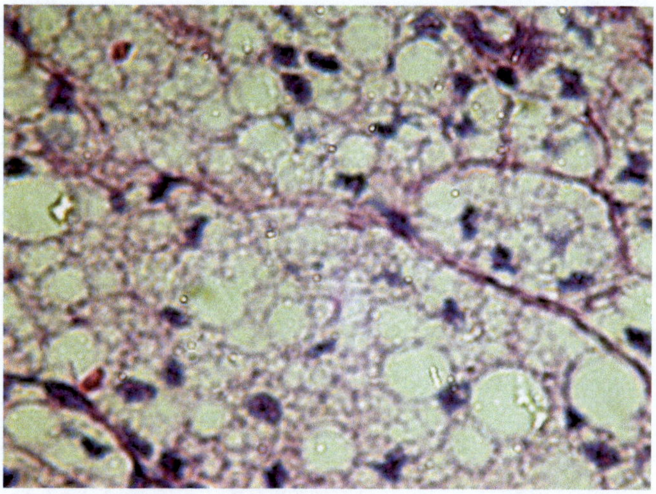

Fig. 7.39. Foamy macrophages filling lymph node sinuses contain flakes and irregular pieces of refractile, non-birefringent silicone leached from breast prosthesis (substage diaphragm partially closed).

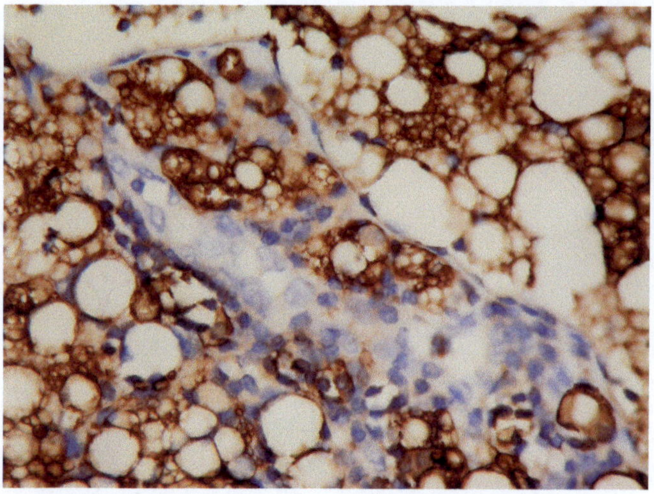

Fig. 7.40. CD68 stains the foam cells in silicone lymphadenopathy.

history. Lipogranulomas develop in draining lymph nodes in patients with gall bladder disease, and other sources of endogenous lipid include hematomas, xanthomatous lesions, tumors, fat emboli, necrotic fat, and cholesterol deposits. Exogenous lipid may be inhaled into the lungs to cause lipoid pneumonia and affect draining lymph nodes. A major source of exogenous lipid is from therapeutic lipid-based reagents as depots to enable slow release of injected drugs, paraffin-based emollients in dermatologic practice, and most commonly, contrast media for lymphangiography and bronchography.

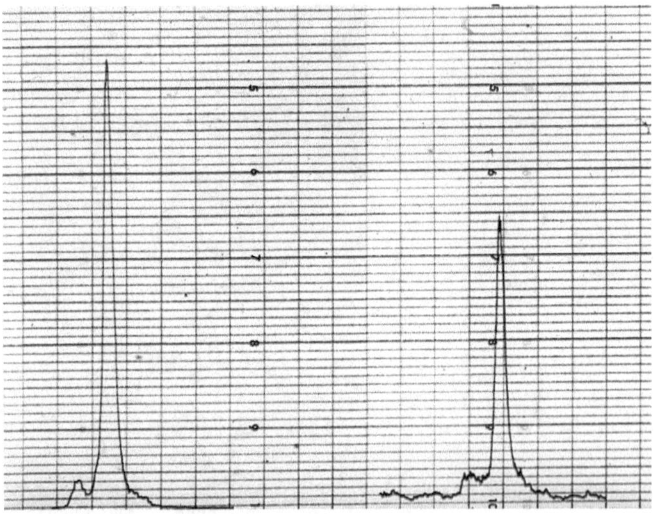

Fig. 7.41. EDXA of pure silicone (*left*) and lymph node tissue with silicone granuloma (*right*). The spectra are similar. A silicon peak identifies the compound silicone. Pure silicon does not occur naturally in the free state. Silicates have other cations like Na, Mg, Al, and K and do not have the optical qualities of silicone.

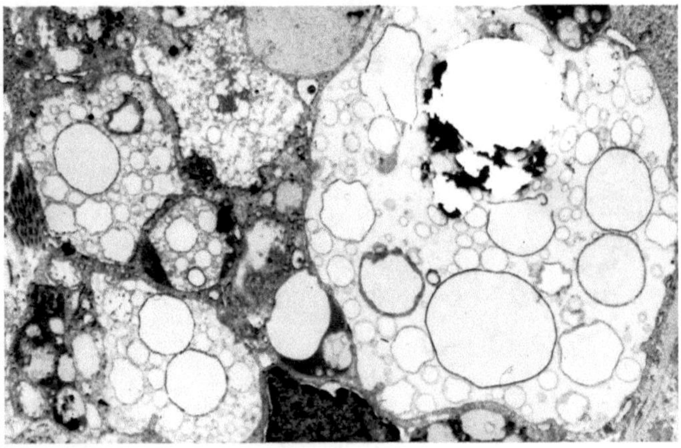

Fig. 7.42. Ultrastructural appearance of silicone in macrophages. The electron lucent compound tears like the epoxy embedding when bombarded with electrons.

Lipid is seen as microcysts and globules of fat, frequently in the subcapsular and medullary sinuses. A granulomatous response of epithelioid cells, macrophages, and giant cells forms around the lipid, and phagocytosed lipid appears as smaller vacuoles that may be stained by Sudan black stains. Lymphocytes, plasma cells, and occasional eosinophils accompany the reaction but discrete granulomas are seldom formed. The distinction from other causes of granulomatous lymphadenopathy is often not difficult (**Table 7.7**; **Fig. 7.45**).

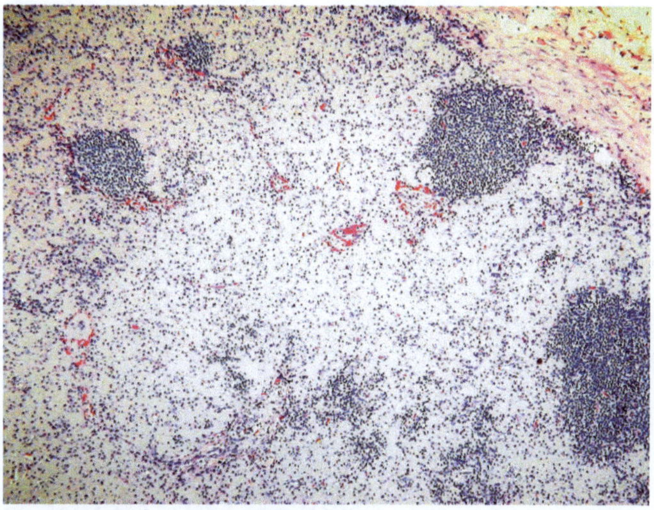

Fig. 7.43. Detritic lymphadenitis. A marked granulomatous response is present. Histiocytes with copious amounts of pale cytoplasm fill the cortex and paracortex with sparing of follicles.

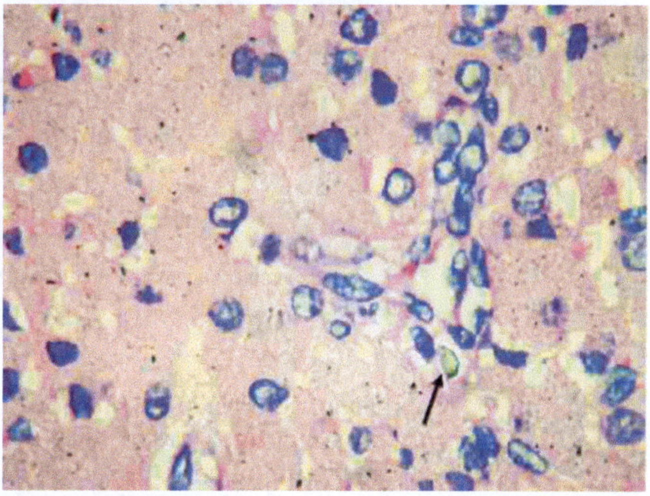

Fig. 7.44. Irregular shards of black cobalt are present in the macrophages and a flake of birefringent polymethylacrylate is seen (*arrow*).

Sinus Pattern

Prominence of the lymph node sinuses may result from a variety of conditions. Non-specific sinus histiocytosis is the most frequent cause of a sinus pattern; much less common etiologies include Rosai–Dorfman disease and incompletely developed examples of conditions described above such as granulomatous lymphadenitis

Table 7.7
Foreign body and lipid granulomatous lymphadenopathy

Silicone – From breast and joint prosthesis; refractile, non-birefringent oily droplets and solid flakes and granules
Detritic material – Commonly cobalt, chromium (both black), polyethylene, ceramic, and poly(methyl methacrylate), all birefringent and refractile
Endogenous lipid – From hematomas, diseased biliary system, xanthomas, cholesterol deposits, tumor, necrotic fat
Exogenous lipid – From lymphangiogram, paraffin-based emollients, lipid-based depots of drugs

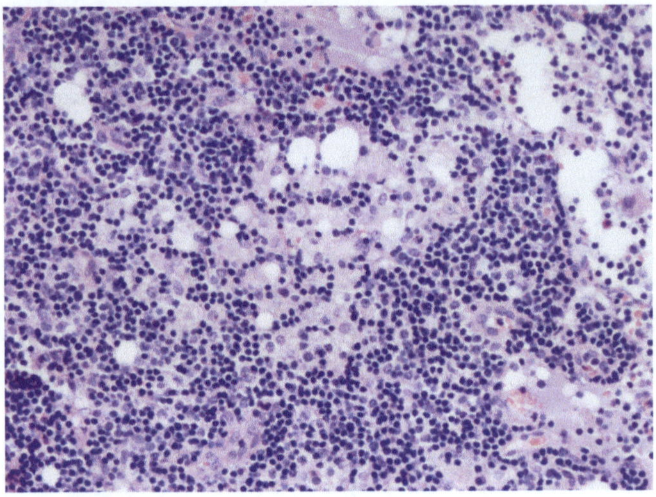

Fig. 7.45. Lipogranulomatous reaction in a lymph node from around the neck of the gallbladder.

and lymphadenopathies. Metastatic carcinoma cells are often distributed in a sinus pattern, while lymphoid malignancies exhibit such a distribution less frequently. Anaplastic large cell lymphoma is the most common such example, and rarely a diffuse large B cell lymphoma may exhibit such a pattern.

Sinus Histiocytosis

Sinus hyperplasia or sinus histiocytosis is a common non-specific reaction found in lymph nodes. It may be the most prominent finding or may be associated with follicular hyperplasia or paracortical hyperplasia. It can be found in lymph nodes draining neoplasms or infectious foci but often the etiology is not known. Histologically it is characterized by expanded sinuses filled with histiocytes (macrophages). The latter are benign-appearing and uniform in appearance with ample quantities of cytoplasm, and oval, sometimes with indented nuclei that contain inconspicuous nucleoli. In thoracic hilar and mediastinal nodes, the histiocytes often contain variable amounts of carbon pigment that can be seen macroscopically. Erythrophagocytosis and hemosiderin pigment may be seen in the histiocytes in patients with hemolytic anemia or after blood transfusion, but the bland cytological appearances, barely discernable nucleoli, and low level of erythrophagocytosis distinguish the histiocytes in this condition from those of Rosai–Dorfman disease (*see* below; **Figs. 7.46** and **7.47**).

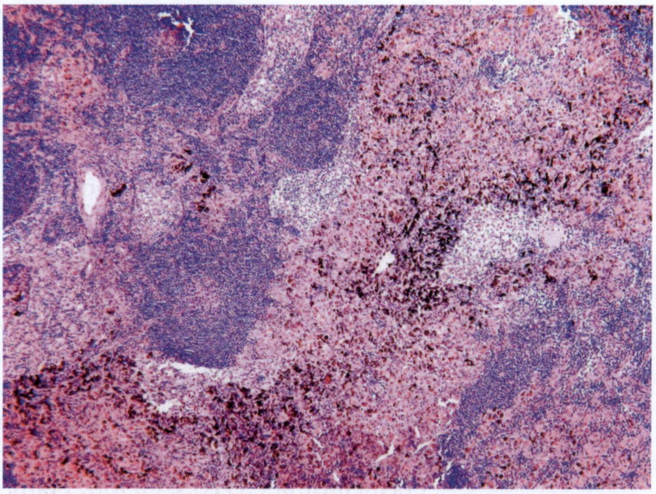

Fig. 7.46. Sinus histiocytosis in a thoracic lymph node. The sinuses are distended by carbon-containing histiocytes/macrophages with intervening small lymphocytes and germinal centers.

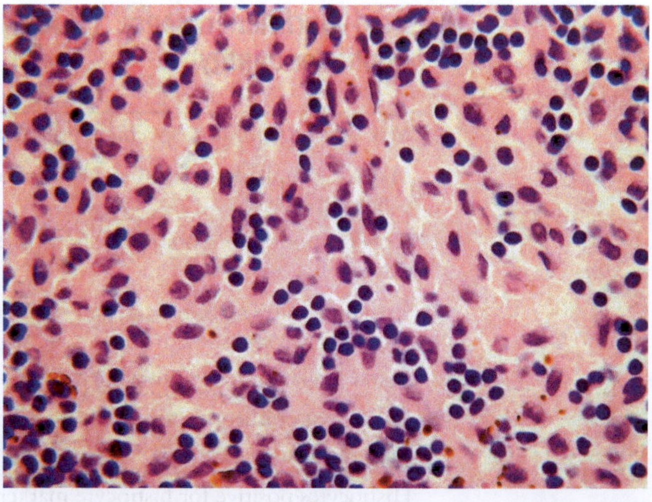

Fig. 7.47. The histiocytes are bland appearing and have oval nuclei with inconspicuous nucleoli and ample cytoplasm.

Rosai–Dorfman Disease (Sinus Histiocytosis with Massive Lymphadenopathy)

Rosai–Dorfman disease or sinus histiocytosis with massive lymphadenopathy (SHML), a disease of unknown etiology, produces massive enlargement of bilateral, mostly cervical lymph nodes. One-third of the patients have involvement of extranodal sites. Virtually any extranodal site may be involved; commonly these include the head and neck, soft tissue, skin, upper respiratory tract, gastrointestinal tract, breast, bones, and central nervous system. The enlarged nodes are painless and the patients may have non-specific febrile illness but are generally well. The disease is self-limited and the nodes eventually recede. Involved nodes are large and matted. There is capsular fibrosis and surrounding connective tissue. The most striking feature is marked dilatation of the sinuses which are filled with histiocytes, lymphocytes, plasma cells, and lymph. The histiocytes have vesicular nuclei containing one distinct nucleolus but do not display mitotic activity. The cytoplasm is eosinophilic and abundant, showing marked phagocytosis of lymphocytes, plasma cells, and erythrocytes. The phagocytosed lymphocytes are contained in vacuoles and usually remain intact and viable, a phenomenon called "emperipolesis" or they may be degraded, appearing as nuclear fragments. The medullary sinuses contain numerous plasma cells, mature lymphocytes, and aggregates of lipid-laden macrophages. Perisinusoidal areas also contain the same cells. The histiocytes stain with histiocytic markers including CD163, CD68, Ham56, and Mac387 as well as with antibodies to S100, lysozyme, and alpha-1-antitrypsin. They may also express CD4 and CD30, a property of macrophages derived from circulating monocytes (**Table 7.8**; **Figs. 7.48**, **7.49**, **7.50**, and **7.51**).

Table 7.8
Rosai–Dorfman disease (sinus histiocytosis with massive lymphadenopathy)

May present with non-specific febrile illness but generally well
Massive lymphadenopathy, painless, may persist for several years, self-limited disease
Cervical nodes commonly affected, one-third have extranodal involvement
Extranodal sites include head and neck, soft tissue, skin, upper respiratory tract, gastrointestinal tract, breast, bones, CNS
Marked dilatation of sinuses by benign-appearing histiocytes
Prominent erythrophagocytosis and emperipolesis
Rare mitosis, no necrosis
Histiocytes positive for histiocyte markers, viz, CD68, CD163, Mac387, Ham56, S100

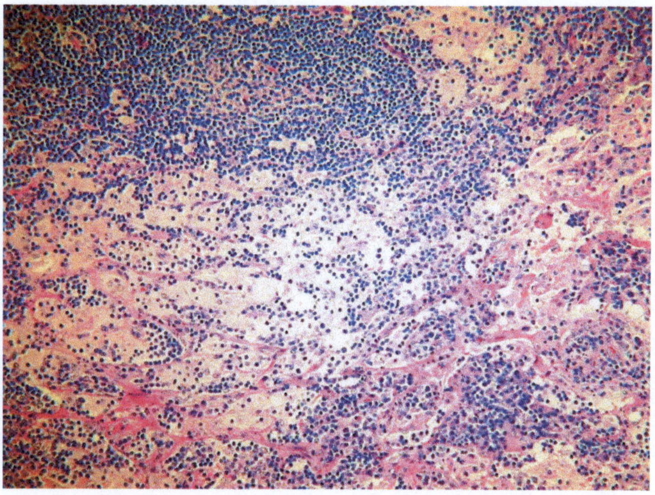

Fig. 7.48. SHML. The sinuses and perisinusoidal tissue contain large cells with abundant pale cytoplasm. Follicles are preserved.

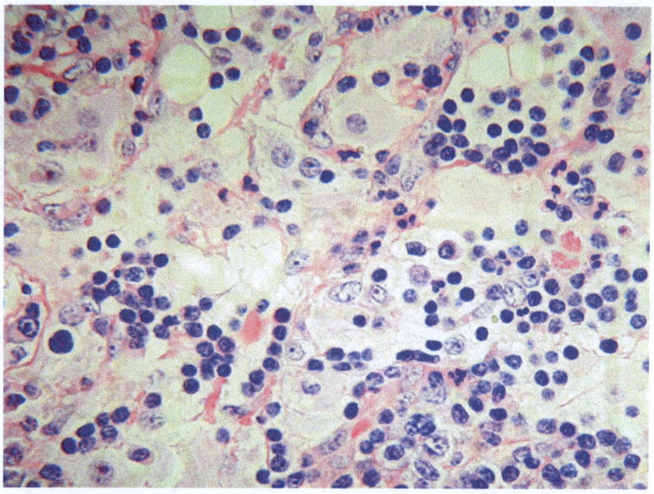

Fig. 7.49. SHML. Background cells are lymphocytes, stimulated cells, and plasma cells. The histiocytes have copious quantities of pale cytoplasm, vesicular nuclei, and small nucleoli. Mitosis is absent.

Necrosis, Apoptosis, and Infarction

At least two forms of cell death can be observed in lymph nodes, namely, necrosis, which is pathological, and apoptosis, which is a form of programmed cell death. While these changes often occur in small foci, they can occasionally be striking and involve multiple foci or larger areas of the lymph node. The changes in the tissue surrounding such areas or foci of necrosis or apoptosis

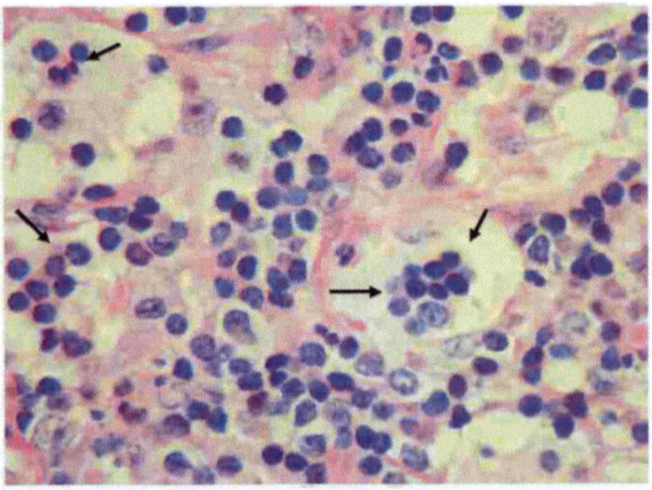

Fig. 7.50. SHML. Lymphocytes and plasma cells are found within the histiocytes (emperipolesis), sometimes in large numbers (*arrows*). The cells are intact and appear viable.

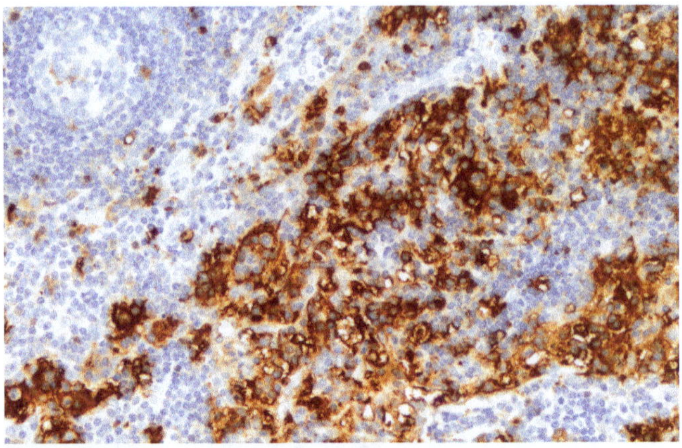

Fig. 7.51. SHML. The histiocytes stain for S100 and also for CD68 and CD163 (not shown). Note the preserved germinal center in the upper left field.

often provide clues to the diagnosis. For example, necrosis occurs within areas of granulomatous response or more discrete granulomas as in the necrotizing granulomatous lymphadenopathies, most of these entities being previously discussed.

Infarction rarely occurs because of the abundant vascularity and anastomoses in lymph nodes. On the rare occasion that infarction occurs, it is due to occlusive vascular thrombosis affecting hilar or intranodal veins and can involve both superficial and deep-seated lymph nodes. Infarction has been described following local trauma from surgery or biopsy. It has been associated with disseminated intravascular coagulation, infectious mononucleosis, systemic lupus erythematosus, cholesterol emboli from atheroma, and intramuscular injection of gold for treatment of rheumatoid arthritis. The most common cause of massive lymph node infarction is due to tumor, most often lymphoma (e.g., DLBCL), followed by metastatic carcinoma, melanoma and granulocytic sarcoma, and vascular impairment from obstruction or compression.

Among the infectious lymphadenitides, *Herpes simplex* is the most common infection to produce extensive necrosis. Less often, extensive necrosis from Kikuchi disease can mimic infarction. In *H. simplex* lymphadenitis, the necrosis can be extensive with only a peripheral rim of lymph node tissue remaining viable. A zone of histiocytes is present at the periphery of the necrotic area which contains numerous apoptotic bodies, some neutrophils, and sheets of degenerating cells. A careful search may reveal the virus in the form of Cowdry nuclear inclusions that stain for viral proteins by immunohistochemistry. It should be noted that immunohistochemistry is often useful even when the tissue is infarcted as antigens are often preserved and can be detected, giving a clue as to the nature of the infarcted tissue (**Figs. 7.52** and **7.53**).

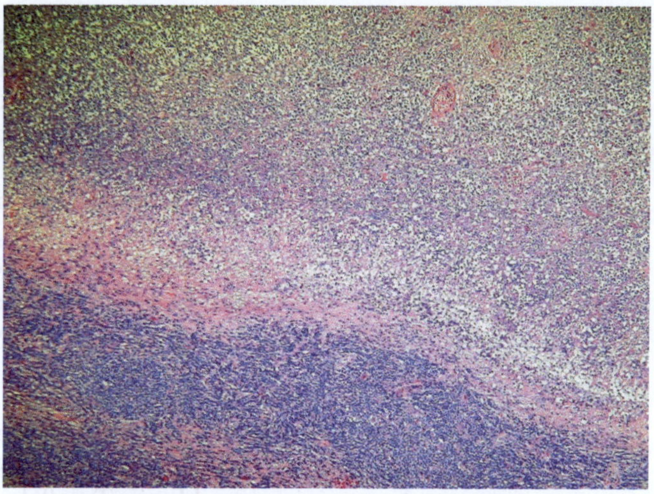

Fig. 7.52. *H. simplex* lymphadenitis. There is extensive necrosis with a zone of histiocytes separating the peripheral rim of preserved lymph node tissue.

Clear Cells

The presence of sheets of cells with moderate quantities of clear or pale cytoplasm and distinct cell outlines can be a striking feature against the dark blue background of lymphoid cells. Aside from monocytoid B cells, which may be especially prominent in toxoplasmosis and HIV lymphadenitis, and macrophages, clear cells with distinct cell outlines that accumulate in sheets are

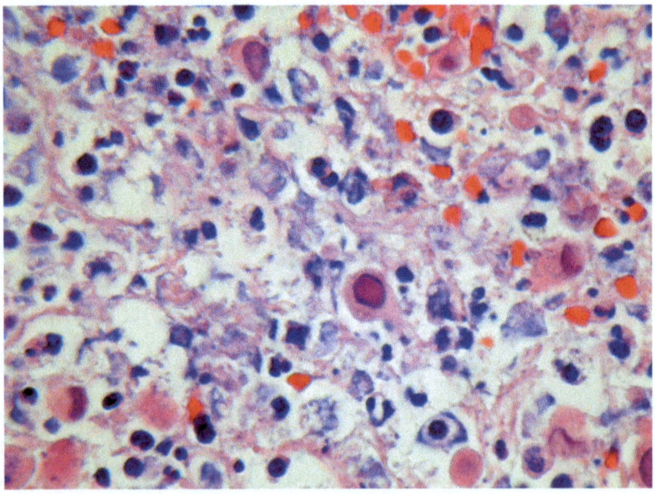

Fig. 7.53. The necrotic areas show degenerating cells, apoptotic bodies, and karyorrhectic debris. Several cells contain Cowdry B viral inclusions.

largely exogenous to the lymph node. They frequently represent metastatic carcinoma with glycogen-rich cytoplasm in which case the nodal architecture is often destroyed by the infiltrating tumor. Among the metastatic tumors that can show clear cell change are those from the lung, kidney, ovary, melanoma, and clear cell sarcoma. A panel of antibodies comprising broad-spectrum cytokeratin, CK20, TTF1, RCA, CD10, and HMB45 will help provide specific identification of the source of the metastasis. Less frequently, mast cells can present as monotonous sheets of clear cells within the lymph node, partially or completely effacing nodal architecture. A similar appearance may be imparted by hairy cell leukemia when it involves the lymph node. Marginal zone B cell lymphomas often exhibit monocytoid cytology at least focally. T cell lymphomas may sometimes display clear cytoplasm (for example, angioimmunoblastic T cell lymphoma), but such cells are often smaller than mast cells, hairy cells, and carcinoma cells.

Mast Cell Disease

The WHO classifies mastocytosis into cutaneous mastocytosis, indolent systemic mastocytosis, systemic mastocytosis with associated clonal hematological non-mast-cell lineage disease, aggressive systemic mastocytosis, mast cell leukemia, mast cell sarcoma, and extracutaneous mastocytoma.

The lymph node may be involved in all forms of mastocytosis but significant lymphadenopathy is uncommon. The mast cell infiltrate may involve any of the lymph node compartments but paracortical areas are most commonly infiltrated either focally or diffusely, rarely totally effacing the architecture. Lymphoid follicles are generally spared and are hyperplastic, vascularity is prominent, and plasmacytosis, eosinophilia, and fibrosis usually accompany mast cell infiltrates. The mast cells may contain basophilic cytoplasmic granules and stain metachromatic with toluidine blue or cresyl violet stains. They are labeled by antibodies to CD45, CD25, CD2, CD117, and mast cell tryptase (**Figs. 7.54**, **7.55**, **7.56**, **7.57**, **7.58**, and **7.59**).

Hairy Cell Leukemia

Lymphadenopathy in hairy cell leukemia (HCL) is uncommon, although in earlier reported series, the incidence was as high as 25–35%. Nodal involvement is perhaps related with high tumor

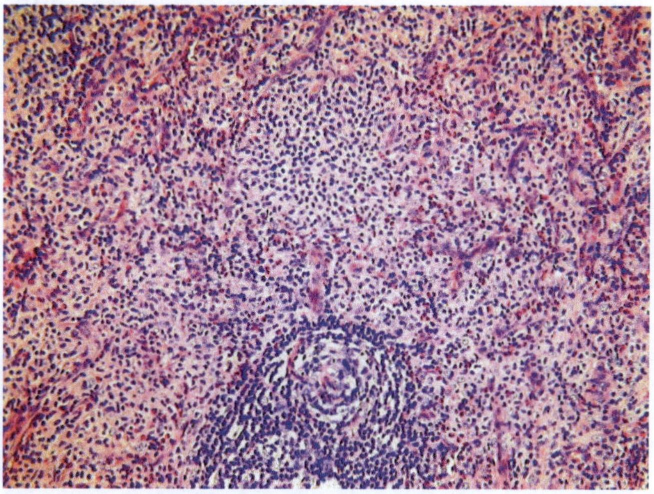

Fig. 7.54. Mastosis. Uniform-appearing cells with moderate quantities of clear cytoplasm infiltrate the cortex diffusely with sparing of the lymphoid follicle. There is prominent vascular proliferation in the paracortex.

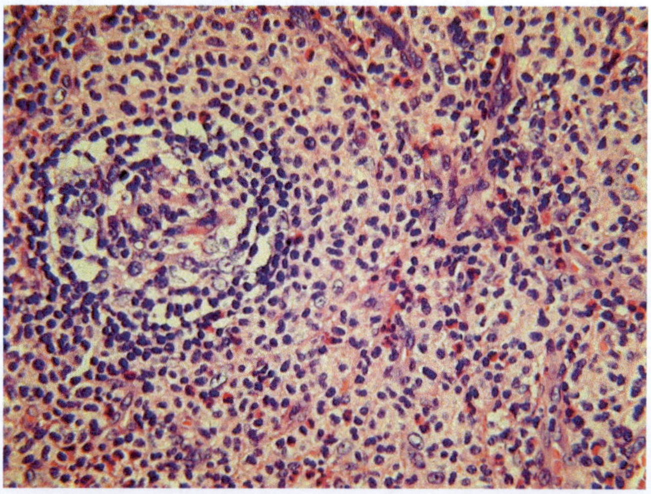

Fig. 7.55. Eosinophils are present among the mast cells that infiltrate around a follicle. Note the prominent vascular background.

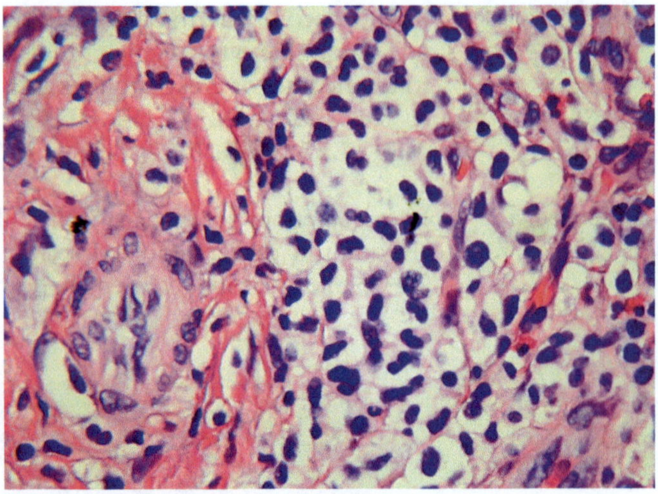

Fig. 7.56. The mast cells have bland kidney-shaped nuclei and moderate amounts of pale cytoplasm. Increased reticulin is evident in the lymph node parenchyma.

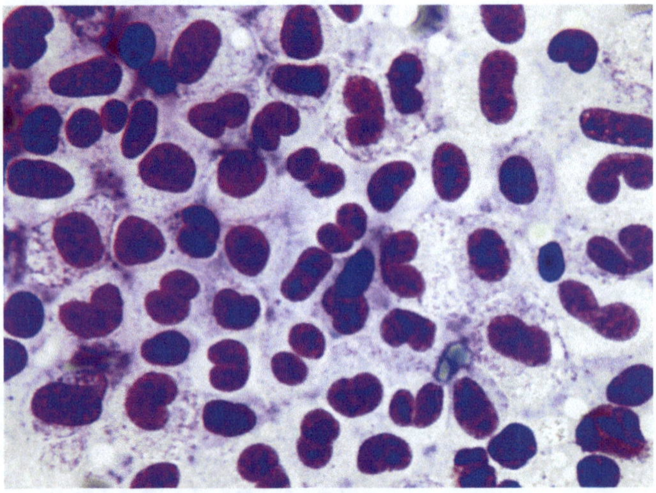

Fig. 7.57. Imprint of mast cells showing bland reniform nuclei with moderate quantities of pale blue cytoplasm. The cells in the lower left field contain azurophilic cytoplasmic granules.

burden or transformation to higher grade disease. Similarly, visceral involvement can also occur in a subset of patients, commonly involving liver, lungs, gastrointestinal tract, pancreas, kidneys, and adrenal glands. Rarely, the meninges, bone, pleura, and skin may be involved. As in the spleen and other viscera, HCL infiltrates diffusely as sheets of bland-appearing, monotonous cells with oval nuclei and moderate quantities of pale blue or clear cytoplasm. Cell membranes are distinct, imparting a fried-egg

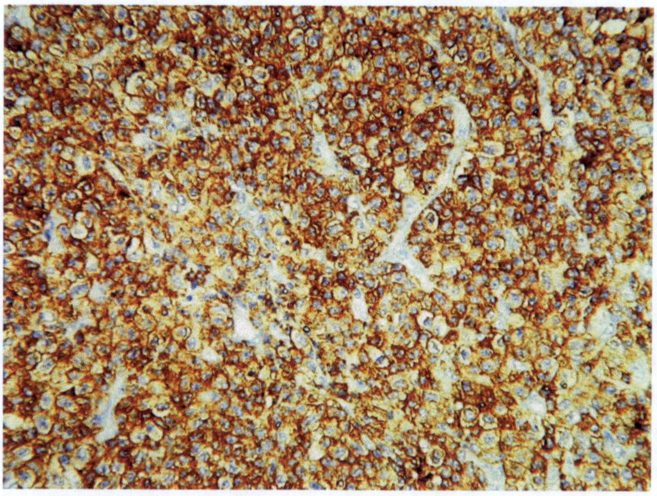

Fig. 7.58. Mast cell tumor in systemic mastocytosis. Mast cells label for CD45.

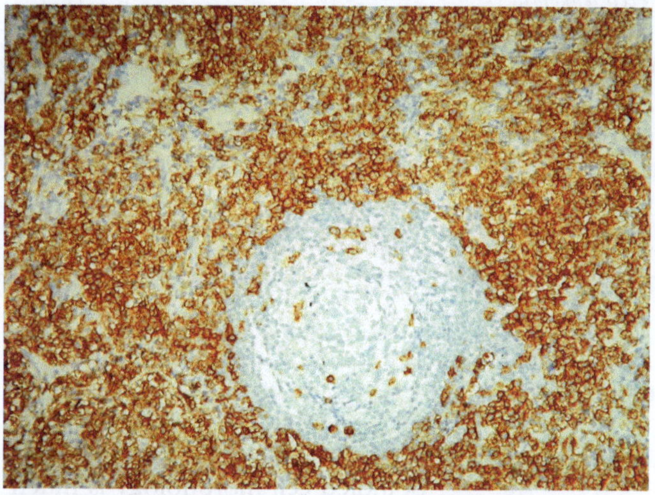

Fig. 7.59. CD117 stains the mast cells and spares the germinal center.

or frogs' spawn appearance. The cell membranes may be frayed especially when the hairy cells are observed in vascular spaces. The chromatin is coarsely clumped and a single small nucleolus may be discernable. The hairy cells stain for tartrate-resistant acid phosphatase, best performed on imprints or smears, and express CD45, CD20, CD79a, CD25, and CD72 (DBA.44). CyclinD1 may be weakly expressed. They are negative for CD5 and CD10. A further description is provided in **Chapter 8** (**Table 7.9**).

Table 7.9
Defining microscopic feature – clear cells

Toxoplasmosis – Monocytoid B cell hyperplasia
HIV lymphadenitis – Monocytoid B cell hyperplasia
Marginal zone B cell lymphoma – Neoplastic B cells with monocytoid features are commonly part of a heterogenous population
Angioimmunoblastic T cell lymphoma – Neoplastic T cells often surrounding vessels
Metastatic tumors
Carcinomas of lung, kidney, ovary, metastatic melanoma, and clear cell sarcoma
Employ immunohistochemistry to identify source of metastasis
Mast cell tumor
Uncommonly occurs in all forms of mastocytosis
Partial involvement of cortex and paracortex with sparing of follicles
Sheets of mast cells with eosinophils, plasma cells, and variable fibrosis
Stain metachromatic with toluidine blue and cresyl violet
CD45+, CD117+, CD25+, and mast cell tryptase+
Hairy cell leukemia
Uncommonly involves lymph nodes, probably related to tumor burden or transformation to high-grade disease
Monotonous sheets of bland-appearing cells with oval nuclei, coarse chromatin, moderate quantities of pale cytoplasm, and distinct cell membranes imparting fried-egg appearance
CD45+, CD20+, CD25+, CD72 (DBA.44)+, TRAP+, cyclinD1+/–
CD5–, CD10–
Ribosome lamella complex, hairy cytoplasmic projections

Spindled Cells

Spindled cell morphology is much more frequently encountered in neoplasms of histiocytic or dendritic cell origin than in lymphomas; neoplasms arising from mesenchymal elements in lymph nodes may also exhibit spindled cell features. Spindled cells may be encountered infrequently in large cell lymphomas such as anaplastic large cell lymphoma and diffuse large B cell lymphoma, while such cell is more prominent in a subset of lymphocyte-depleted classical Hodgkin lymphoma cases. Rarely, peripheral T cell lymphomas may show areas of spindling. In contrast, spindled cells are typical of follicular dendritic cell (FDC) sarcoma and interdigitating dendritic cell (IDRC) sarcoma, and they may also be encountered in histiocytic sarcoma; these entities and their immunohistochemical distinction have been described in detail previously. Rare examples of metastatic carcinoma may exhibit sarcomatoid morphology. In rare cases of *Mycobacterium avium-intracellulare*, the histiocytes adopt a spindled morphology and form bundles in lymph nodes ("pseudotumors").

Inflammatory Myofibroblastic Tumor

Inflammatory myofibroblastic tumor, previously known as inflammatory pseudotumor, can occur in many extranodal sites including lung, liver, spleen, intestines, pancreas, urinary bladder, orbit, and skin and is rarely associated with involvement of draining lymph nodes. It represents an exaggerated inflammatory process with proliferation of myofibroblasts and fibroblasts in a background of inflammation and prominent vessels. It is associated with non-specific systemic symptoms including fever, and Epstein–Barr virus has been found in the spindle cells in half to two-thirds of extranodal cases. The pathological changes are progressive and commence with replacement of the lymphoid tissue by inflammatory cells and fibroblastic and vascular proliferation in regions where there is most connective tissue including the hilum, trabeculae, and capsule. These changes eventually subside to give way to dense sclerosis and hyalinization, with residual pockets of inflammation. The fibroblastic proliferation is admixed with lymphocytes, plasma cells, and neutrophils, but eosinophils are neither seen nor is there necrosis. The endothelial cells lining the proliferating vessels are flattened or low cuboidal in shape, and occasional giant cells and epithelioid histiocytes may be present. The spindle cells are mostly myofibroblasts and express smooth muscle actin and are ensheathed by thin fragmented basal lamina as outlined with type-IV collagen or laminin. They may stain for ALK protein. The perinodal tissue shows changes of panniculitis and focal vasculitis if frequently present (**Figs. 7.60**, **7.61**, **7.62**, and **7.63**).

Palisaded Myofibroblastoma

Palisaded myofibroblastoma is an asymptomatic intranodal proliferation of spindled myofibroblastic cells with stellate deposits of collagen and areas of hemorrhage. The majority have been described in groin nodes, although other sites have been reported. Grossly, areas of hemorrhage may be visible and the node characteristically shows several features that include partial or complete replacement by a proliferation of crisscrossing spindled cells with thin tapered nuclei which are often aligned to produce palisades, compressed lymph node tissue at the periphery, intraparenchymal hemorrhage and extravasation of red cells, intracellular and extracellular fuchsinophilic bodies, and so-called amianthoid fibers which occurs in almost all cases. The latter are deposits of eosinophilic collagen with circular or stellate outlines and a central core of homogenous densely eosinophilic collagen bundles that radiate out as hair-like spokes surrounded by a peripheral zone of weakly eosinophilic or pale zone. The radiating fibers resemble amianthoid fibers thought to represent

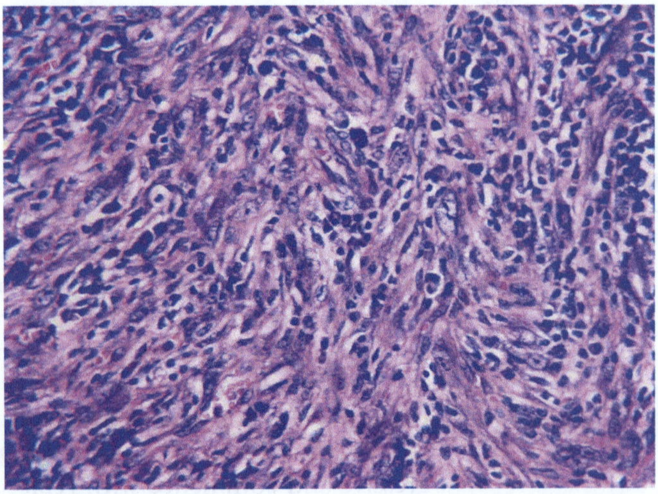

Fig. 7.60. Inflammatory myofibroblastic pseudotumor, axillary node. There is a mixed cellular proliferation of inflammatory cells, vessels, and fibroblasts.

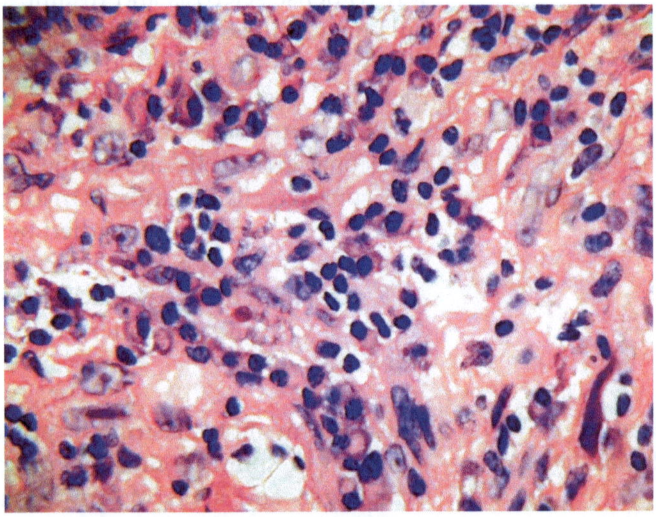

Fig. 7.61. Close-up appearance showing groups of lymphocytes, plasma cells, and histiocytes in between proliferating fibroblasts.

degenerate or so-called crystalline collagen. However, electron microscopy has not confirmed the presence of amianthoid characteristics and the fibers display characteristics of collagen. The tumor nodule is separated from compressed lymph node tissue by a thick pseudocapsule. The spindle cells stain for smooth muscle actin which also highlights the fuchsinophilic bodies. They also show strong expression of cyclinD1 and a low Ki67 count and are S100–, CD34– and GFAP–. Electron microscopy demonstrates thin fragmented basal lamina investing the spindle cells, well-developed rough endoplasmic reticulum, and cytoplasmic dense

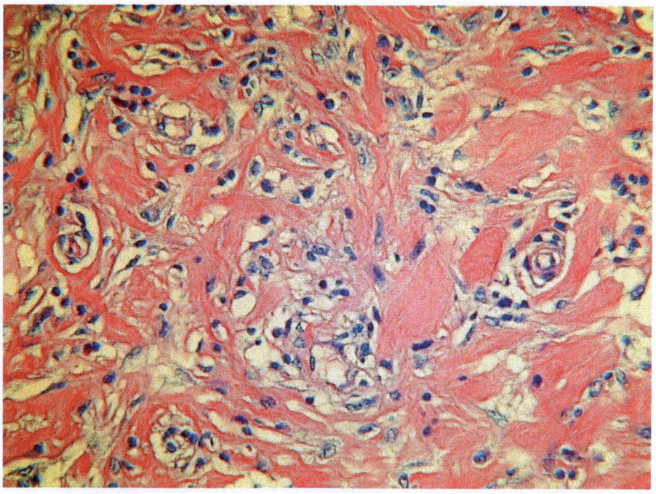

Fig. 7.62. In more advanced areas, the fibrosis is dense and hyalinized with small collections of intervening lymphoid cells and vessels.

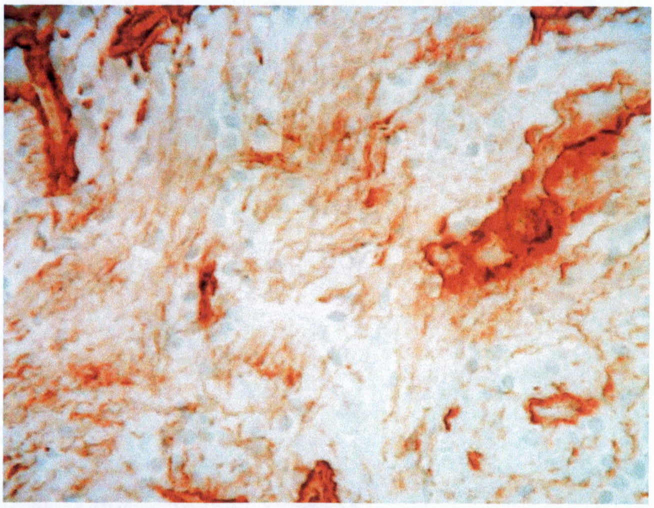

Fig. 7.63. Thin-fragmented basal lamina invests the spindle cells, a feature of myofibroblasts which also stain for alpha-smooth muscle actin (not shown).

bodies, characteristics of myofibroblasts (**Figs. 7.64**, **7.65**, **7.66**, and **7.67**).

Kaposi Sarcoma

Kaposi sarcoma is a vascular tumor encountered rarely and sporadically among immunocompetent individuals outside of central Africa (a region of endemicity), but much more frequently in immunocompromised populations. The incidence is especially high among people with AIDS and is also increased, although to a lesser degree, in transplant recipients. Most cases of Kaposi sarcoma are multicentric, with involvement of skin, lymph nodes,

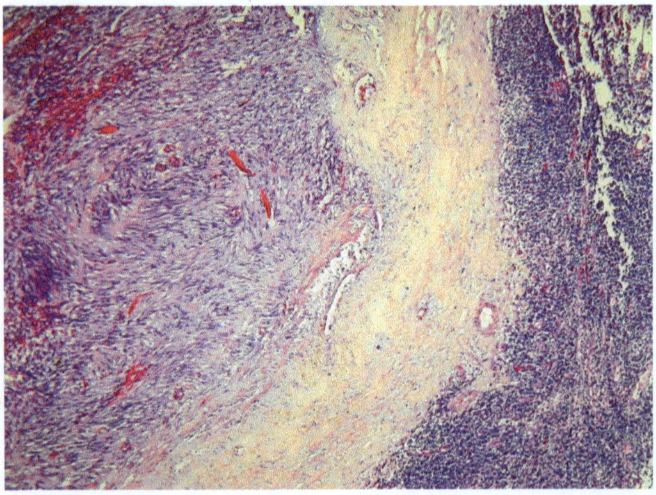

Fig. 7.64. Palisaded myofibroblastoma in inguinal node. A thick pseudocapsule separates the spindle cell proliferation from the compressed lymph node tissue. Areas of hemorrhage are present but necrosis is not evident.

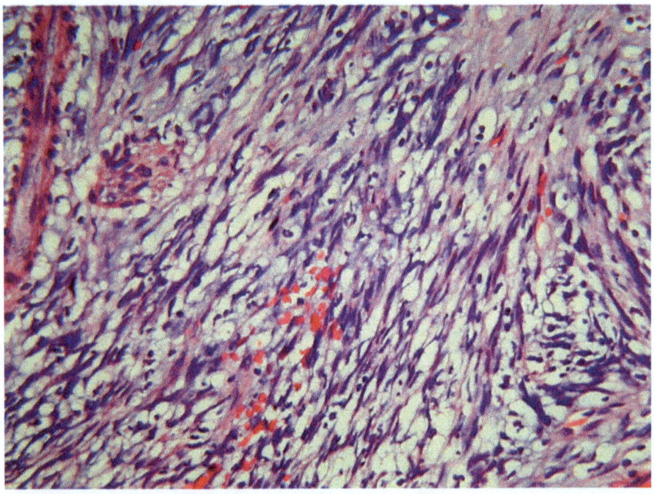

Fig. 7.65. The spindle cells have thin-tapered nuclei that do not display atypia or mitosis. There are extravasated red cells present.

and viscera, and most demonstrate detectable human herpesvirus 8 (HHV-8).

Affected lymph nodes show capsular involvement by a proliferation of spindled cells that form nodules with slit-like vascular spaces containing erythrocytes. Variation in vascular morphology may be observed within and between cases, and this is thought potentially to reflect the degree of differentiation. Nodal involvement typically progresses along trabeculae to the medulla.

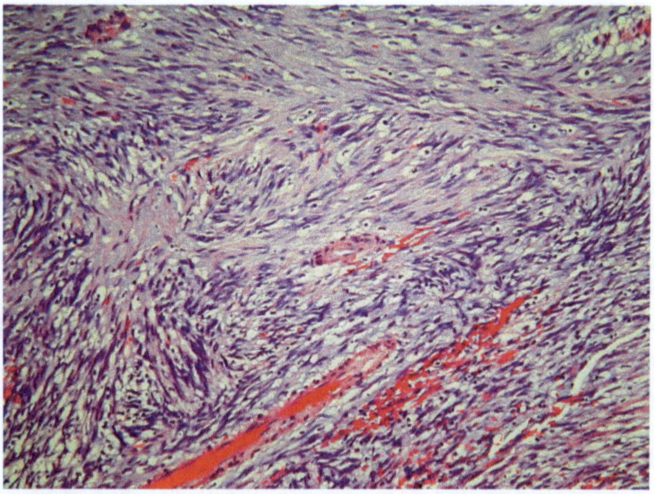

Fig. 7.66. The spindled tumor shows focal areas with a storiform pattern and focal hemorrhage is present.

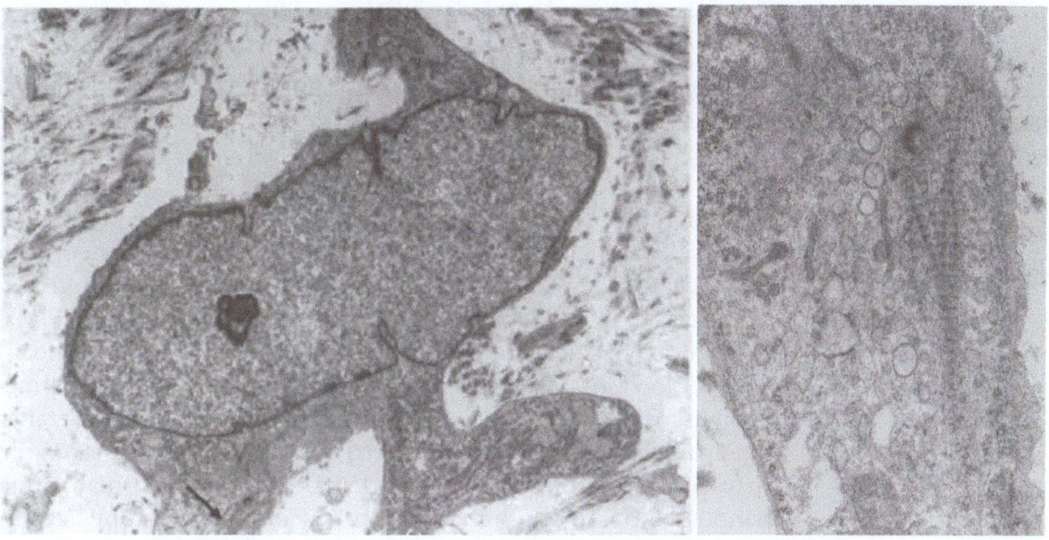

Fig. 7.67. Electron micrograph of palisaded myofibroblastoma showing dense body (*arrow* and *inset*) and abundant rough endoplasmic reticulum, scanty mitochondria, and thin-fragmented basal lamina investing the cell.

Cytologic atypia and mitotic activity are modest, and plasmacytic proliferation is common, as is preservation of reactive follicles. Immunohistochemistry shows positivity of the spindled cells for endothelial markers such as CD31 and CD34, as well as for vimentin and (variably) factor-VIII-related antigen. The presence of HHV-8 may be confirmed by immunohistochemical staining for latent nuclear antigen (**Table 7.10**).

Table 7.10
Defining microscopic feature – spindled cells

Large cell lymphoma – Rare ALCL, DLBCL with spindled cells; lymphocyte-depleted classical Hodgkin lymphoma may have a prominent component
Follicular dendritic cell sarcoma – Small nucleoli, mild cytologic atypia; may arise in association with Castleman disease (hyaline–vascular)
Interdigitating dendritic cell sarcoma – Prominent nucleoli, storiform pattern; interdigitating cell junctions seen using electron microscopy
Mycobacterium avium-intracellulare – Rarely, the organism-containing histiocytes feature spindled morphology and form bundles ("pseudotumors")
Inflammatory myofibroblastic tumor – Constitutional symptoms; EBV association in many cases; fibroblastic and vascular proliferation accompanied by a mixed leucocytic infiltrate; ALK detectable immunohistochemically
Palisaded myofibroblastoma – Asymptomatic, usually involving groin nodes; nodule composed of spindled cells with admixture of collagen deposits (amianthoid fibers)
Kaposi sarcoma – Vascular tumor; HHV-8 associated; may be sporadic but much more frequently seen in the settings of AIDS, other immunocompromised states; spindled cell proliferation with vascular slits containing erythrocytes; capsular involvement with progression to trabeculae; plasmacytic proliferation; CD31, CD34 expressed

Vascular Prominence

A spectrum of reactive and neoplastic conditions may give rise to increased vascularity of the lymph node. The lymphoid neoplasm most closely associated with vascular proliferation is angioimmunoblastic T cell lymphoma, in which arborizing small vessels are often surrounded by neoplastic T cells with abundant clear cytoplasm. Hyalinized small blood vessels are sometimes prominent in mantle cell lymphoma. Vascular neoplasms ranging from benign (hemangioma) to malignant (Kaposi sarcoma) may also arise infrequently. Castleman disease and rheumatoid lymphadenopathy both may feature vascular proliferation accompanied by plasmacytosis, but the latter lacks follicles exhibiting hyaline–vascular changes. Vascular proliferation accelerates with progression of HIV lymphadenitis. The Azzopardi phenomenon in which basophilic DNA material is seen in vessel walls accentuates blood vessels in lymphadenopathy associated with systemic lupus erythematosus. In Kimura disease, marked eosinophilic infiltration accompanies the vascular changes, while syphilis lymphadenopathy features a lymphoplasmacytic infiltrate surrounding the new vessels in the capsule and perinodal adipose tissue (which also show vasculitic changes). Bacillary angiomatosis and vascular transformation of lymph node sinuses are also among the reactive lesions associated with vascular proliferation.

Bacillary Angiomatosis

Occurring almost exclusively in HIV-positive individuals, bacillary angiomatosis is caused by *Bartonella henselae*, which is also the etiologic agent of cat-scratch disease in immunocompetent people. While characterized predominantly by cutaneous proliferations of variably sized blood vessels, in some cases lymph nodes are found to contain similar nodular proliferations of pleomorphic vessels. The endothelial cells are often plump and sometimes form clusters lacking well-formed vascular lumens. Warthin–Starry stain reveals bacterial forms between the newly developed capillaries.

Vascular Transformation of Lymph Node Sinuses

The striking vascular proliferation characteristic of vascular transformation of lymph node sinuses involves the node only partially, as it is restricted to the sinuses and spares the parenchyma. This rare entity is usually an incidental finding and has been associated with lymphatic and/or venous obstruction by tumor or thrombus or as a result of surgery or radiotherapy. Similar changes have been produced by experimental occlusion of efferent lymphatics and veins, but obstruction may not be the sole cause, as such changes have been seen in cases lacking obvious impediments to vascular drainage. Small proliferating vessels with hyperplastic endothe-

Table 7.11
Defining microscopic feature – vascular prominence

Angioimmunoblastic T cell lymphoma – Clear cells (neoplastic T cells) surrounding arborizing blood vessels
Mantle cell lymphoma – Hyalinized small blood vessels
Kaposi sarcoma – Slit-like vascular spaces containing erythrocytes; plasmacytic proliferation; capsular involvement; commonly associated with AIDS, other immunocompromised states
Castleman disease – Vascular proliferation accompanied by plasmacytosis and hyaline–vascular changes of some of the follicles
Rheumatoid lymphadenopathy – Similar to Castleman disease, save for the follicular changes
SLE lymphadenopathy – Fibrinoid necrosis of blood vessels with deposition of basophilic material giving rise to the Azzopardi phenomenon
HIV lymphadenitis – Paracortical vascular proliferation accompanies follicular involution with progression of disease
Syphilis – Lymphoplasmacytic cuffing of proliferating vessels within and outside of the capsule; accompanied by vasculitis
Kimura disease – Marked eosinophilic infiltration in addition to vascular proliferation
Bacillary angiomatosis – Nodular proliferation of capillaries in lymph nodes draining skin with similar lesions; predominantly affects HIV-infected people; Warthin–Starry staining highlights causative organism (*Bartonella henselae*)
Vascular transformation of lymph node sinuses – Distended sinuses due to proliferation of small vessels; capsular sparing; may be attributable to impairment of efferent lymphatic and blood vessel drainage

lial cells distend sinuses throughout the lymph node, and while there is no vascular proliferation within the cortical and para-cortical areas, compression may result from the expansion of the sinuses. Unlike Kaposi sarcoma, the lymph node capsule is not involved. Staining with CD34 and CD31 shows intense staining of the cells lining the dilated spaces, often revealing focal layering of the hyperplastic cells. In contrast, staining for D2-40, which is believed to stain lymphatic endothelial cells specifically, displays a single layer of D2-40+ cells lining some of the dilated spaces, suggesting that there is also proliferation of lymphatic sinuses (**Table 7.11**; **Figs. 7.68**, **7.69**, **7.70**, and **7.71**).

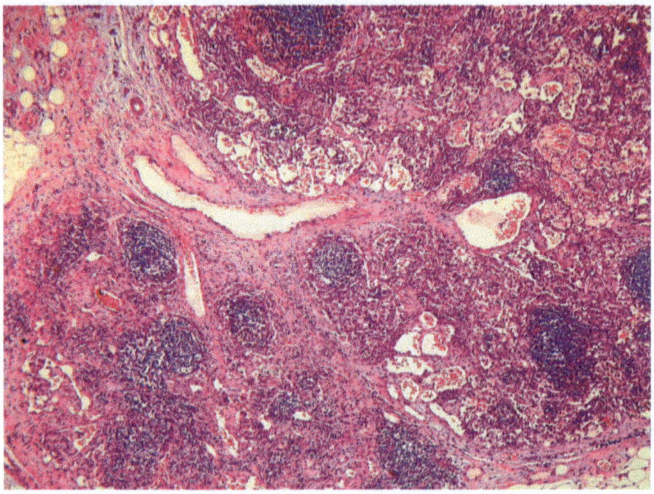

Fig. 7.68. Vascular transformation of sinuses. Subcapsular sinuses are distended and partly filled with blood. Cortex with follicles and paracortex are spared.

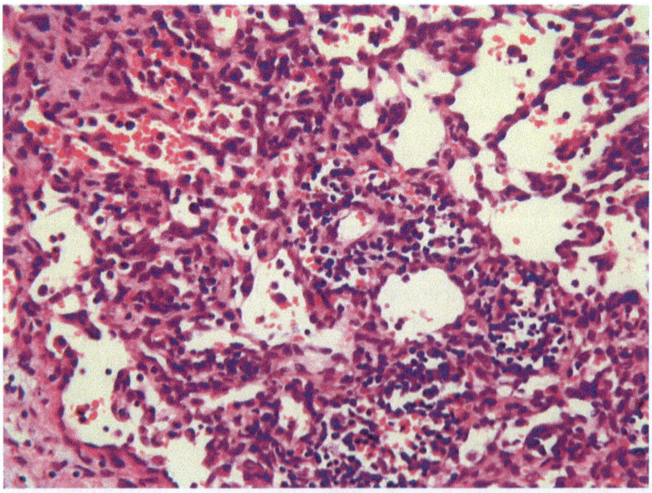

Fig. 7.69. The small vascular spaces are lined by hyperplastic endothelial cells. Plasma cells are present in the medullary perisinusoidal tissue.

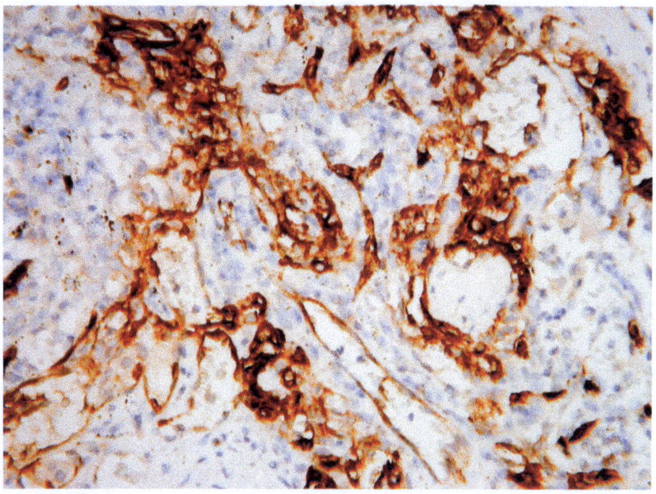

Fig. 7.70. The cells lining the dilated spaces label with CD34 which reveals focal piling up of endothelial cells.

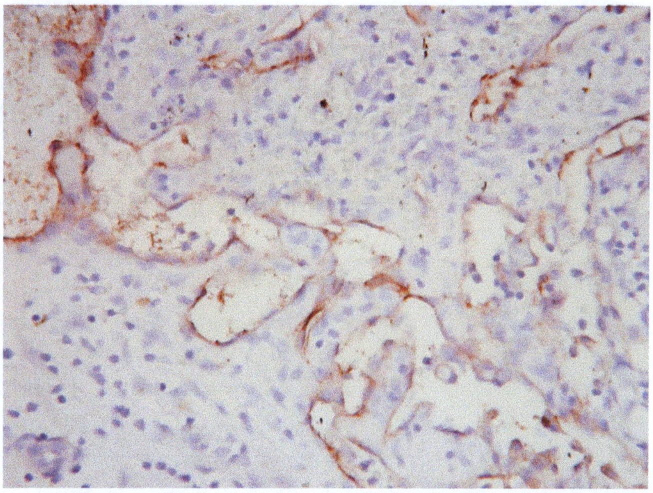

Fig. 7.71. D2-40 stains endothelial cells lining the dilated spaces suggesting that some of the spaces may be lymphatic. Unlike CD34+ cells, D2-40+ cells appear to be a single layer.

Hemorrhage

Parenchymal hemorrhage is encountered infrequently. Paracortical foci of hemorrhage may be seen in HIV lymphadenitis. Hemorrhage may be grossly discernible on sectioning of lymph nodes with involvement by bacillary angiomatosis or palisaded myofibroblastoma. Metastatic carcinoma may also be associated with hemorrhage (**Table 7.12**).

Table 7.12
Defining microscopic feature – hemorrhage

HIV lymphadenitis
Bacillary angiomatosis
Palisaded myofibroblastoma
Metastatic carcinoma

Starry Sky Pattern

The presence of tingible body macrophages amidst the monomorphous population of neoplastic B cells in Burkitt lymphoma produces the prototypic "starry sky" pattern, but this motif is not specific with respect to etiology. The pink histiocytes typical of mantle cell lymphoma may give rise to a similar appearance, as may tingible body macrophages in a subset of large B cell lymphomas with high-proliferative rates (including plasmablastic lymphoma), in lymphoblastic lymphoma, and in the blastoid variant of mantle cell lymphoma (**Table 7.13**).

Table 7.13
Defining microscopic feature – starry sky pattern

Burkitt lymphoma
Mantle cell lymphoma – Pink histiocytes in typical cases or tingible body macrophages in blastoid variant
Large B cell lymphomas (including plasmablastic lymphoma)
Lymphoblastic lymphoma

Mottled Pattern

Variation in color discernible at scanning magnification may result from heterogeneity among benign lymphoid cells, the presence of neoplastic cells amidst a reactive background, or from the presence of collections of abnormal cells. In cases of reactive lymphoid hyperplasia, the paracortex is susceptible to acquiring a moth-eaten appearance attributable to increased numbers of large cells amidst the background of small lymphocytes. In viral lymphadenitides such as that associated with infectious mononucleosis, proliferation of immunoblasts may yield this appearance, while in dermatopathic lymphadenopathy, increased numbers of Langerhans cells and interdigitating dendritic cells may have a similar effect. Mottled nodules may result from the infiltration of germinal centers by small B cells and T cells in progressive transformation of germinal centers or reflect the presence of neoplastic large B cells ("L&H cells" or "popcorn cells") in nodules comprised predominantly of small B and T cells in nodular lymphocyte-predominant Hodgkin lymphoma. Nodal involvement by the former is typically focal, in contrast to the more extensive architectural disruption associated with the latter. Paraimmunoblasts and prolymphocytes make up the pale proliferation centers that produce the typical variegated low-magnification appearance of small lymphocytic lymphoma; perivascular clustering of neoplastic T cells with abundant clear cytoplasm in angioimmunoblastic T cell lymphoma likewise produces pale nodules (**Table 7.14**).

Table 7.14
Defining microscopic feature – mottled pattern

Reactive paracortical hyperplasia (e.g., viral lymphadenitis) – Immunoblasts amidst small lymphocytes
Dermatopathic lymphadenopathy – Langerhans cells and interdigitating dendritic cells among small lymphocytes
Progressive transformation of germinal centers – Mottled nodules; small B cells and T cells infiltrate germinal centers; often focal or involving scattered follicles
Nodular lymphocyte-predominant Hodgkin lymphoma – Mottled nodules; neoplastic "L&H cells" within nodules composed of small B and T cells; nodal infiltration typically nodular and extensive
Small lymphocytic lymphoma – Pale proliferation centers (consisting of paraimmunoblasts and prolymphocytes) in a dark background of small neoplastic B cells
Angioimmunoblastic T cell lymphoma – Pale collections of neoplastic T cells with clear cytoplasm

Fibrosis/Hyalinization

Fibrosis may occur with resolution of a variety of lymphadenitides; examples include healing of granulomas in *M. tuberculosis* and sarcoidosis. Capsular thickening is seen in syphilitic lymphadenitis and is accompanied by broad collagenous bands traversing lymph node parenchyma in nodular sclerosis classical Hodgkin lymphoma (CHL). The fibrosis encountered in lymphocyte depleted and mixed cellularity CHL, in contrast, is generally more diffuse. Fibrosis may be accompanied by hyalinization of follicles in late HIV lymphadenitis; hyalinized germinal centers are integral to the diagnosis of the hyaline–vascular variant of Castleman disease (**Table 7.15**).

Table 7.15
Defining microscopic feature – fibrosis/hyalinization

Resolving lymphadenitis – Mycobacterium tuberculosis
Sarcoidosis – Fibrosis of some resolving granulomas
Syphilitic lymphadenitis – Fibrous capsular thickening
Classical Hodgkin lymphoma, nodular sclerosis subtype – Thickened capsule with broad collagenous bands extending into lymph node parenchyma
Classical Hodgkin lymphoma, mixed cellularity, and lymphocyte-depleted subtypes – Diffuse fibrosis in some cases
HIV lymphadenitis – Fibrosis and hyalinization of follicles in advanced disease
Castleman disease – Hyalinized germinal centers in hyaline–vascular variant

Signet Ring Cells

While nuclear eccentricity due to cytoplasmic vacuolation is most readily associated with adenocarcinoma cells from anatomic sites, such as stomach and breast, such morphology may rarely be seen in lymphoid neoplasms. Described first and most frequently in follicular lymphoma, signet ring morphology has subsequently been reported in examples of various B cell and T cell non-Hodgkin lymphomas, including diffuse large B cell lymphoma and anaplastic large cell lymphoma – ALK positive. In case of B cell lymphomas, the cytoplasmic vacuoles often represent inclusions of immunoglobulin, whereas, in T cell lymphomas the uncommon signet ring appearance is suggested to be due to endocytosed membrane receptors. Rare metastatic melanomas may also exhibit signet ring morphology. Signet ring sinus histiocytosis is encountered rarely and generally in association with underlying malignancy. Distinction among these lesions is facilitated by correlation with clinical history and use of appropriate immunohistochemical stains (**Table 7.16**).

Table 7.16
Defining microscopic feature – Signet ring cells

Metastatic adenocarcinoma – From stomach, breast
Non-Hodgkin lymphoma – Follicular lymphoma, DLBCL, PTCL, ALCL
Metastatic melanoma
Signet ring sinus histiocytosis – Generally associated with underlying malignancy

Bizarre or Multinucleated Cells

The presence of large abnormal cells that are multinucleated or exhibit other bizarre morphologic features is not specific with respect to etiology. Such cells may be seen in viral lymphadenitides (e.g., Warthin–Finkeldey multinucleated giant cells in measles or HIV lymphadenitis), other reactive conditions (e.g., Kimura disease), and in various lymphoid neoplasms (e.g., classical Hodgkin lymphoma, anaplastic large cell lymphoma, peripheral T cell lymphoma NOS, diffuse large B cell lymphoma) (**Table 7.17**).

Table 7.17
Defining microscopic feature – bizarre or multinucleated cells

Viral lymphadenitis – Warthin–Finkeldey cells in measles or HIV lymphadenitis
Other reactive lymphadenopathies – Kimura disease
Lymphoma – CHL, ALCL, PTCL- NOS, DLBCL

Extramedullary Hematopoiesis

The presence of marrow elements in lymph nodes is uncommon after the neonatal period and should prompt a search for underlying hematologic disease. Myeloproliferative neoplasms and recent receipt of hematopoietic growth factors are leading considerations in the differential diagnosis in adults, while in children, benign disorders of erythrocytes (e.g., thalassemia) or of marrow stroma are more frequent causes. Marrow elements may be seen in the lymph node sinuses.

Prominent Eosinophils

Conspicuous nodal infiltration by eosinophils may represent a component of the inflammatory response to an antigenic challenge, as in parasitic infections or drug reactions. Eosinophils may also comprise a portion of the reactive leucocytic infiltrate accompanying neoplasms such as classical Hodgkin lymphoma (nodular sclerosis and mixed cellularity), diffuse large B cell lymphoma, peripheral T cell lymphoma NOS, and Langerhans cell histiocytosis (**Table 7.18**).

Table 7.18
Defining microscopic feature – prominent eosinophils

Parasitic infection (e.g., filariasis)
Drug reaction
Classical Hodgkin lymphoma (nodular sclerosis, mixed cellularity)
Diffuse large B cell lymphoma
Peripheral T cell lymphoma NOS
Langerhans cell histiocytosis

Prominent Neutrophils

As at other anatomic sites, a neutrophilic infiltrate may be associated with bacterial infection (e.g., cat-scratch disease, lymphogranuloma venereum). Neutrophils are also present in necrotic foci in herpes simplex virus-associated lymphadenopathy; they are conspicuously absent, in contrast, in systemic lupus erythematosus and Kikuchi–Fujimoto lymphadenopathy. Their presence between the proliferating vascular structures in bacillary angiomatosis may assist in distinguishing this lesion from Kaposi sarcoma. Neutrophils may also comprise a minor portion of the reactive leucocytic background in classical Hodgkin lymphoma (nodular sclerosis and mixed cellularity) (**Table 7.19**).

Table 7.19
Defining microscopic feature – prominent neutrophils

Bacterial infection – Cat-scratch disease, lymphogranuloma venereum, bacillary angiomatosis
HSV infection
Classical Hodgkin lymphoma (nodular sclerosis)

Prominent Plasma Cells

Plasma cells may comprise a portion of the reactive leucocytic background in lymphoid neoplasms, represent a subset of the neoplastic cells, or proliferate in the setting of particular reactive lymphadenopathies. The plasma cell variant of Castleman disease features sheets of interfollicular plasma cells, as in the case of rheumatoid arthritis-associated lymphadenopathy and syphilitic lymphadenitis. A lesser degree of plasmacytic proliferation is seen in HIV lymphadenitis; increased numbers in the medullary cords accompany dermatopathic lymphadenopathy. Clusters of clonal plasma cells occur in lymphoplasmacytic lymphoma, while the plasma cells seen in some cases of classical Hodgkin lymphoma (nodular sclerosis and mixed cellularity subtypes) and peripheral T cell lymphoma NOS are polytypic. They also comprise a portion of the leucocyte population in inflammatory myofibroblastic tumor (**Table 7.20**).

Table 7.20
Defining microscopic feature – prominent plasma cells

Castleman disease – Sheets of plasma cells in plasma cell variant; lesser numbers may be seen in hyaline-vascular variant
Rheumatoid lymphadenopathy
Syphilitic lymphadenitis
Dermatopathic lymphadenopathy – Prominent in medullary cords
Lymphoplasmacytic lymphoma – Clusters of clonal plasma cells
Classical Hodgkin lymphoma (nodular sclerosis and mixed cellularity) – Polytypic plasma cells in the inflammatory background
Peripheral T cell lymphoma NOS – Polytypic plasma cells in the inflammatory background
Inflammatory myofibroblastic tumor

Infiltration of Pericapsular Fat

While extension of neoplastic B cell populations through the lymph node capsule is common in lesions such as follicular lymphoma, small lymphocytic lymphoma, lymphoplasmacytic lymphoma, and lymphoblastic lymphoma, infiltration of extranodal adipose tissue is not specific for malignant processes. A variety of reactive conditions, including Kikuchi–Fujimoto lymphadenopathy, rheumatoid arthritis-associated lymphadenopathy, and infectious mononucleosis, exhibit transgression of the capsule by proliferating lymphocytes (**Table 7.21**).

Table 7.21
Defining microscopic feature – infiltration of pericapsular fat

Follicular lymphoma
Small lymphocytic lymphoma
Lymphoplasmacytic lymphoma
Lymphoblastic lymphoma
Kikuchi–Fujimoto lymphadenopathy
Rheumatoid lymphadenopathy
Infectious mononucleosis

Extraneous Cells – Pigmented Cells, Epithelial Cells, Foreign Material, Dermatopathic Lymphadenitis, Hemosiderin

Inclusions of Benign Extraneous Cells

A variety of extraneous cells, epithelial cells being by far the most common, may be encountered in the lymph node, and the problem lies in the identification of the nature of such cells and distinguishing them from metastatic deposits.

The nature of the inclusion varies with the site of the lymph node.

Cervical lymph nodes may contain inclusions of salivary gland tissue and there may be an associated follicular hyperplasia. The salivary gland material may be acini or ducts, some lined by metaplastic squamous epithelium and others forming keratin-filled cysts or solid nests of epithelium. The nature of benign-appearing thyroid follicles, characteristically close to the subcapsular sinus, is still controversial. These deposits show no nuclear atypia, papillary structures, or psammoma bodies. Opinion has vacillated between benign inclusions and metastatic deposits of follicular thyroid carcinoma as the explanation for such thyroid follicles.

Heterotopic breast ducts and dilated spaces lined by low cuboidal epithelium may be seen in axillary lymph nodes. The epithelium shows no evidence of atypia and may be of apocrine or squamous type, and less frequently be ciliated. There is no associated desmoplastic response to the epithelium.

Mediastinal nodes may contain cystic deposits in the subcapsular region that are thought to represent either benign respiratory epithelium or mesothelial cells of the pleura. The nature of the cells can be confirmed by immunohistochemistry.

Pelvic and abdominal lymph nodes may contain benign glandular tissue, which when accompanied by endometrial stroma represents endometriosis. In the absence of the latter, these glands

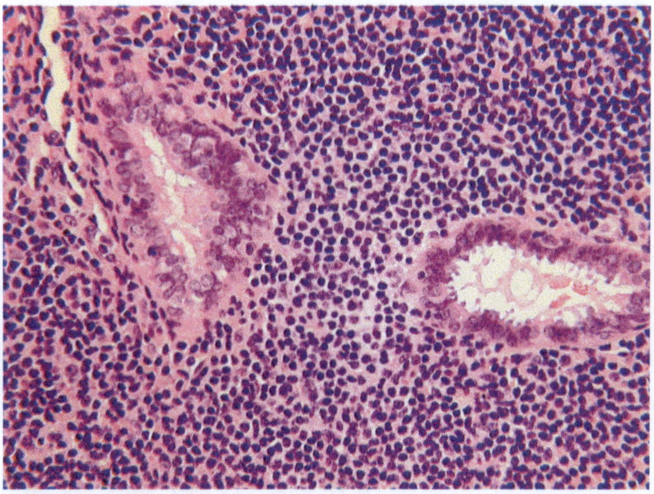

Fig. 7.72. Pelvic lymph node with benign glandular inclusions lined by ciliated epithelium of endosalpingiosis type with luminal secretions.

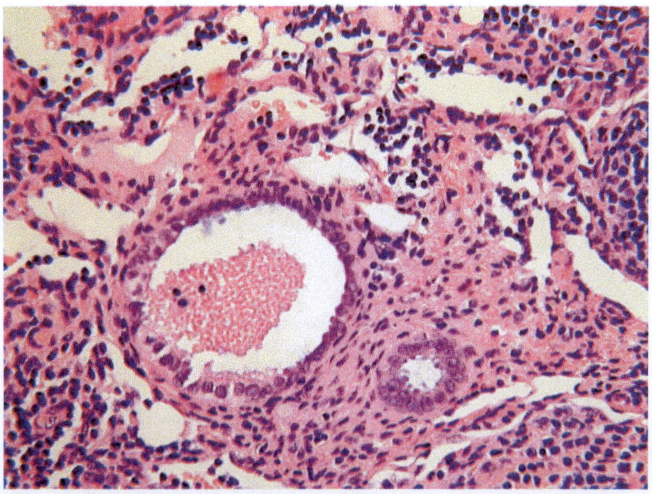

Fig. 7.73. Benign Mullerian deposits in abdominal lymph node surrounded by non-desmoplastic stroma.

which are lined by cuboidal or tall columnar, sometimes pseudostratified and ciliated cells with no evidence of malignant features represent deposits of Mullerian tissue. Occasional intraluminal mucin may be present.

Benign nevus cells may be found in the capsule of peripheral lymph nodes from a variety of sites. Such deposits show no evidence of atypia or desmoplasia. Their nature can be confirmed with stains for S100, Melan A, or tyrosinase (**Figs. 7.72, 7.73, 7.74**, and **7.75**; **Table 7.22**).

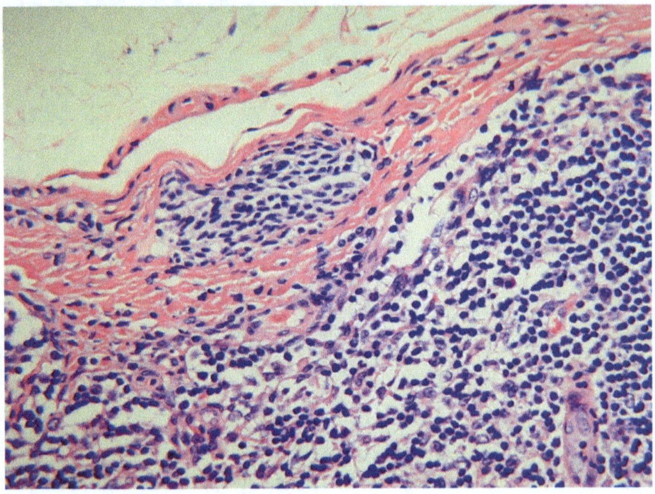

Fig. 7.74. Axillary node with a capsular deposit of nevus cells that shows no evidence of cytological atypia or desmoplasia.

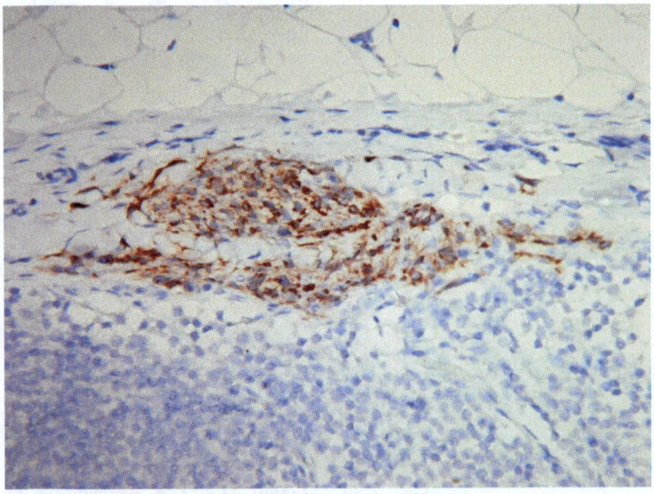

Fig. 7.75. The nevus cells stain for Melan A.

Table 7.22
Defining microscopic feature – benign inclusions of extraneous cells

No atypia in inclusions, no associated desmoplasia
Inclusions vary with site of lymph node:
Cervical nodes – Salivary gland inclusions; thyroid follicles (uncertain etiology)
Axillary nodes – Heterotopic mammary epithelium
Mediastinal nodes – Cysts of respiratory epithelium; mesothelial inclusions
Abdominal and pelvic nodes – Endosalpingiosis; Mullerian-type inclusions; endometriosis
Peripheral lymph nodes – Benign nevus cells

Chapter 8

Nodal Involvement by Leukemias and Extranodal Lymphomas

Key words: Primary myelofibrosis, chronic myelomonocytic leukemia, cell prolymphocytic leukemia, T cell prolymphocytic leukemia, NK cell disorders/leukemia, extranodal lymphomas, hairy cell leukemia.

Nodal Involvement by Leukemia

A number of leukemias can show secondary involvement of lymph nodes. Aside from chronic lymphocytic leukemia, lymphoblastic leukemia, and adult T cell leukemia/lymphoma which have been previously discussed in detail, involvement of lymph nodes is only infrequently seen in the other leukemias and often only in advanced stages of the disease (**Table 8.1**).

Leukemic infiltrates in the lymph node show a variable pattern and there is often infiltration of the paracortex and interfollicular areas with preservation of the follicles. There is a propensity to involve lymph node sinuses, and in severe cases, partial effacement of the lymph node by the leukemic infiltrate may be observed.

Myeloid Leukemia/Myeloid Sarcoma

Myeloid leukemia involving lymph nodes or extramedullary sites is known as myeloid sarcoma and can arise in patients with myelodysplastic syndromes and chronic myeloproliferative diseases. The presence of myeloperoxidase, a peroxidative enzyme, imparts a distinctive green color which accounts for the term *chloroma* applied to this tumor. The color fades within hours of exposure to air but can be restored by applying hydrogen peroxide. Exposure of these tumors to ultraviolet light produces a

A.S.-Y. Leong, *A Pattern Approach to Lymph Node Diagnosis*,
DOI 10.1007/978-1-4419-7176-0_8, © Springer Science+Business Media, LLC 2011

Table 8.1
Lymph node involvement by leukemias

Myeloid leukemia/myeloid sarcoma
Primary myelofibrosis
Chronic myelomonocytic leukemia, blast phase
B cell prolymphocytic leukemia
T cell prolymphocytic leukemia
Chronic lymphoproliferative disorder of NK cells
Aggressive NK cell leukemia

bright red fluorescence due to the presence of abundant protoporphyrins.

The infiltrate is diffuse, and in partially involved nodes, sheets of myeloblasts infiltrate the paracortex, sinuses, and medulla with sparing of the follicles. Myeloid sarcoma can be divided into *differentiated, immature*, and *blastic* tumors that are composed respectively of promyelocytes and more mature neutrophils, myeloblasts and promyelocytes, and predominantly of myeloblasts with no evidence of granulocytic differentiated.

In distinction to diffuse large cell lymphoma which infiltrates in a destructive manner, myeloid sarcoma preserves the normal tissue planes and architecture. Both conditions often produce coagulative necrosis. While the cells of large cell lymphoma have thick nuclear membranes and prominent nucleoli, those of myeloid sarcoma display small or inconspicuous nucleoli and delicate nuclear membranes. The presence of eosinophilic myeloblasts is particularly useful for the identification of myeloid sarcoma.

In air-dried smears and imprints, chloroacetate esterase enzyme activity can be found in meyloid cells and their precursors. In formalin-fixed tissue sections, the Leder stain or naphthyl–ASD–chloroacetate stain produces a bright red cytoplasmic precipitate in myeloid precursors and granulocytes.

Immunohistological stains are particularly helpful in identifying myeloid sarcomas which are positive for lysozyme, CD117, CD34, and CD43. Various myelomonocytic markers such as CD68, CD15, Mac387, and HAM56 stain the tumors. More specific markers such as myeloperoxidase and neutrophil elastase label more mature cells (**Table 8.2**; **Figs. 8.1**, **8.2**, **8.3**, **8.4**, **8.5**, and **8.6**).

Primary Myelofibrosis

In primary myelofibrosis, extramedullary hematopoiesis is most commonly seen in the liver and spleen; nodal involvement is rare, manifesting as nodular aggregates of megakaryocytes mixed with less conspicuous numbers of erythroid and granulocytic cells.

Table 8.2
Myeloid sarcoma – morphology and immunohistology

Differentiated subtype: composed of pro-myelocytes and more mature neutrophils
Immature subtype: composed of promyelocytes and myeloblasts
Blastic subtype: composed mostly of myeloblasts, no evidence of granulocytic differentiation
Tumor cells infiltrate along tissue planes with preservation of architecture
Myeloblasts have oval to irregular nuclei with thin nuclear membranes and small nucleoli
Immunohistology: positive for lysozyme, CD117, CD43, CD34.
More specific markers expressed – myeloperoxidase, neutrophil elastase
Express myelomonocytic markers – CD68, CD15, Mac387, Ham56

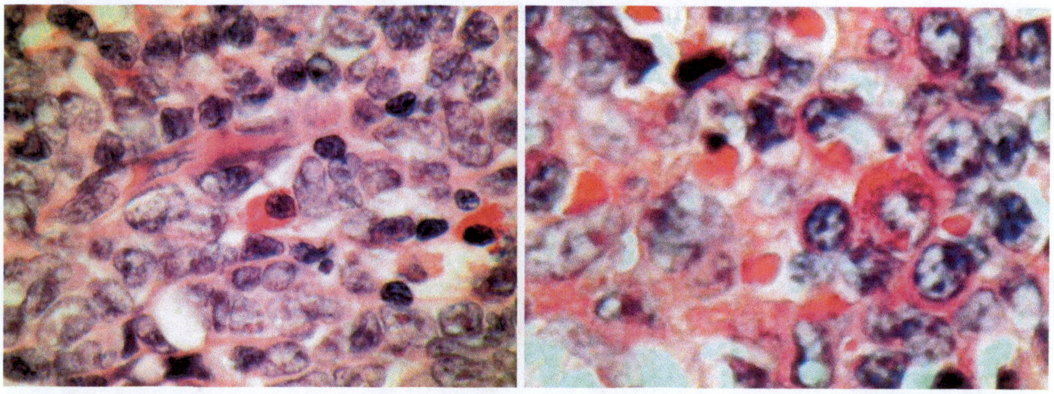

Fig. 8.1. Myeloid sarcoma, immature type, with myeloblasts, promyelocytes, and two eosinophil precursors. The myeloblasts display delicate nuclear membranes, vesicular nuclei with one or more small eosinophilic nucleoli. *Inset:* eosinophilic myeloblast.

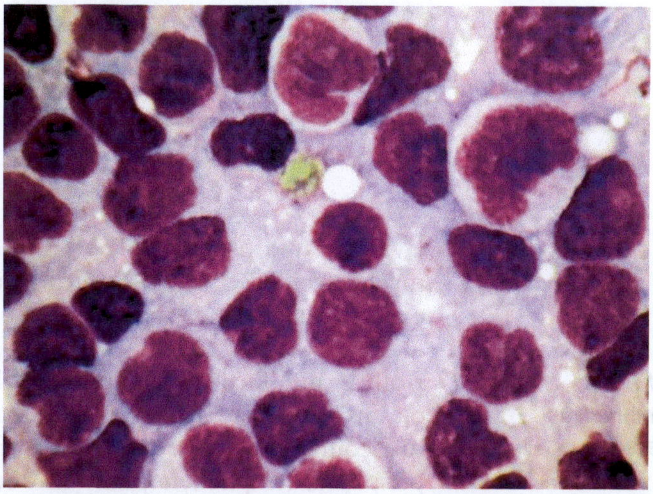

Fig. 8.2. Imprint showing myeloblasts and promyelocytes with thin nuclear membranes and several small nucleoli. No cytoplasmic granules are seen.

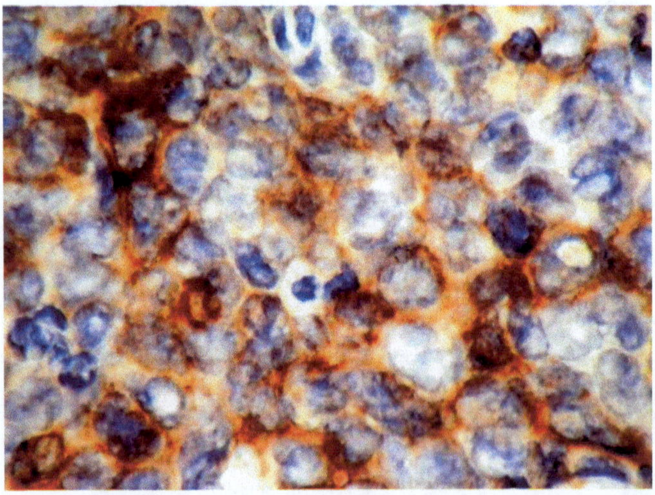

Fig. 8.3. Myeloid sarcoma. The tumor cells stain for CD117.

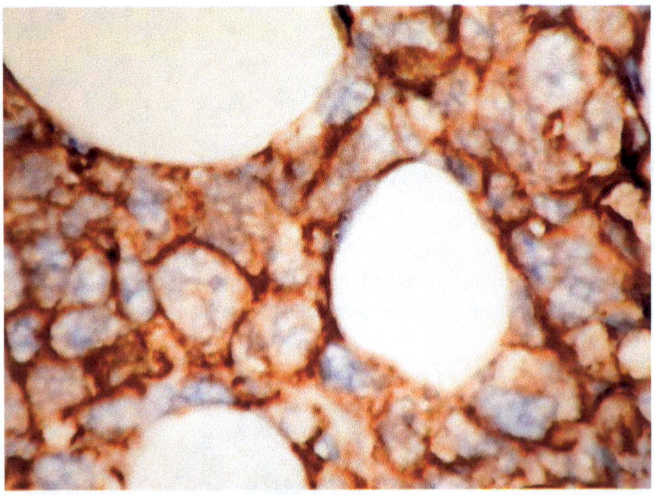

Fig. 8.4. The tumor also stains for CD43 and showed weaker staining for CD34 (not shown).

FVIII-related protein, CD34, and other myeloid antigens (e.g., myeloperoxidase, CD43) are helpful in confirming such foci of extramedullary hematopoiesis.

B and T Cell Prolymphocytic Leukemias

Both B and T cell prolymphocytic leukemias are aggressive neoplasms of mature B and T cells that do not have a known normal counterpart. They primarily affect the peripheral blood, and peripheral lymphadenopathy in both forms of leukemia is minimal. The cytologic features of both leukemias are very similar except that T cell prolymphocytic leukemia cells may display more striking nuclear convolutions. The medium-sized cells have round

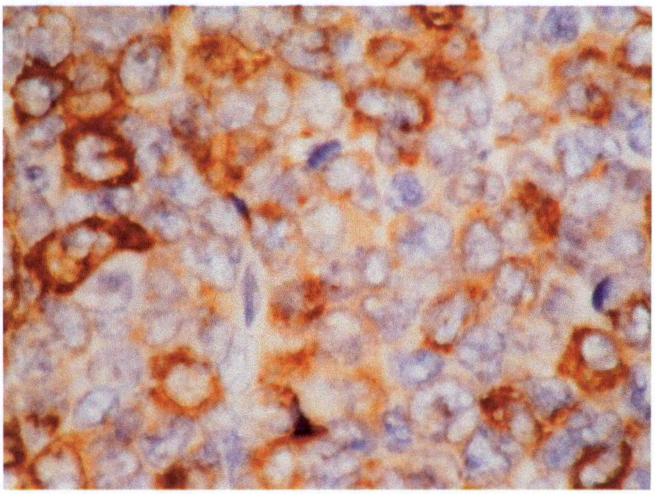

Fig. 8.5. Myeloblasts and promyelocytes stain for myeloperoxidase.

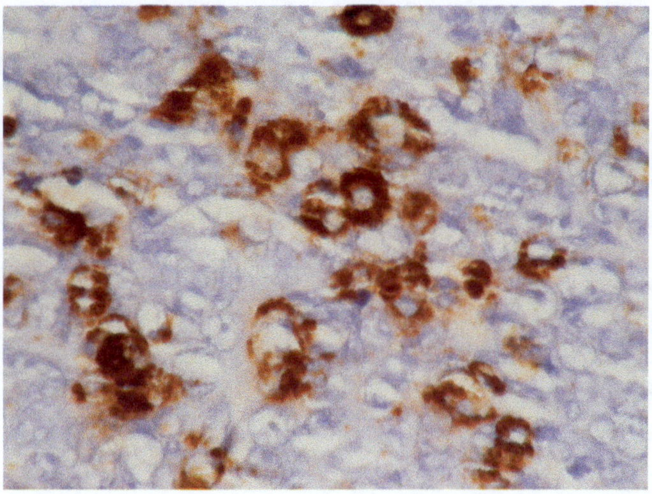

Fig. 8.6. More mature forms in the myeloid sarcoma stain for neutrophil elastase.

nuclei with a prominent central nucleolus and small amounts of basophilic cytoplasm. Prognosis in both conditions is poor.

The morphology of nodal infiltration in B cell prolymphocytic leukemia is not well known and has been confused by other conditions including leukemic variants of mantle cell lymphoma and CLL with increased numbers of prolymphocytes. Differentiation requires immunophenotypic or genetic studies. Nodal involvement may be vaguely nodular but proliferation centers are absent, and distinction from blastoid mantle cell lymphoma may be difficult. The cells of B cell prolymphocytic leukemia are strongly positive for sIgM and sIgD and show mature B cell antigens including CD20 and CD79a. CD5 and CD23 expression is seen in less than 30% of cases and about half are ZAP-70 and CD38 positive.

T cell prolymphocytic leukemia involvement of lymph nodes is diffuse and tends to predominate in paracortical areas with prominent high-endothelial vessels that contain the neoplastic cells. Follicles may be spared. The diagnosis is best made on peripheral blood films which show small- to medium-sized lymphoid cells with granular cytoplasm and round, oval, or markedly irregular nuclei and visible nucleoli. Some cases may comprise smaller cells and nucleoli may not be visible and others may have very irregular nuclear outlines. The cells show post-thymic T cell antigens such as CD3, CD7, and CD2, and 60% of cases are CD4+/CD8–, 25% CD4+/CD8+, and 15% CD4–/CD8+. The neoplastic cells are CD1a– and TdT– (**Table 8.3**; **Figs. 8.7, 8.8, 8.9, 8.10, 8.11**, and **8.12**).

Table 8.3
B and T Cell prolymphocytic leukemia – morphology and immunohistology

B cell prolymphocytic leukemia
Nodal involvement infrequent
Diffuse or vaguely nodular pattern; proliferation centers absent
Medium-sized cells, round nuclei, condensed chromatin, central nucleolus, scanty pale basophilic cytoplasm
CD20+, CD79a+, sIgM+/D+
CD23+ and CD5+ in <30% of cases
CD38+ and ZAP-70+ in about 50%
T cell prolymphocytic leukemia
Nodal involvement infrequent
Paracortical involvement, may spare follicles, prominent high-endothelial vessels
Medium-sized cells, oval or markedly irregular nucleus, visible nucleolus, scanty basophilic cytoplasm
CD3+, CD7+, CD2+
CD4+/CD8– (60%), CD4+/CD8+ (25%), and CD4–/CD8+ (15%)

NK Cell Lymphoproliferative Disorders

Chronic lymphoproliferative disorders of NK cells are rare and heterogenous, and nodal involvement is infrequent. Diagnosis is based on the recognition of the circulating NK cells and immunohistochemistry is necessary for identification. The same requirements apply for aggressive NK cell leukemia.

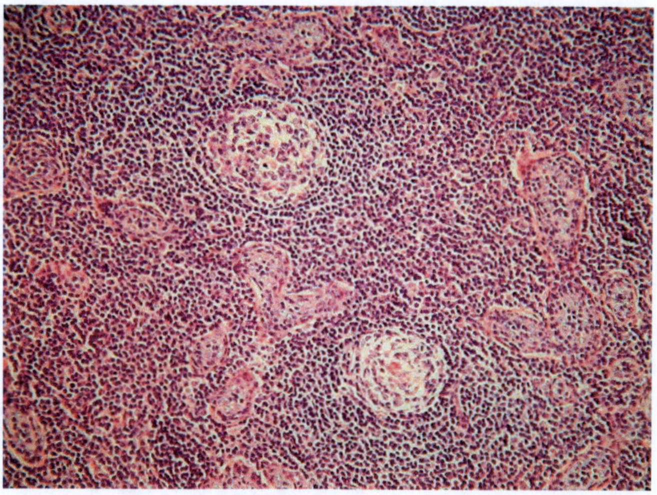

Fig. 8.7. T cell prolymphocytic leukemia infiltrating the paracortex with sparing of follicles.

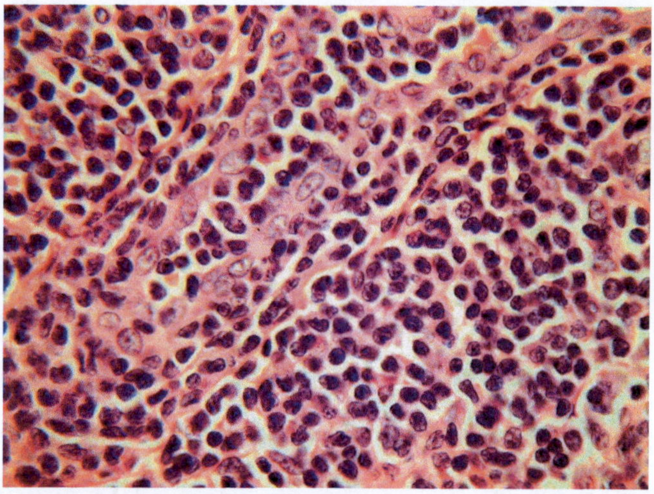

Fig. 8.8. The neoplastic cells in the paracortex infiltrate the wall of the high-endothelial venule and are also seen within the lumen.

Nodal Involvement by Extranodal Lymphomas

A number of extranodal lymphomas can involve lymph nodes secondarily but are uncommon and involvement is often localized. Such extranodal lymphomas include splenic B cell marginal zone lymphoma, advanced stage hairy cell leukemia, heavy-chain disease, plasma cell neoplasms, mucosa-associated lymphoid tissue (MALT) lymphoma, cutaneous DLBCL, leg type, lymphomatoid

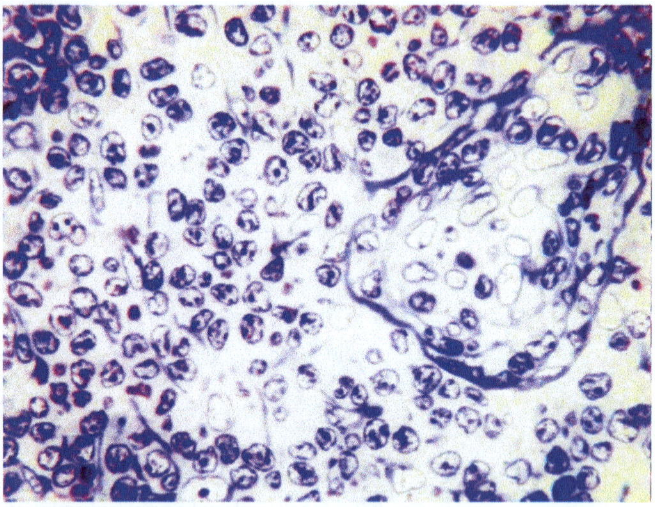

Fig. 8.9. Plastic-embedded section of lymph node showing medium-sized lymphoid cells with scant cytoplasm and central nucleoli. Some cells show prominent nuclear folds. The leukemic cells infiltrate the wall of the high-endothelial vessel.

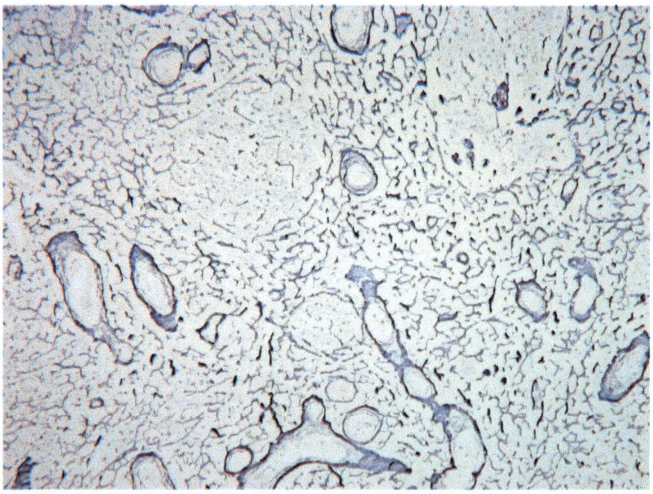

Fig. 8.10. Reticulin stain showing prominent high-endothelial vessels in the paracortex and preserved follicles (*arrows*).

granulomatosis, and extranodal NK cell lymphoma – nasal type (**Table 8.4**).

Splenic B Cell Marginal Zone Lymphoma

Nodal infiltration in splenic B cell marginal zone lymphoma is very uncommon and limited to splenic hilar lymph nodes that show dilatation of sinuses with lymphoma cells surrounding and replacing germinal centers. Unlike primary MZL of lymph nodes, there is a more intimate mixture of the lymphoma cells and mantle cells so that a distinct marginal zone is not

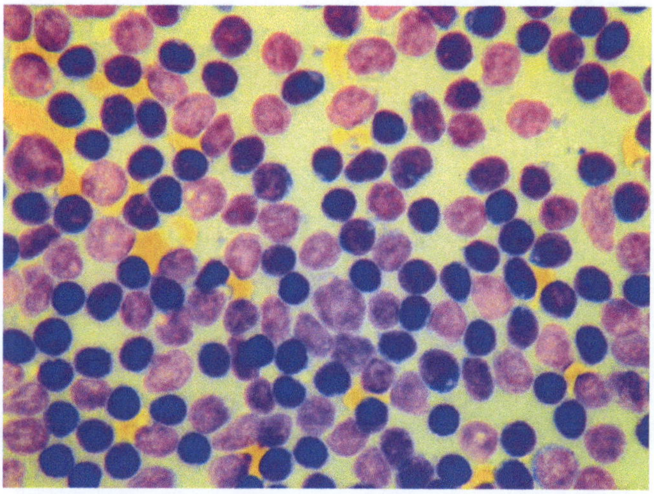

Fig. 8.11. Buffy coat smear of peripheral blood showing the T-prolymphocytic leukemia cells.

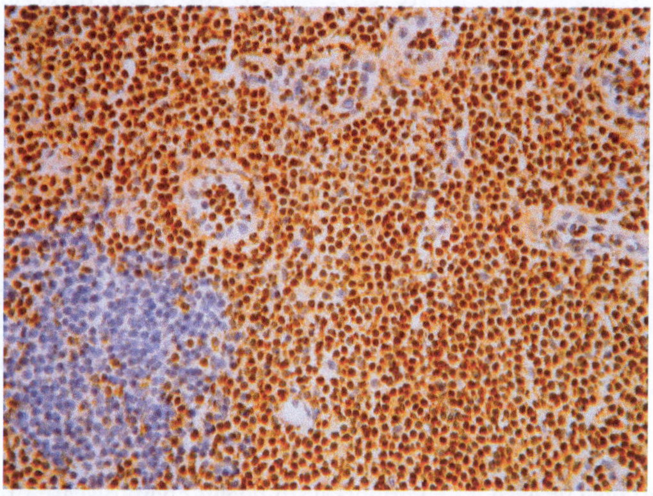

Fig. 8.12. CD3+ leukemic cells are present in the paracortex and within the lumen of high-endothelial venules. The follicle is not stained. The leukemic cells co-expressed CD4 and CD8 (not shown).

discernable. The neoplastic cells are CD20+/CD79a+/CD23–/CD10–/Bcl6–/CD43–/cyclinD1–. CD5 is often negative.

Hairy Cell Leukemia (HCL)

Hairy cell leukemia (HCL) is primarily a disease of the spleen and bone marrow with peripheral blood involvement. It is an indolent neoplasm of small mature B-lymphoid cells with oval nuclei and abundant cytoplasm that is thrown into "hairy" projections when they circulate in the peripheral blood. HCL may involve splenic hilar lymph nodes in advanced stage disease and rarely other abdominal nodes show infiltration.

Table 8.4
Extranodal lymphoma that infrequently involve lymph nodes

Splenic B cell marginal zone lymphoma – Very uncommon nodal involvement
Hairy cell leukemia – Rarely involves lymph nodes in advanced stage
Heavy chain disease
Monoclonal gammopathy of undetermined significance and extraosseous plasmacytoma
MALT lymphoma – Localized nodes, regional nodes
Cutaneous DLBCL, leg type – Regional nodes
Lymphomatoid granulomatosis – Very rare nodal involvement
Extranodal NK cell lymphoma, nasal type – Uncommon nodal involvement
Blastic plasmacytoid dendritic cell neoplasm (blastic NK cell lymphoma)

Infiltration is variably interfollicular or paracortical with sparing of follicles; sinuses are distended with neoplastic cells that are CD20+/CD103+/DBA.44+ and weakly cyclinD1 positive. There is often bright monotypic sIg expression. CD10, Bcl6, and CD5 are negative. The neoplastic cells also characteristically produce acid phosphatase isoenzyme that is resistant to tartaric acid (TRAP) so that TRAP staining, although not specific, used to be extensively employed for the identification of HCL. TRAP can also be seen in CLL/SLL, splenic marginal zone lymphoma, Sézary syndrome, and other disorders. Electron microscopic appearances are distinctive with hairy cytoplasmic projections and with the presence of ribosome lamella complexes. Hairy cell leukemia is highly sensitive to either α interferon or nucleosides, and less commonly there is prolonged remission following splenectomy (**Figs. 8.13**, **8.14**, **8.15**, **8.16**, **8.17**, **8.18**, **8.19**, **8.20**, and **8.21**).

Heavy-Chain Disease

Patients with heavy-chain disease present with systemic symptoms such as anorexia, weight loss, weakness, or recurrent bacterial infections and often show autoimmune manifestations including rheumatoid arthritis, autoimmune hemolytic anemia or thrombocytopenia or both, vasculitis, Sjogren syndrome, systemic or cutaneous lupus erythematosus, myasthenia gravis, or thyroiditis. The disease is generalized and includes hepatosplenomegaly, lymphadenopathy, and involvement of Waldeyer ring, skin and subcutaneous tissue, salivary glands, thyroid, and gastrointestinal tract. Peripheral blood circulating plasma cells, lymphocytes, and eosinophilia may be present. Lymph nodes show a polymorphous infiltration of lymphocytes, plasmacytoid lymphocytes, plasma cells, immunoblasts, histiocytes, and eosinophils, and can mimic Hodgkin lymphoma, angioimmunoblastic T cell lymphoma, lymphoplasmacytic lymphoma, and CLL. The neoplastic cells are

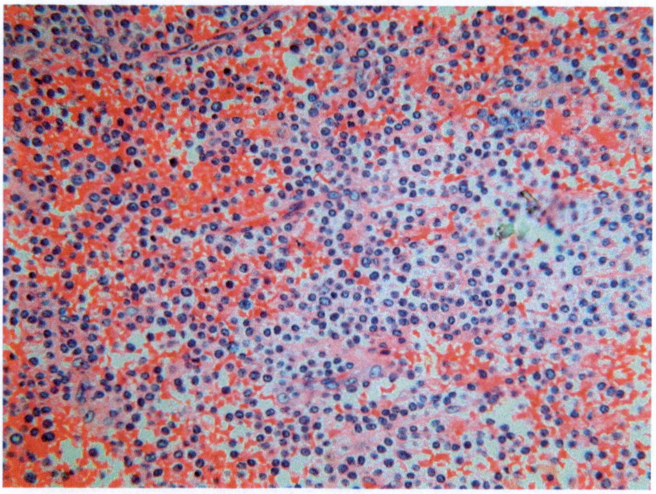

Fig. 8.13. HCL in axillary lymph node with associated skin nodule over forearm. Splenectomy performed for HCL 2 years previously. Sheets of monotonous oval cells produce a frog spawn appearance. Blood-filled spaces are present.

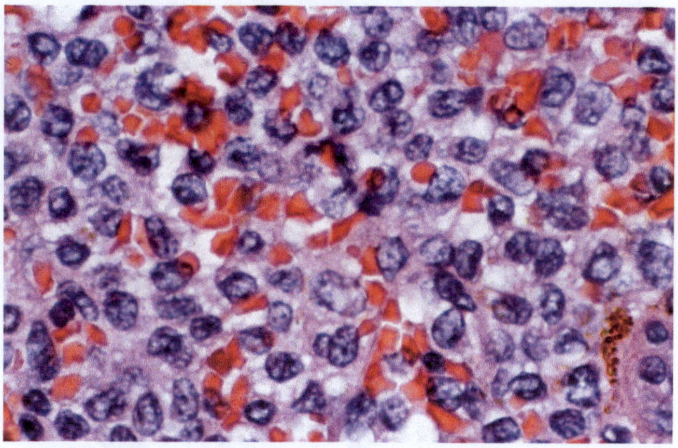

Fig. 8.14. The cells are bland and uniform-appearing with coarsely clumped chromatin and moderate quantities of pale cytoplasm.

CD79a+/CD20+/CD38+/CD138+. They are CD10–, Bcl6–, and CD5–. There is monotypic cytoplasmic staining for gamma heavy chain in gamma heavy-chain disease and for mu heavy chain in mu heavy-chain disease.

Plasma Cell Neoplasms

Some plasma cell neoplasms can involve lymph nodes and present as sheets of differentiated plasma cells that may be accompanied by blastic forms which contain nucleoli. Variable quantities of immunoglobulin secretion may be seen in the form of Mott cells and Russell bodies. There is monotypic cIg heavy- and light-chain

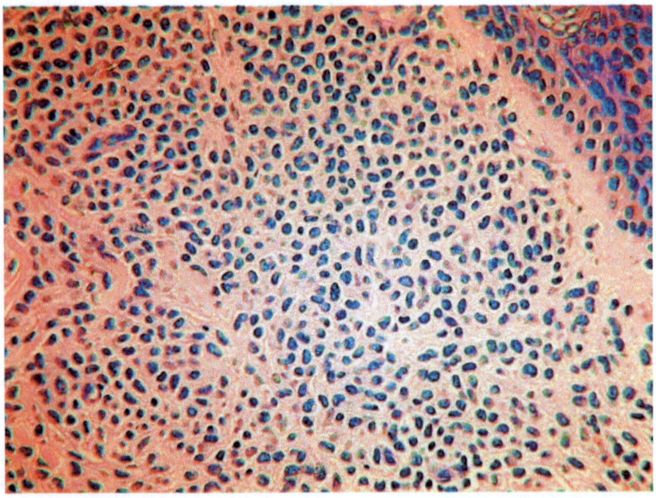

Fig. 8.15. The associated skin nodule in the forearm shows an infiltrate of similar cells in the dermis.

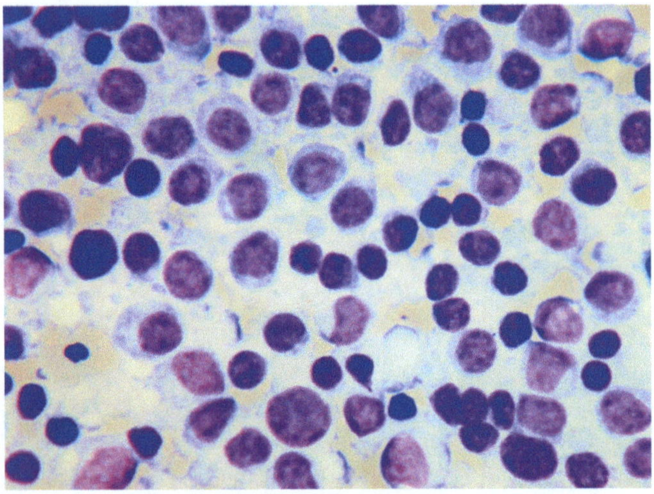

Fig. 8.16. Imprint of the lymph node shows the bland-appearing cells with moderate quantities of pale blue cytoplasm. A single nucleolus is visible in some cells.

expression. These changes may be seen in monoclonal gammopathy of undetermined significance and extraosseous plasmacytoma.

Mucosa-Associated Lymphoid Tissue (MALT) Lymphoma

The gastrointestinal tract is the most common site of MALT lymphoma, other sites being salivary gland, head and neck, lung, ocular adnexa, skin, thyroid, and breast. Occasional draining lymph nodes may be involved but multifocal nodal involvement by MALT lymphoma is very uncommon. Nodal marginal zone lymphoma and MALT lymphoma involving lymph nodes are

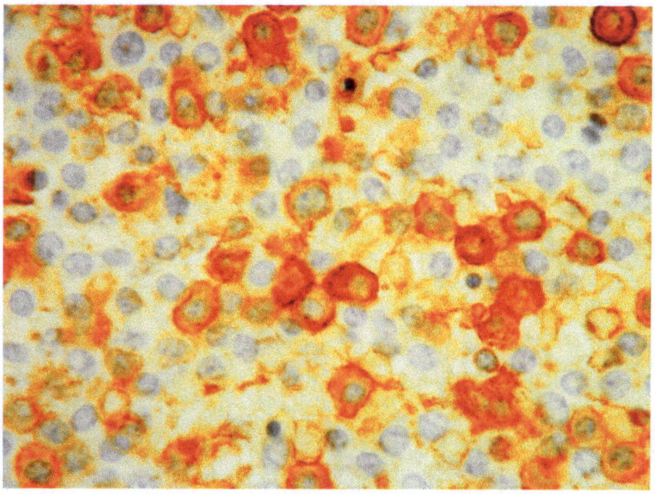

Fig. 8.17. The neoplastic cells in the lymph node stain for DBA.44.

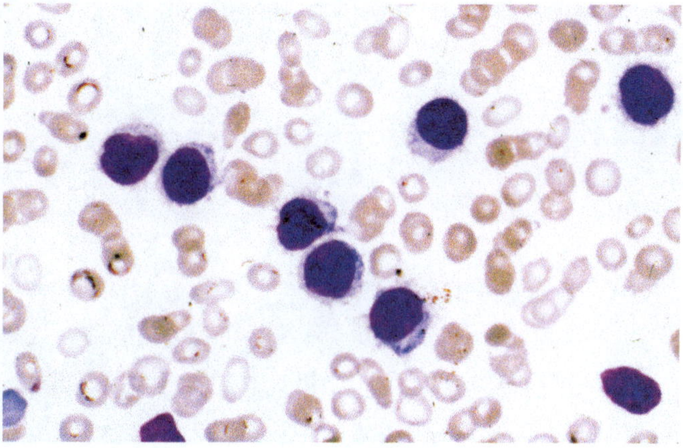

Fig. 8.18. Imprint of lymph node showing cells with oval nuclei, dense chromatin, inconspicuous nucleoli, and moderate quantities of pale blue cytoplasm.

histologically and immunophenotypically indistinguishable (nodal marginal zone lymphoma is discussed in **Chapter 5**). Arbitrarily, nodal marginal zone lymphoma is diagnosed when there is no evidence of extranodal or splenic disease. The lymphoma cells invade the marginal zone of the nodes with subsequent interfollicular expansion. Discrete accumulations of monocytoid B cells may be present in a parafollicular and perisinusoidal distribution, and both plasma cell differentiation and colonization of follicles may be seen. The lymphoma cells are CD20+, CD79a+, CD5–, CD10–, Bcl6–, CyclinD1–, CD23–, CD43+/–, and infrequently CD5+. As there is currently no specific marker for MALT lymphoma, staining for FDC to show

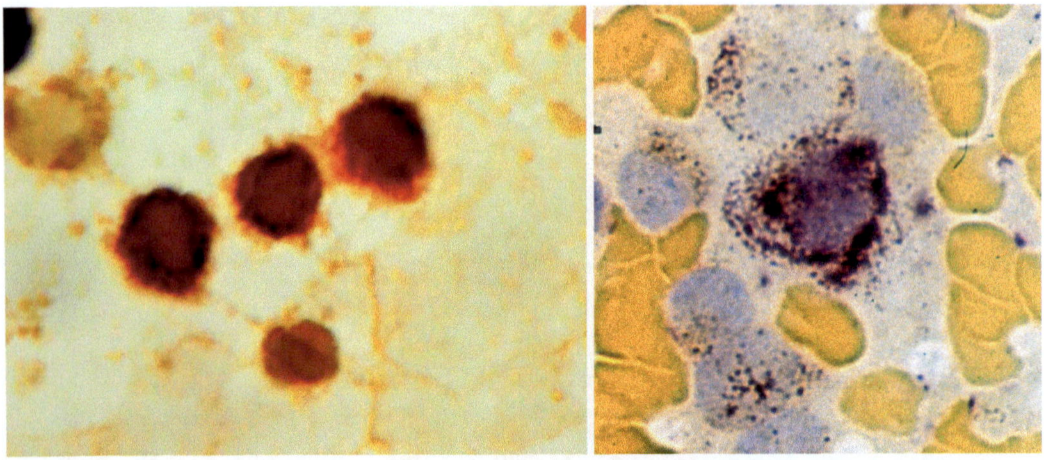

Fig. 8.19. Strong acid phosphatase expression in the hairy cells (*left panel*) which is resistant to tartaric acid (*right panel*).

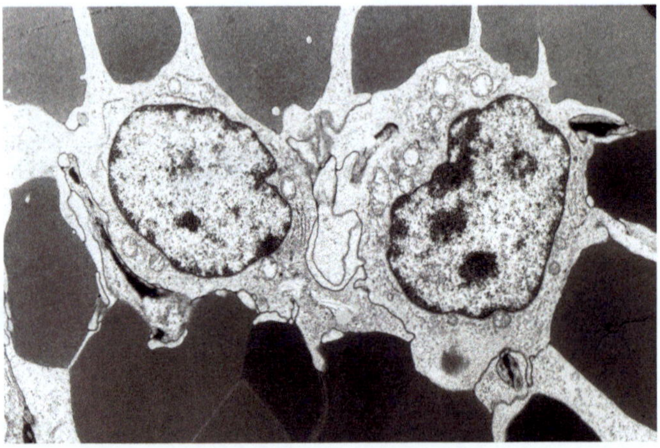

Fig. 8.20. Electron micrograph of tissue imprint showing hairy cells with long cytoplasmic processes flanked by red cells. There is interdigitation of cytoplasmic processes in between the two cells.

the lymphoma cells within FDC meshworks is useful for diagnosis (**Figs. 8.22**, **8.23**, **8.24**, and **8.25**).

Primary Cutaneous Diffuse Large B Cell Lymphoma (DLBCL) – Leg Type

Primary cutaneous DLBCL, leg type, is a lymphoma composed exclusively of large transformed B cells. It occurs in the lower legs and frequently disseminates to extracutaneous sites including regional lymph nodes which show striking sheets of centroblasts and immunoblasts infiltrating in a diffuse manner. The lymphoma cells are CD20+, CD79a+, and nearly always express Bcl2 and IRF4/MUM1. Bcl6 positivity is seen in most cases but not in CD10.

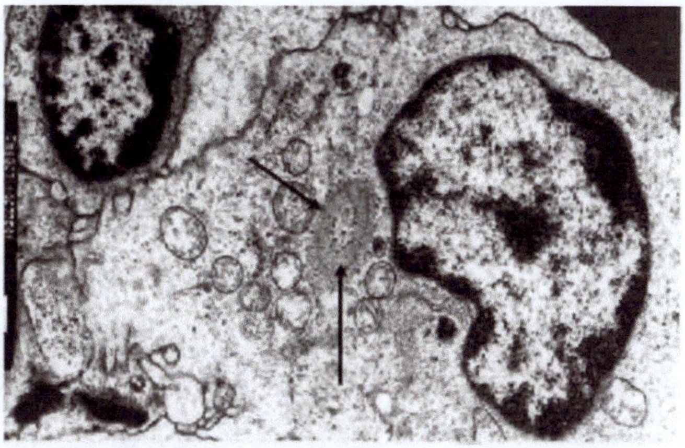

Fig. 8.21. Electron micrograph of hairy cell with distinctive ribosome lamellar complex (*arrows*).

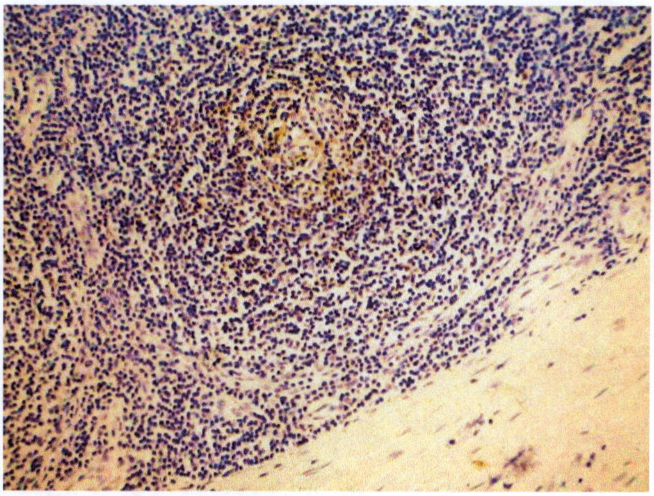

Fig. 8.22. Gastric node secondarily involved by gastric MALT lymphoma. The infiltrate is perifollicular with a central atrophic germinal center.

Lymphomatoid Granulomatosis

Lymphomatoid granulomatosis is an angiocentric and angiodestructive lymphoproliferative disease that involves extranodal sites, most commonly the lungs in over 90% of cases, with the brain, kidney, liver, and skin as other sites. Involvement of lymph nodes is very rare.

Extranodal NK/T Cell Lymphoma – Nasal Type

Among the extranodal NK/T cell lymphomas, the nasal type may show secondary involvement of regional lymph nodes. The histological features in lymph nodes are not unlike those in other sites. The lymphomatous infiltrate is diffuse and permeative with angiodestruction being frequently present. Coagulative necrosis and apoptosis are very common and the morphologic spectrum

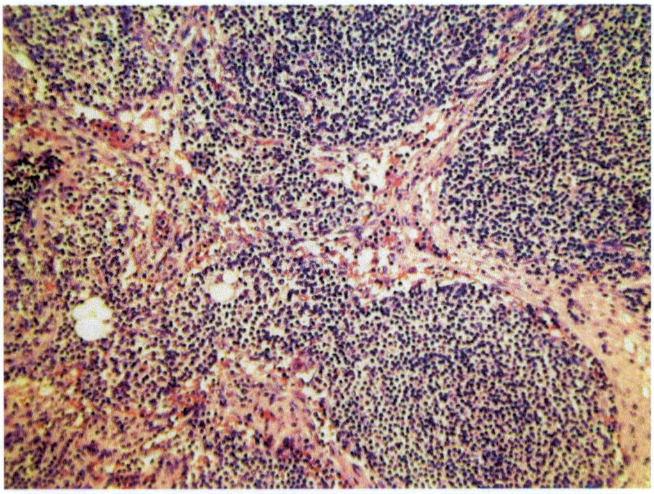

Fig. 8.23. Lymph node involvement by gastric MALT lymphoma shows a nodular pattern as a result of perifollicular infiltration of uniform-appearing small cells.

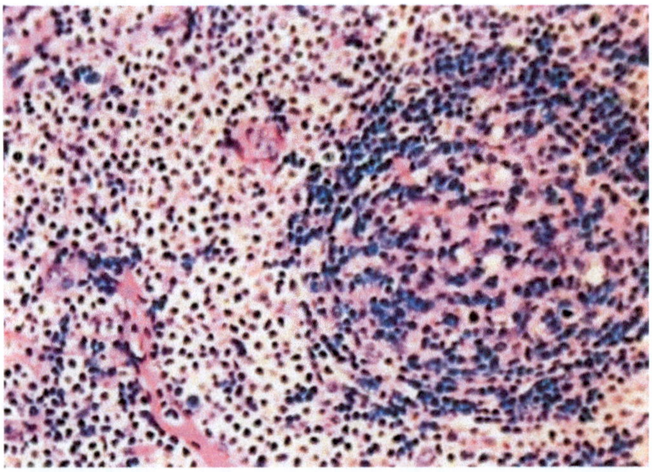

Fig. 8.24. A monotonous population of monocytoid cells with abundant pale cytoplasm and dark nuclei surround a follicle which shows colonization by the neoplastic cells.

of the lymphoma cells is often very broad, with a range of cells sizes. The cells often display irregular, folded nuclei that can be elongated, generally have granular chromatin, inconspicuous nucleoli, and often moderate amounts of pale or clear cytoplasm. Azurophilic cytoplasmic granules are seen in Giemsa-stained touch preparations. The cells are CD56+/CD2+/CD3ε+, and CD3−. They stain for cytotoxic molecules and other T and NK cell-associated antigens are negative.

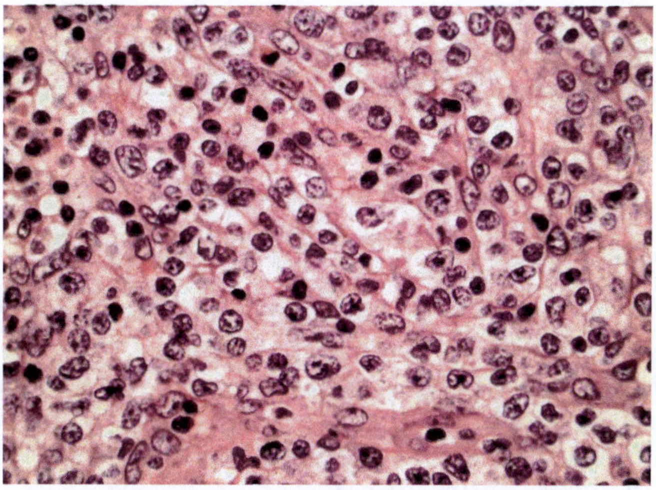

Fig. 8.25. Monocytoid neoplastic cells infiltrate the sinusoids and interfollicular regions.

Blastic Plasmacytoid Dendritic Cell Neoplasm

Blastic plasmacytoid dendritic cell neoplasm (BPDCN), previously known as blastic NK cell lymphoma and CD4+/CD56+ hematodermic neoplasm, is a rare, aggressive tumor derived from the precursors of plasmacytic dendritic cells. It is longer regarded as a lymphoma but instead it represents a unique precursor hematopoietic neoplasm that responds to acute leukemia treatment regimens and bone marrow transplantation. BPDCN occurs mostly in elderly patients with a high frequency of cutaneous and bone marrow involvement and leukemic dissemination. Regional lymph node involvement occurs in lesser frequency. A fulminant leukemic phase ultimately develops. Some cases are associated with myelodysplasia but there is no association with Epstein–Barr virus. Diffuse lymph node infiltration in a leukemic manner is seen in the interfollicular areas and medulla. The infiltrate comprises monomorphous medium sized cells resembling lymphoblasts, with irregular nuclei, fine chromatin, and one or more small nucleoli. The cytoplasm is scant and lacks granules unlike that of NK cell tumors. They show an immunophenotype similar to that of plasmacytoid dendritic cells and are frequently CD4+/CD43+/CD5RA+/CD56+. They express CD123, the IL-3 receptor α chain, and HLA-DR. In addition, other lymphoid- and myeloid-associated antigens such as CD7, CD2, and CD33 may be expressed, and CD68 in the form of small cytoplasmic dots is seen in about half the cases. There is variable positivity for Tdt. T and B cell receptor genes are usually germline (**Table 8.5**).

Table 8.5
Secondary lymph node involvement by extranodal lymphomas morphology and immunohistology

Splenic marginal zone lymphoma
- Uncommon, limited to splenic hilar nodes
- Dilatation of sinuses, lymphoma cells surrounding and replacing germinal centers
- Marginal zone often not discernable
- CD20+, CD79a+, CD23–, CD10–, Bcl6–, CD43–, cyclinD1–, CD5 often negative

Hairy cell leukemia
- Splenic hilar nodes involved in advanced stage
- Partial involvement
- Sinuses, cortex, and medullar infiltrated by neoplastic cells; follicles may be spared
- TRAP+, CD20+, CD13+, DBA.44+
- Bright monotypic sIg
- CD10–, Bcl6–, CD5–

Heavy-chain disease
- Systemic symptoms, autoimmune disease
- Lymphadenopathy associated with hepatosplenomegaly, involvement of skin, Waldeyer ring, salivary glands, thyroid, gastrointestinal tract, and peripheral blood
- Infiltrate of lymphocytes, plasmacytoid lymphocytes, plasma cells, immunoblasts, histiocytes, and eosinophils
- CD79a+, CD20+, CD38+, CD138+
- Monotypic cIgγ or cIgμ
- CD10–, Bcl6–, CD5–

Plasma cell neoplasms
- Groups and sheets of plasma cells with blast forms in lymph node
- Monotypic cIg heavy- and light-chain expression

MALT lymphoma
- Invade marginal zone of lymph node with interfollicular expansion
- Discrete accumulations of monocytoid cells in parafollicular and perisinusoidal areas
- Plasma cell differentiation and colonization of follicles may be seen
- No specific markers for MALT lymphoma
- CD20+, CD79a+, Bcl2+, IRF4/MUM1+, Bcl6 mostly positive but CD10–

Lymphomatoid granulomatosis
- Nodal involvement very rare
- Angiocentric and angiodestructive process

Extranodal NK/T cell lymphoma, nasal type
- Regional nodes may be involved
- Diffuse and permeative process with angiodestruction
- Broad morphologic spectrum, range of cell sizes, often irregular folded nuclei, sometimes elongated, moderates amounts of pale or clear cytoplasm
- CD56+, CD2+, CD3ε+, CD3–
- Cytotoxic molecules TIA-1, granzyme B and perforin positive
- T and NK cell-associated antigens negative

Table 8.5 (continued)

Blastic plasmacytoid dendritic cell neoplasm
• Skin, bone marrow and leukemic presentation with local node infiltration in about 50%
• A rare precursor hemopoietic neoplasm that responses to acute leukemic therapies
• Cells mimic lymphoblasts, have agranular cytoplasm and infiltrate in a leukemic pattern
• CD4+/CD56+/CD43+/CD123+/HLA-DR+; less frequently CD2+/CD7+/CD33+/CD68+

EBV-Associated T Cell Lymphoproliferative Disorders

There are two rare types of T cell lymphoproliferative disorders that are associated with Epstein–Barr virus (EBV) infection which are difficult to diagnose and deserve mentioning. One occurs mostly in childhood and represents a fulminant progression of an EBV infection which may involve lymph nodes, and the other is a primary cutaneous infection that may progress to systemic disease with involvement.

EBV-Positive T Cell Lymphoproliferative Disorders of Childhood

While two major types of Epstein–Barr virus (EBV)-associated T cell lymphoproliferative disorders (LPD) affecting children and young adults have been described, in neither are the lymph nodes the primary site of involvement. Awareness of the clinical setting in which the lymph node biopsy has been obtained and familiarity with their patterns of nodal involvement are critical to recognition of these entities.

Systemic EBV-Positive T Cell Lymphoproliferative Disease of Childhood

The severe, frequently life-threatening illnesses belonging in this diagnostic category include cases that have previously been classified under a variety of terms, including sporadic fatal infectious mononucleosis, fulminant hemophagocytic syndrome, and severe chronic active EBV infection. The varied terminology used historically is reflective of the fact that this disease can occur in more than one setting; while primary active EBV infection may precede involvement, other cases arise in the context of chronic active EBV infection (CAEBV). In both settings, progression to multiorgan failure is characteristically rapid, with death often resulting within days or weeks of onset. This T cell LPD, which shows no apparent predilection with respect to sex, is encountered most frequently in eastern Asia, especially Japan and Taiwan, and is distinctly uncommon in Western nations.

Clinical

Cases arising in the setting of primary EBV infection present acutely with constitutional symptoms (fever, lethargy) in otherwise healthy young people. Rather than resolving spontaneously over a period of many weeks, however, the illness progresses with development of hepatic failure accompanied by hepatosplenomegaly and, on occasion, lymphadenopathy. Hemophagocytic syndrome often develops, along with pancytopenia, a coagulopathy, sepsis, and multi-organ failure.

The same constellation of findings may be seen in cases occurring after CAEBV has developed. CAEBV is defined by persistence of infectious mononucleosis-like symptoms for six or more months accompanied by high-titer early antigen and viral capsid antigen antibodies (EA-IgG and VCA-IgG, respectively), as well as histologic evidence of lymphadenitis or infection of other tissue with demonstration of EBV in such tissue. In some cases, EBV infects T cells or NK cells instead of B cells, and a monoclonal T cell population becomes detectable; this is the scenario in which progression to an overt LPD occurs, and it is important to characterize such cases as systemic EBV-positive T cell LPDs of childhood and not merely as CAEBV.

Morphology

The lymph node findings in these cases are not nearly as striking as those in the liver and spleen, where conspicuous lymphoid proliferations are more likely to be encountered. In general, nodal architecture remains intact and sinuses patent. Evidence of erythrophagocytosis may be noted, along with sinus histiocytosis, but recognition of the EBV-infected T cells may require use of ISH for EBV-encoded RNA (EBER). Such a histologic picture contrasts starkly with the prominent paracortical immunoblastic proliferation observed in typical cases of infectious mononucleosis.

Immunohistology

The neoplastic cells express pan-T cell markers such as CD3, as well as cytotoxic molecules such as TIA-1. Negativity of the cells for CD56 contrasts with aggressive NK cell leukemia. The heterogeneity of cases in this category is highlighted by the tendency for the malignant cells to express CD4 or CD8 and to be associated with the type of EBV infection in which the LPD originated. Those arising in a background of CAEBV are usually CD4+, while CD8 expression is typical of those occurring subsequent to primary acute EBV infection. As noted above, ISH for EBER highlights the neoplastic T cells.

Genetics

Recurrent karyotypic abnormalities are lacking, but clonal TCR gene rearrangement is characteristic.

The disparity between the severe, acute clinical syndrome and the comparatively non-descript H&E lymph node morphology is striking, and proper diagnosis requires pertinent clinical history and familiarity with this diagnostic entity.

Hydroa Vacciniforme-Like Lymphoma

Hydroa vacciniforme-like lymphoma is an EBV-associated cutaneous T cell lymphoma that in some cases progresses to systemic disease that may feature lymphadenopathy. Occurring predominantly in children from Asia, Native Americans and those from Mexico, Central America, or South America, this lesion is related to mosquito bite hypersensitivity.

Clinical

A papulovesicular eruption develops on the face or another sun-exposed site; progression to ulceration with subsequent scarring is common. Recurrent lesions may occur over a period of several years, and late in the clinical course, constitutional symptoms, hepatosplenomegaly, and lymphadenopathy may occur. Progression becomes more rapid once systemic involvement takes place.

Morphology

Involved lymph nodes typically show diffuse infiltration, ranging from predominantly paracortical to near-total effacement, by a population of intermediate to large cells with abundant eosinophilic cytoplasm and pleomorphic nuclei that range from round to oval to irregular. Multinucleated cells may be seen, as can vacuolated cells and areas exhibiting spindle cell morphology. Hemophagocytosis, while sometimes present, is generally inconspicuous. The neoplastic cells are accompanied by a mixed leucocytic infiltrate that may include lymphocytes, plasma cells, eosinophils, neutrophils, and reactive histiocytes. Resemblance to other lesions such as large cell lymphomas of B or T cell lineage, melanoma, or carcinoma may be striking and emphasizes the necessity of immunohistochemical staining.

Immunohistology

A cytotoxic T cell immunophenotype is most common, with an NK cell phenotype less frequently exhibited. ISH for EBER is consistently positive.

Genetics

Clonal TCR gene rearrangement is typical of CD8+ cases but not for those cases with an NK cell phenotype.

Chapter 9

Needle Core Biopsies and Aspirates

Key words: Diagnostic approach, mantle cell lymphoma, Langerhans cell histiocytosis, inflammatory myofibroblastic tumor, anaplastic large cell lymphoma, Hodgkin lymphoma, diffuse large B cell lymphoma, follicular lymphoma, peripheral T cell lymphoma, malignant germ cell tumor, flow cytometry, fine-needle aspiration.

Needle Core Biopsies

It used to be the requirement that for proper examination of lymph nodes, a fresh intact specimen was required because fragmentation produced crushing with distortion of architecture and cytology of the fragile lymphoid cells contained within. The advent of techniques including immunohistochemistry, flow cytometry, and molecular analysis to supplement morphological examination has contributed significantly to the ability to diagnose fragmented pieces of lymph node tissue and material removed piecemeal, although this is far from ideal.

Advantages of Needle Core Biopsies

Radiologists, with the aid of image guidance, can now obtain needle core biopsies of lymph node and lymphoid tissue from deep-seated sites, enabling them to target material that appears most pathological rather than most accessible, opening up a new dimension in the diagnosis of lymph node pathology. Computed tomography (CT)-guided needle core biopsies allow access to lesions in the abdomen, thorax, pelvis, and retroperitoneum that would otherwise require access by invasive methods such as laparotomy or thoracostomy. Other advantages include the ease and speed of needle core biopsies, ability to repeat the non-invasive procedure should unsatisfactory material be obtained the first time, tolerance of the procedure by debilitated patients in whom diagnostic material may otherwise not be obtainable, and

A.S.-Y. Leong, *A Pattern Approach to Lymph Node Diagnosis*,
DOI 10.1007/978-1-4419-7176-0_9, © Springer Science+Business Media, LLC 2011

the ability to commence appropriate chemotherapy immediately without having to wait for recovery from invasive surgical procedures. Besides the ability to perform needle core biopsies on an outpatient basis without hospitalization and its low morbidity, the diagnostic material is also suitable in staging and followup for recurrences. Additional cores can be obtained for flow cytometry, cytogenetics, molecular analysis, and other investigations as necessary.

Disadvantages of Needle Core Biopsies

Disadvantages of needle core biopsies include the lesser amount of material available for examination, loss of some topographical and architectural features, the risk of sampling error, and the danger that it may be employed inappropriately to replace the biopsy of complete lymph nodes. The latter should remain the method of choice for superficial lymph nodes in patients who are fit for surgical procedure.

As it appears inevitable that needle core biopsies will increasingly be employed for the diagnosis of lymphoid lesions, it would be useful to provide a short discussion of the approach to the examination and diagnosis of such material, the potential pitfalls, and limitations.

Handling of Needle Core Biopsies

In the handling of needle core biopsies, it is important that they are immediately and adequately fixed. In this regard, the radiologist/clinician should be reminded to immerse the thin core of tissue immediately into 10% buffered formalin and not allow it to dry out under bright lights. Fixation is rapid because of the small size of the sample, and a minimum of 4–6 h is often all that is required.

The lesser amount of material available requires that care be taken to conserve tissue as the biopsy may be cut through before all necessary immunohistochemical stains have been completed. As such, it should be the routine to initially cut multiple sections onto silanized slides in anticipation of immunohistochemistry. If multiple cores have been obtained for histologic examination, it is best to process each biopsy in a separate cassette, as imperfect alignment of multiple cores during embedding may result in wastage of valuable tissue. It needs to be emphasized that with needle core samples, flow cytometry plays an invaluable role. As such, a separate core should be sent unfixed for flow cytometry. Should other investigations be anticipated, an additional core can be appropriately apportioned.

Diagnostic Approach to Needle Core Biopsies of Lymph Nodes and Potential Pitfalls

In diagnosing needle core biopsies, the same principles and pattern approach employed for intact lymph node specimens are applicable. However, while it is possible to recognize many specific entities in needle core biopsies, it should be emphasized that the nature of the specimen and its size may not allow the appreciation of architectural alteration, which is an important criterion for the identification of neoplastic infiltrates. Sampling, furthermore, is a problem, and failure to detect variation that might otherwise be seen in an intact lymph node, such as high-grade transformation or a diffuse component in a follicular lymphoma, remains a possibility. The fragile lymphoid lesions may be traumatized, especially with traction artifacts imposed by fibrous issue. Because of these deficiencies, there is a greater reliance on the results of immunohistochemistry and flow cytometry.

One approach to the diagnosis of needle core biopsies is to ask a series of sequential questions as with lymph node biopsies.

Does the Sample Represent Lymph Node Tissue?

It may not be possible to answer this question, as lymph node architecture may not be identifiable; however, it should at least be ascertained that the material is lymphoid in nature.

Is Lymph Node Architecture Destroyed?

Employ stains for FDC to outline follicles. If necessary, use other stains such as reticulin to examine for sinuses.

Is the Process Lymphoid?

Stain for cytokeratins to exclude metastatic carcinoma, especially small cell mimics such as small cell carcinoma and lobular carcinoma of the breast. HMB45, Melan A, and/or tyrosinase positivity will identify metastatic melanoma. CD45 positivity confirms the lymphoid nature of the infiltrate, although lymphoblastic lymphomas and T cell lymphomas (e.g., ALCL) may be CD45 negative, and Hodgkin and Reed–Sternberg cells characteristically do not express this marker.

If Lymphoid, Is the Process Follicular/Nodular or Diffuse?

Staining for FDC will help resolve this question. Additionally, as with sections of excisional biopsy specimens, partially closing the microscope condenser diaphragm may enhance recognition of subtle nodularity.

If Follicular, Is It Reactive or Neoplastic?

The appearance of FDC meshwork will help identify neoplastic follicular proliferations which can be further subtyped; the pattern of Ki67 positivity is often of less utility in small-core biopsy samples than in larger sections due to the lesser number of evaluable follicles. CyclinD1 positivity identifies mantle cell lymphoma, and positivity for Bcl2 and MT2 (CD45RA), in conjunction with appropriate morphologic features, and expression of markers of germinal center differentiation (i.e., Bcl6, CD10) identifies follicular lymphomas. The layers of the follicles and hues help identify mantle cell and marginal zone lymphomas.

If There Are Nodules, Are They Homogenous or Heterogenous in Composition?

If heterogenous, exclude growth centers of CLL/SLL and Hodgkin lymphoma by immunostaining for CD23, CD45, CD15, and CD30. Colonization of follicles by DLBCL produces heterogenous nodules/follicles. PTGC and NLPHL produce large heterogenous nodules with prominent FDC meshworks.

If homogenous, exclude lymphoblastic lymphoma by staining for Tdt, CD3, CD4 and CD8, and paracortical T cell nodules by demonstrating DRC meshworks with S100, CD1a, and langerin (CD207).

Do All of the Follicles Appear Hyperplastic? If So, Does This Ensure That the Process Is Reactive?

Ensure that the sample is representative; it is possible, that the primary pathology has not been sampled. Examine interfollicular regions especially carefully; subtle interfollicular involvement by neoplasia can be difficult to recognize even in excisional biopsy specimens, when let alone with smaller quantities of tissue. If, after correlation with clinical data, it seems most likely that the process truly is reactive, can a specific diagnosis be made?

If the Infiltrate Is Diffuse, Is It Homogenous or Heterogenous, and What Is the Cell Size?

Heterogenous diffuse infiltrates are more difficult to diagnose, and CD79a and CD3 stains may help identify if the cells are overwhelmingly predominantly B or T (this is aided by flow cytometry). If predominantly T cell, then a T cell lymphoma should be considered. The presence of large pleomorphic cells raises the possibility of ALCL, and CD30 and ALK staining are required. Hodgkin lymphoma should also be considered.

Homogenous lymphoid infiltrates suggest lymphoma, and subtyping for B and T cell lymphoma is required.

Examples of core biopsies are provided below.

CASE 1: 62-year-old man with retroperitoneal mass, 50 x 40 x 40 mm.

Diagnosis: Mantle cell lymphoma (**Figs. 9.1**, **9.2**, **9.3**, and **9.4**).

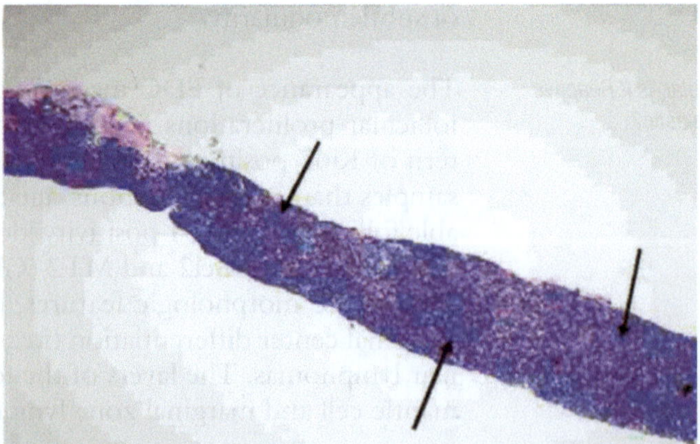

Fig. 9.1. Mantle cell lymphoma, retroperitoneum. The image-guided needle core is cellular and shows a vaguely nodular pattern (*arrows*).

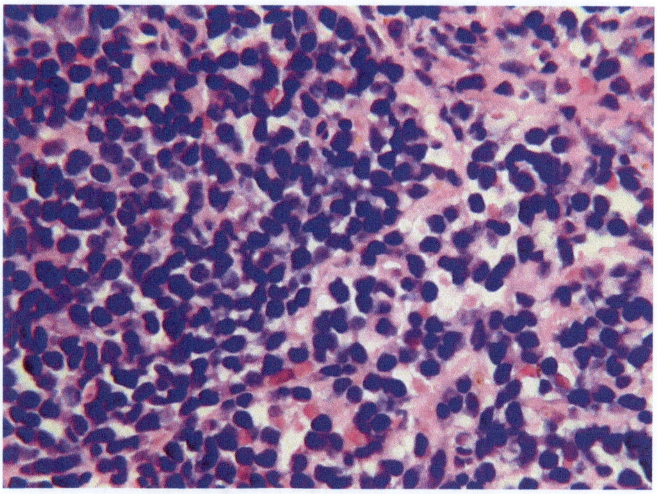

Fig. 9.2. The infiltrate is homogenous and composed of small lymphocytes with coarse chromatin and mildly irregular nuclei. Cytoplasm is scanty.

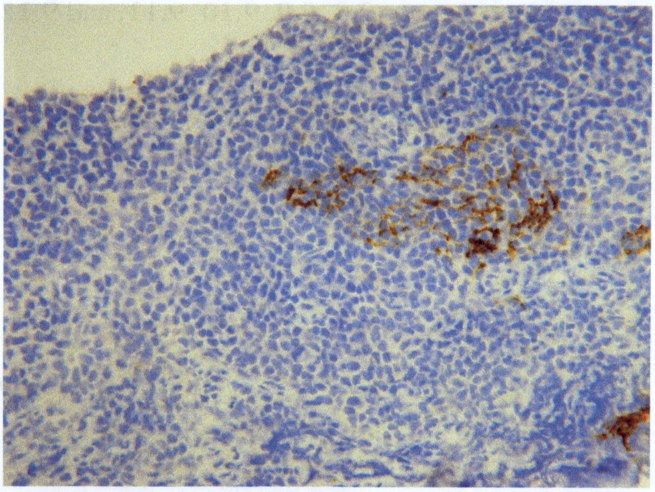

Fig. 9.3. CD23 reveals residual FDC meshworks in the center of several of the nodules but there is no staining of the lymphoma cells.

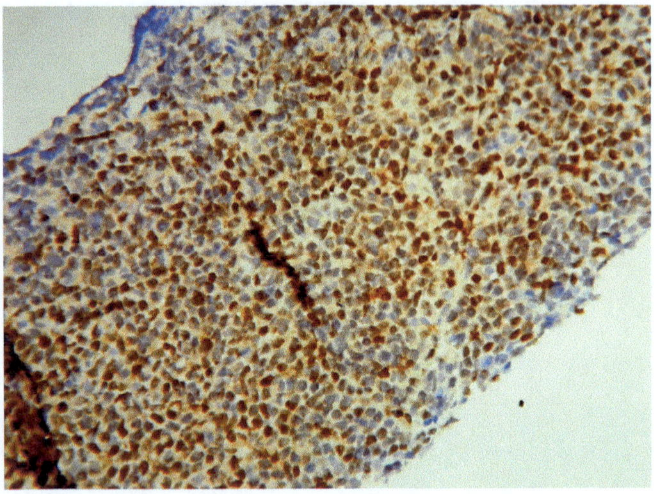

Fig. 9.4. Strong nuclear staining for cyclinD1 is observed in the lymphoma cells which are also CD20+/CD43+ and variably CD5+ (not shown).

CASE 2: 18-year-old man, largely asymptomatic 30 x 30 x 20 mm mass behind the right sternomastoid muscle.

Diagnosis: Langerhans cell histiocytosis (**Figs. 9.5**, **9.6**, **9.7**, **9.8**, **9.9**, **9.10**, **9.11**, and **9.12**).

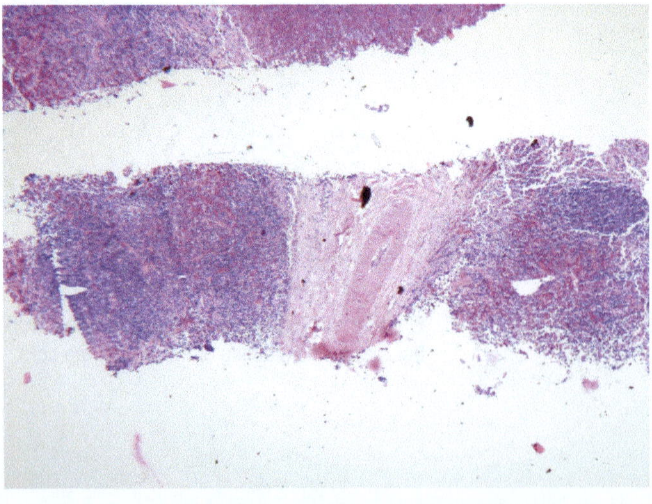

Fig. 9.5. Langerhans cell histiocytosis, cervical node. The infiltrate is polymorphous and displays areas of eosinophilia mixed with blue/grey hues. The former represents areas of eosinophil infiltration and the latter contains Langerhans cells, histiocytes, and small lymphocytes.

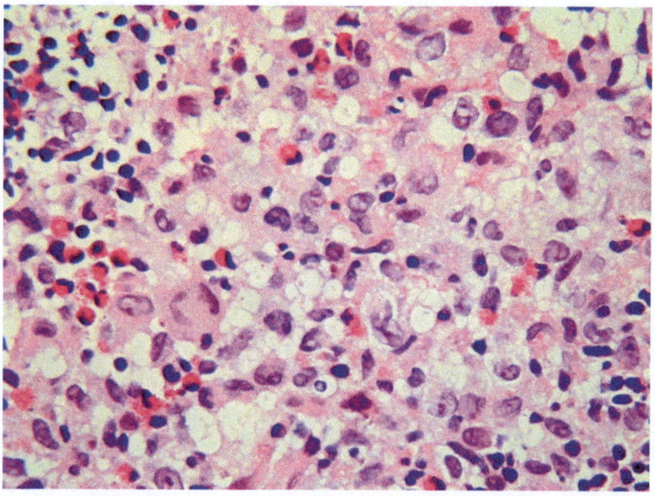

Fig. 9.6. The eosinophilic infiltrate contains large cells with folded, convoluted nuclei, small barely discernable nucleoli, and abundant eosinophilic cytoplasm. These Langerhans cells are mixed with eosinophils, macrophages, and small lymphocytes.

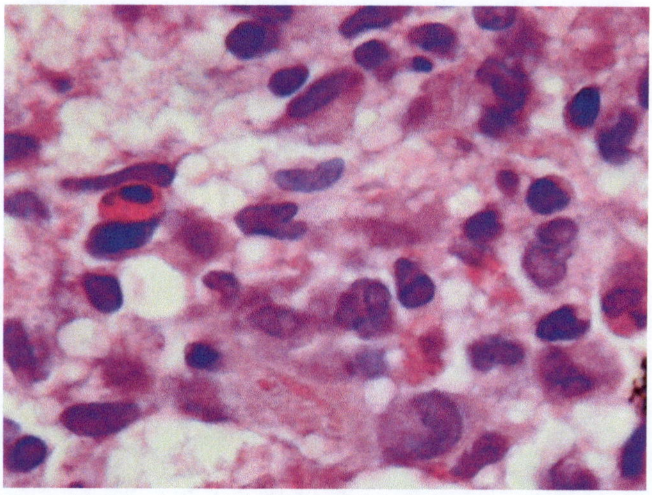

Fig. 9.7. Close-up appearance of Langerhans cells with their markedly folded and lobated nuclei, occasional small nucleoli, and abundant cytoplasm. Eosinophils are present.

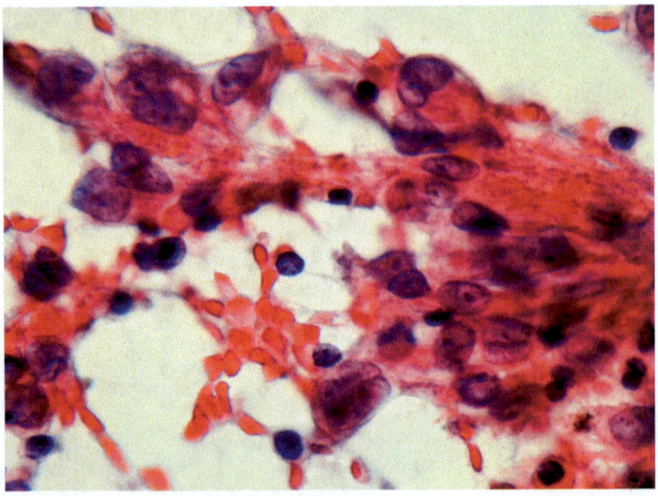

Fig. 9.8. An aspiration biopsy obtained in a separate pass shows the cytological appearance of the Langerhans cells (Papanicolaou stain).

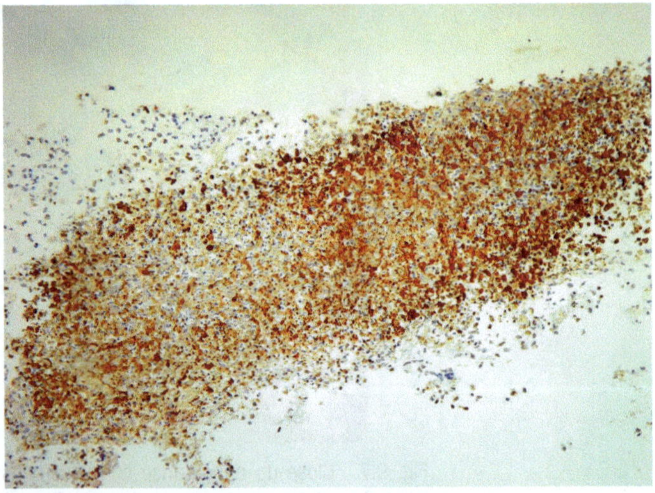

Fig. 9.9. The Langerhans cells stain for S100 protein.

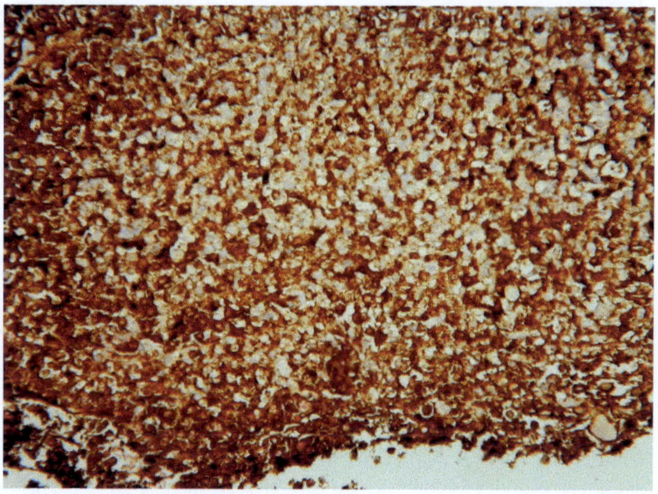

Fig. 9.10. There is strong staining for CD1a. The intermixed large cells that do not stain are macrophages.

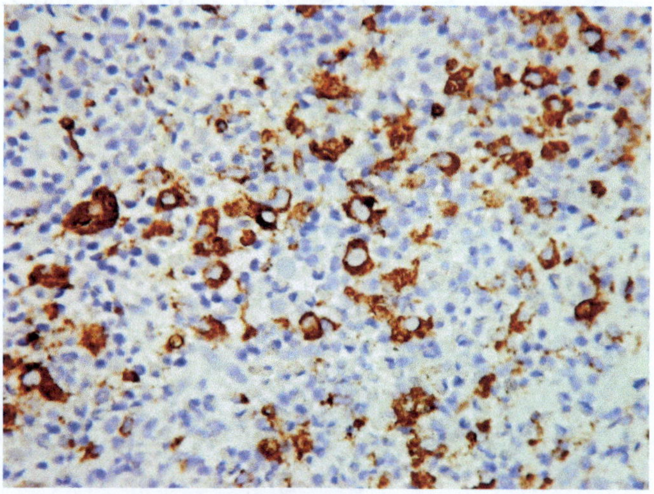

Fig. 9.11. CD68 labels macrophages present among the infiltrating cells. Other unstained large cells represent Langerhans cells.

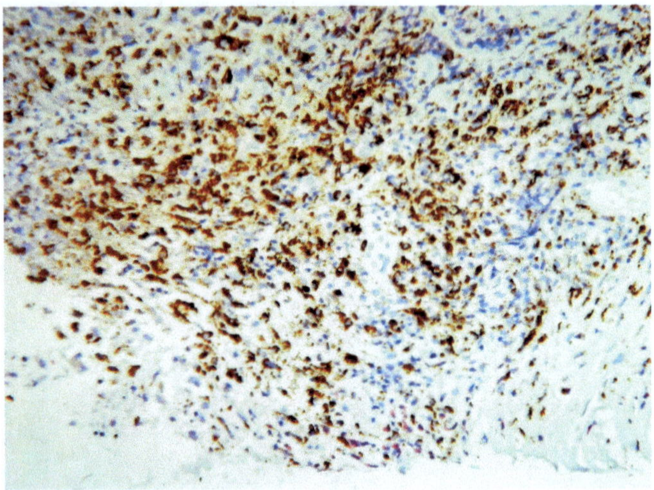

Fig. 9.12. The Langerhans cells stain for langerin.

CASE 3: 40-year-old man with history of fever and night sweats and anemia. A core biopsy was obtained from a tender localized left axillary mass of 30 mm diameter.

Diagnosis: Inflammatory myofibroblastic tumor (**Figs. 9.13, 9.14, 9.15, 9.16, 9.17**, and **9.18**).

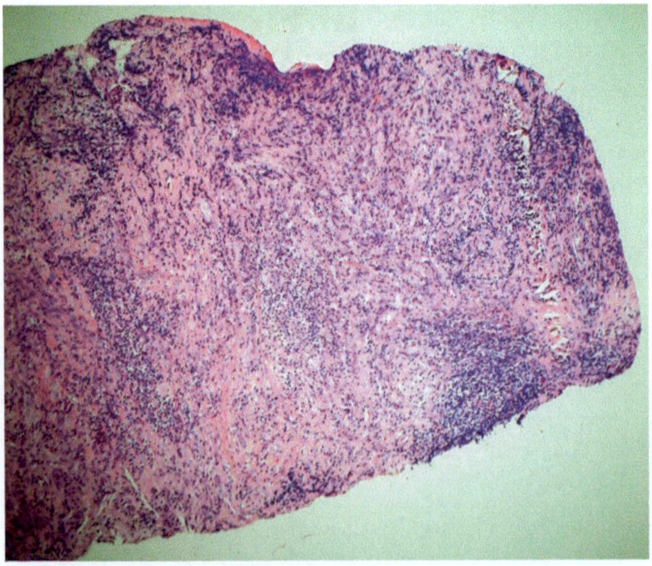

Fig. 9.13. Inflammatory myofibroblastic tumor. One end of the core shows a polymorphous infiltrate in fibrous tissue.

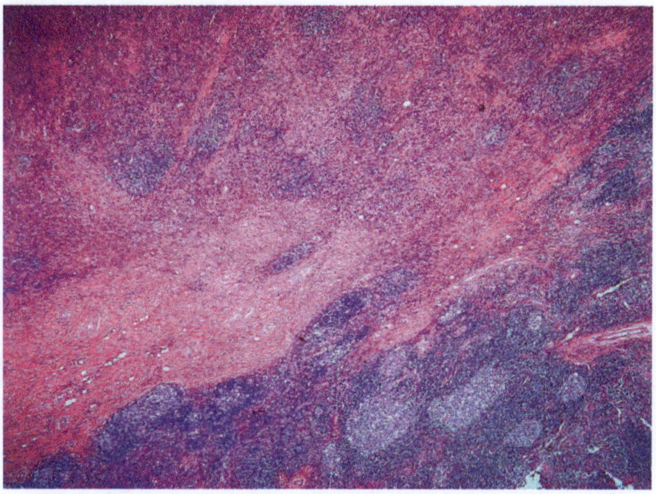

Fig. 9.14. At the other end of the core lymphoid tissue is evident and a polymorphous infiltrate is present in the adjacent fibrous tissue.

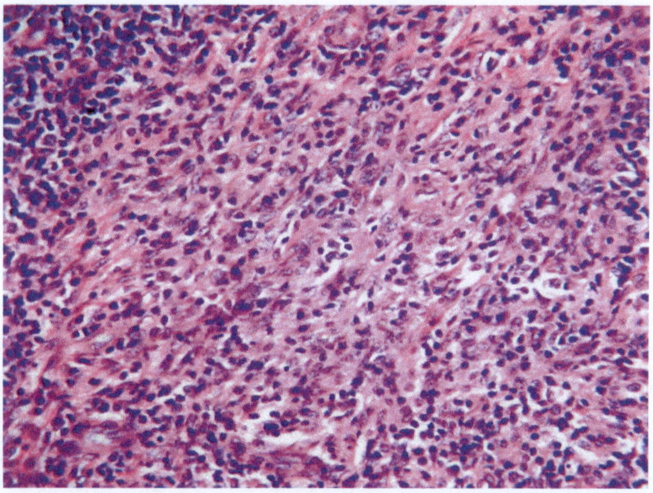

Fig. 9.15. A polymorphous infiltrate of plasma cells, stimulated lymphoid cells, histiocytes, and scattered eosinophils infiltrates the spindle cell stroma.

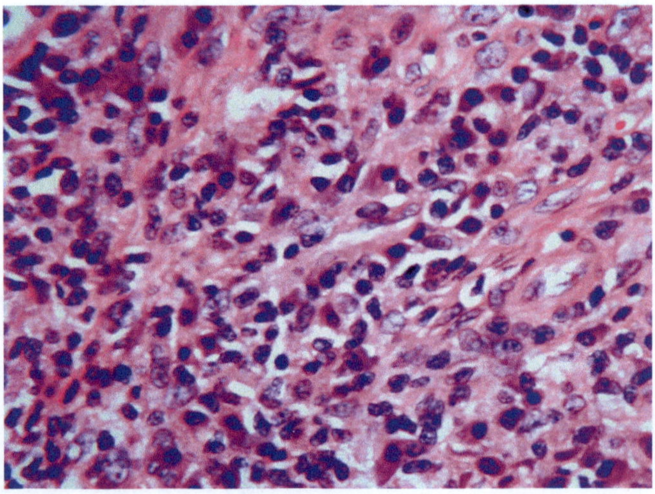

Fig. 9.16. Close up of the polymorphous inflammatory infiltrate. Th larger vesicular nuclei with small eosinophilic nucleoli (*arrows*) belong to the spindle cells. No atypia is present.

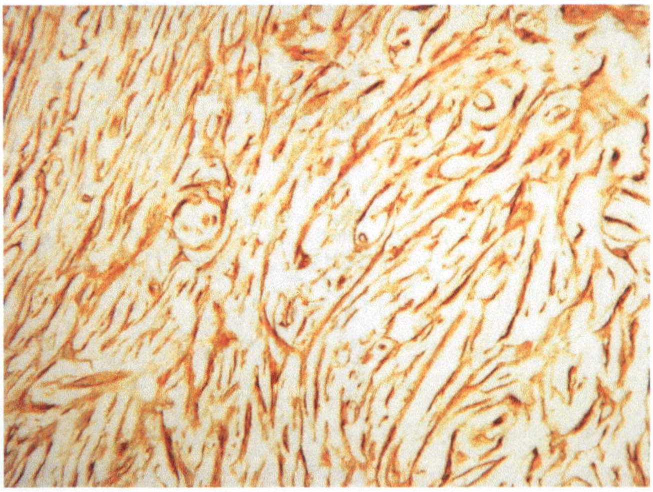

Fig. 9.17. Inflammatory myofibroblastic tumor. The spindle cells stain for smooth muscle actin.

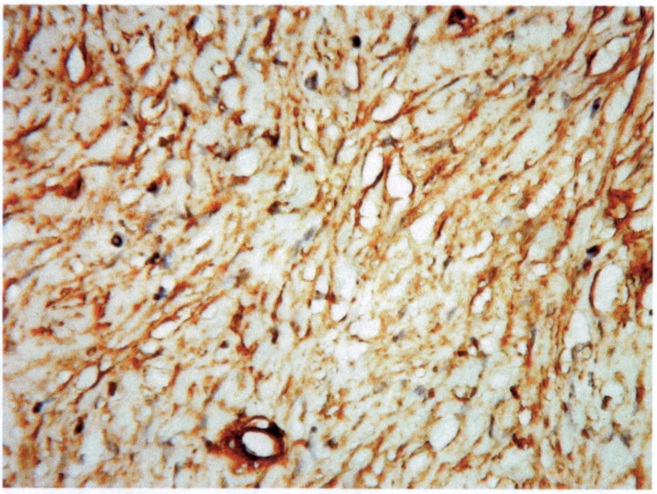

Fig. 9.18. Staining for type-IV collagen shows thin fragmented basal lamina investing the spindle cells, a pattern expressed by myofibroblasts.

CASE 4: 51-year-old man with axillary lymphadenopathy (2–3 cm), progressive anorexia, and night sweats. CT revealed extensive retroperitoneal adenopathy.

Diagnosis: Anaplastic large cell lymphoma, ALK positive (**Figs. 9.19**, **9.20**, **9.21**, and **9.22**).

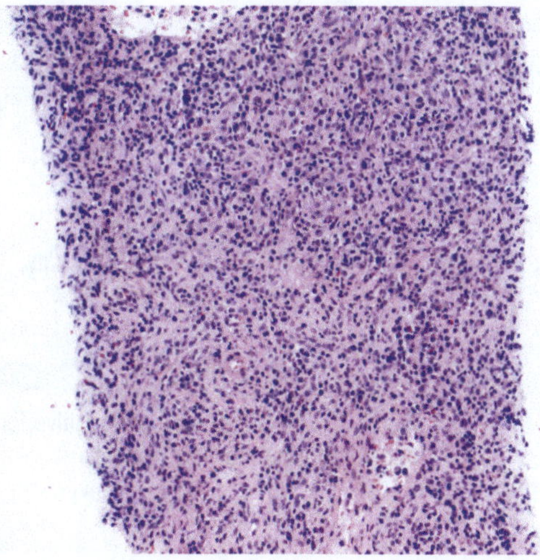

Fig. 9.19. ALCL, ALK+, in axillary lymph node. Core biopsy shows a diffuse, heterogenous infiltrate.

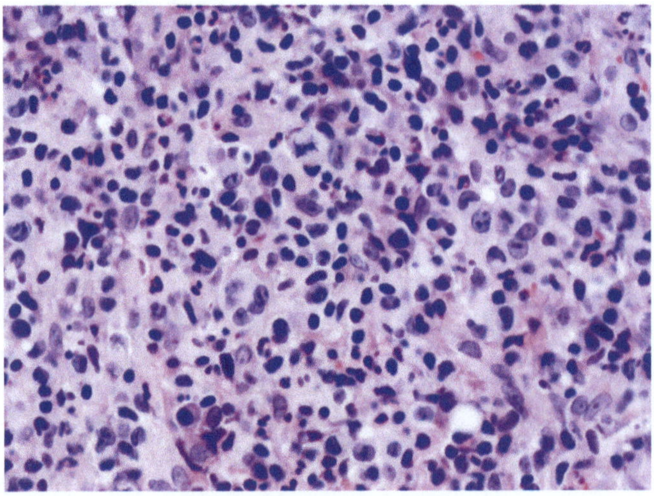

Fig. 9.20. Large abnormal lymphoid cells with irregular nuclei are accompanied by small lymphocytes, histiocytes, neutrophils, and plasma cells.

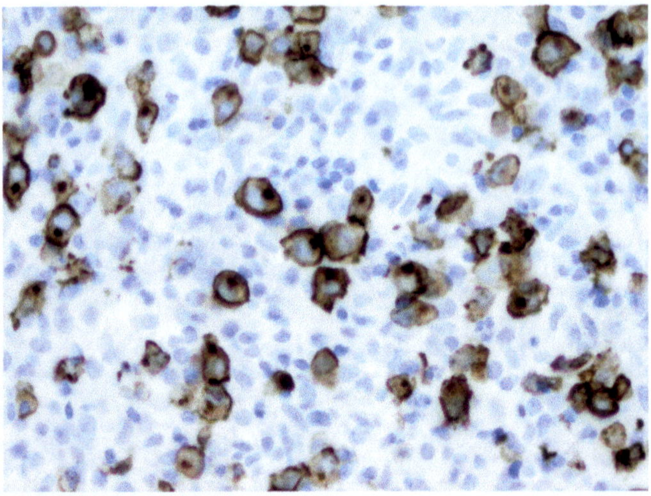

Fig. 9.21. The large cells are positive for CD30, staining with the typical membranous and paranuclear dot-like pattern.

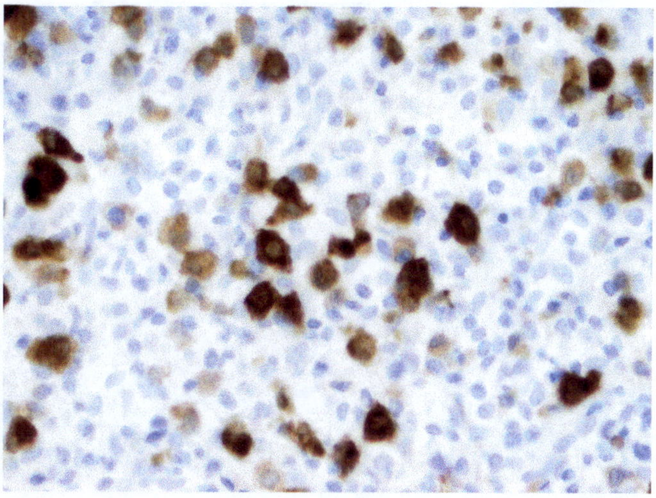

Fig. 9.22. ALK positivity within the large neoplastic cells is nuclear and cytoplasmic.

CASE 5: 44-year-old man with a 3-month history of abdominal pain. CT scan showed diffuse abdominal lymphadenopathy, and the patient underwent CT-guided biopsy of a mesenteric lymph node.

Diagnosis: Anaplastic large cell lymphoma, ALK negative (**Figs. 9.23**, **9.24**, **9.25**, **9.26**, and **9.27**).

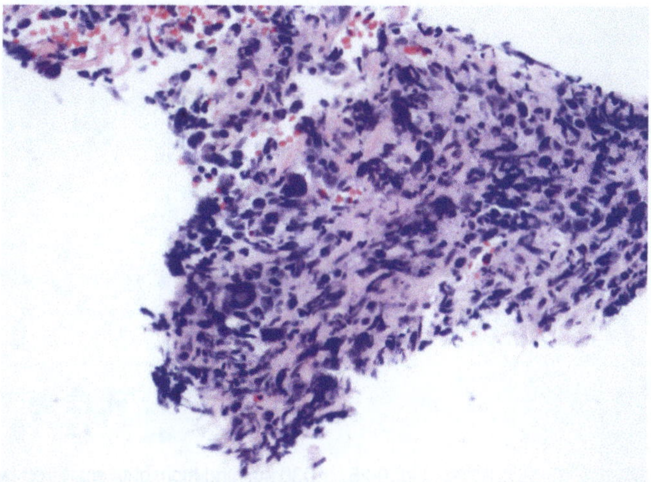

Fig. 9.23. Anaplastic large-cell lymphoma, ALK negative, in a mesenteric lymph node. Crush artifact is prominent, but even at low power a large cell process may be suspected.

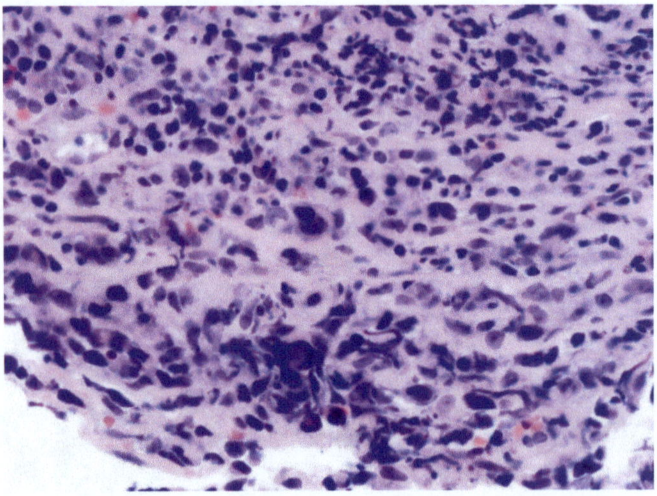

Fig. 9.24. At higher magnification, the presence of large abnormal cells among a greater number of small lymphocytes is discernible.

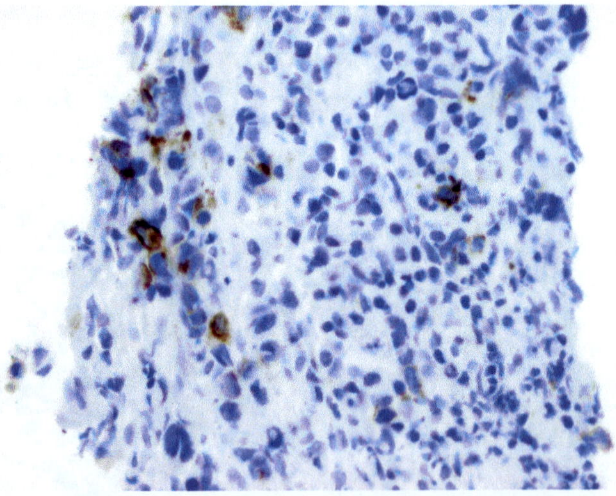

Fig. 9.25. CD30 staining highlights scattered large abnormal lymphocytes.

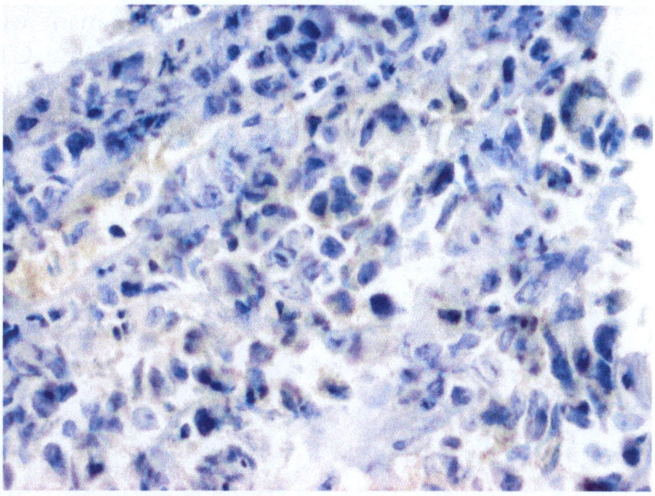

Fig. 9.26. The neoplastic lymphocytes are negative for ALK.

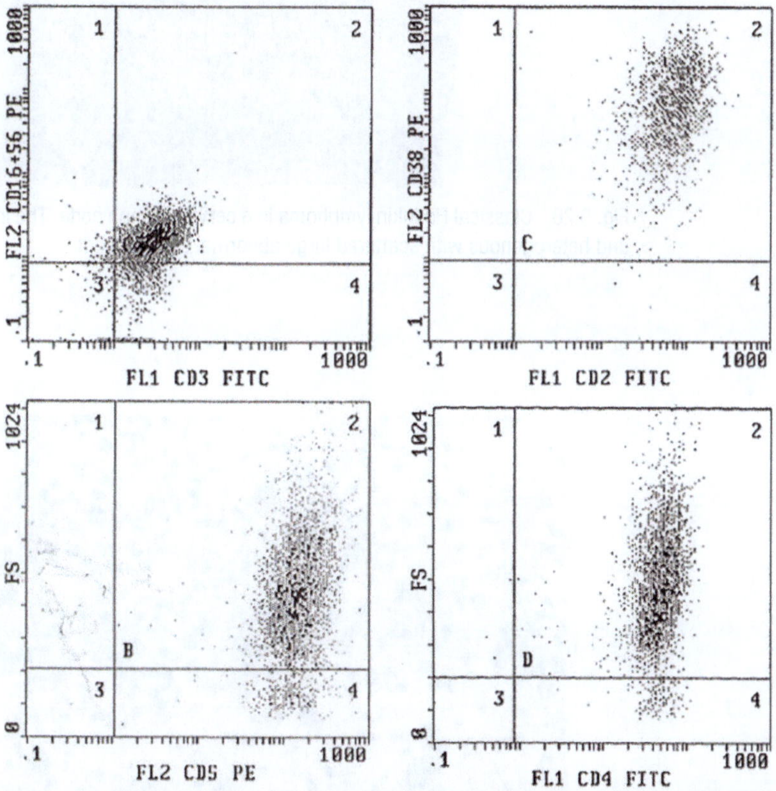

Fig. 9.27. Flow cytometric analysis of a concurrent fine-needle aspirate specimen shows a predominance of T cells with dim CD3, bright CD2, and bright CD5 expression. The cells express CD4 but not CD8, and they are large by light scatter criteria. Together with the morphologic and immunohistological findings, ALCL, ALK– was the most likely diagnosis.

CASE 6: 30-year-old man with progressive axillary and cervical lymphadenopathy. CT scan revealed diffuse thoracic and abdominal lymphadenopathy, and ultrasound-guided biopsy of an enlarged left cervical lymph node was performed.

Diagnosis: Classical Hodgkin lymphoma (**Figs. 9.28**, **9.29**, **9.30**, **9.31**, **9.32**, **9.33**, **9.34**, and **9.35**).

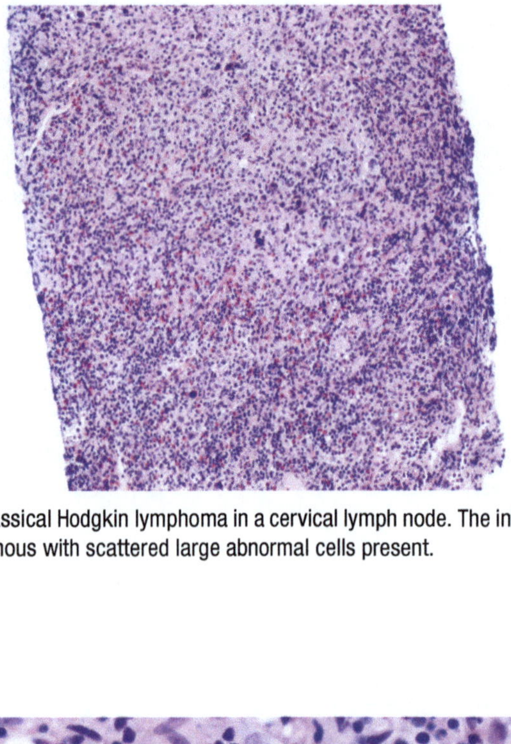

Fig. 9.28. Classical Hodgkin lymphoma in a cervical lymph node. The infiltrate is diffuse and heterogenous with scattered large abnormal cells present.

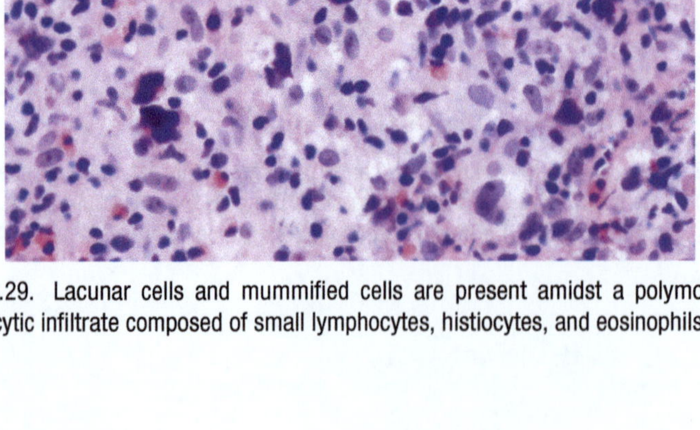

Fig. 9.29. Lacunar cells and mummified cells are present amidst a polymorphous leucocytic infiltrate composed of small lymphocytes, histiocytes, and eosinophils.

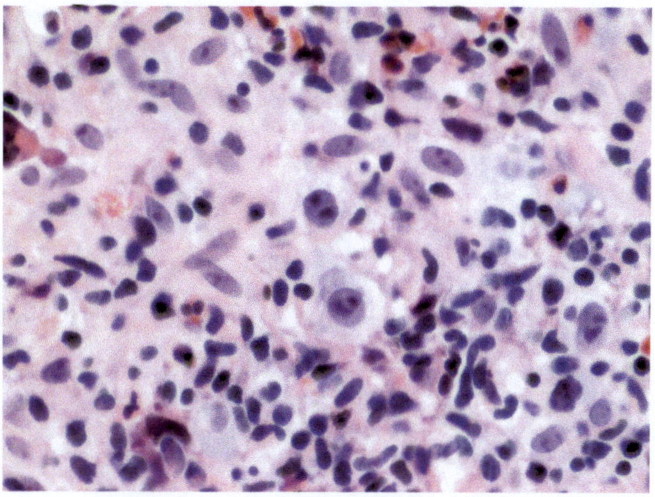

Fig. 9.30. The lacunar cells show irregular nuclei, prominent nucleoli, and abundant pale cytoplasm. The milieu is typical of classical Hodgkin lymphoma.

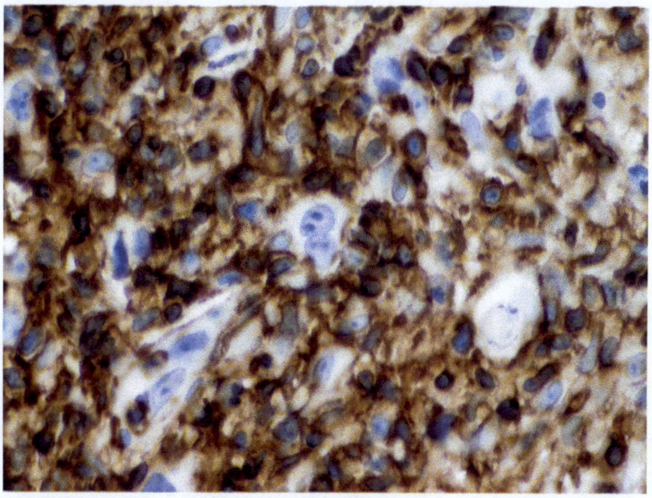

Fig. 9.31. The lacunar cells lack CD45 expression.

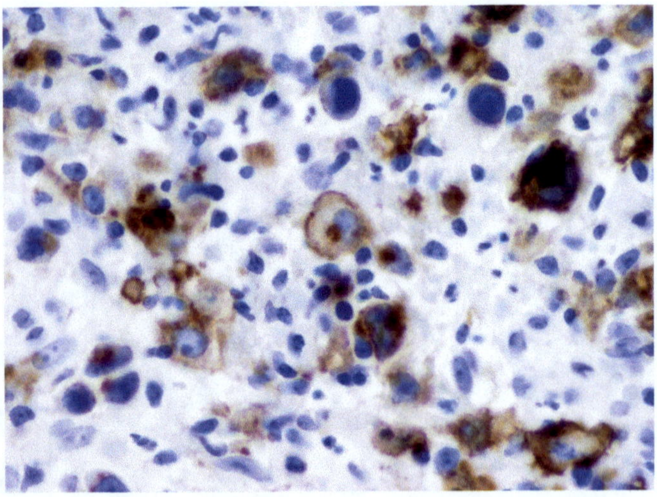

Fig. 9.32. CD30 is present in a membranous and paranuclear pattern in the large cells.

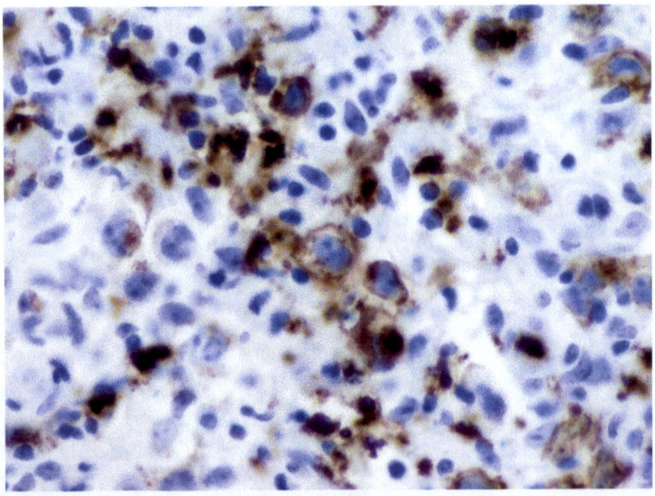

Fig. 9.33. Staining for CD15 shows immunoreactivity in a similar pattern. Eosinophils also stain for CD15.

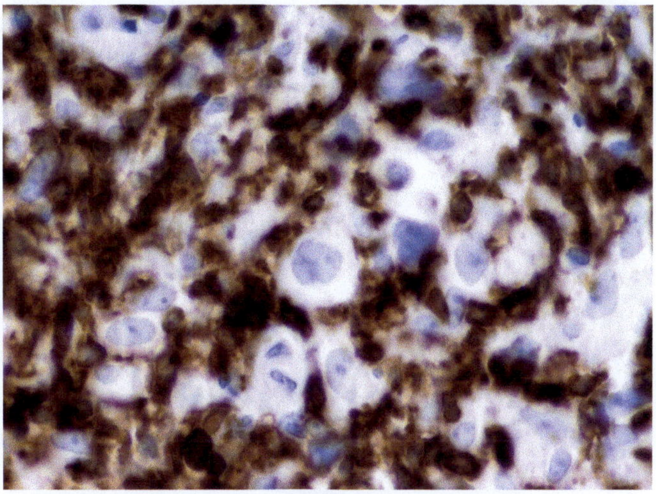

Fig. 9.34. CD3 highlights numerous small T cells in the background.

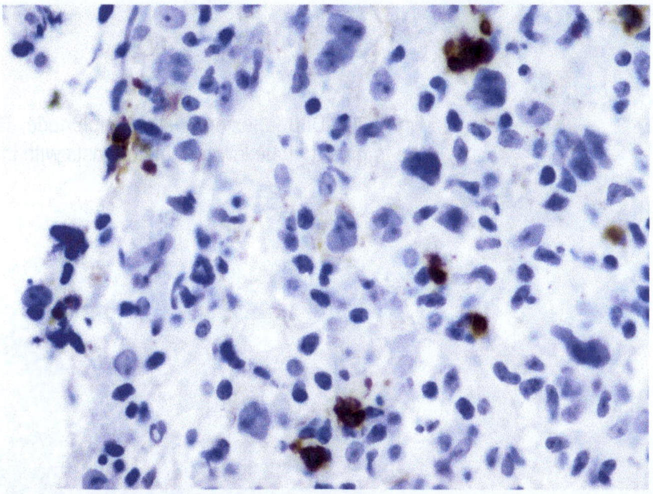

Fig. 9.35. CD20 outlines only less numbers of small B cells and shows only very weak, variable positivity of the large cells.

CASE 7: 63-year-old man with painless swelling of right lower extremity. Deep venous thrombosis was ruled out, and a subsequent CT scan showed multiple large abdominal and pelvic masses (up to 11 cm). Core biopsy of an external iliac lymph node was performed.

Diagnosis: Diffuse large B cell lymphoma (DLBCL) (**Figs. 9.36**, **9.37**, **9.38**, **9.39**, **9.40**, **9.41**, and **9.42**).

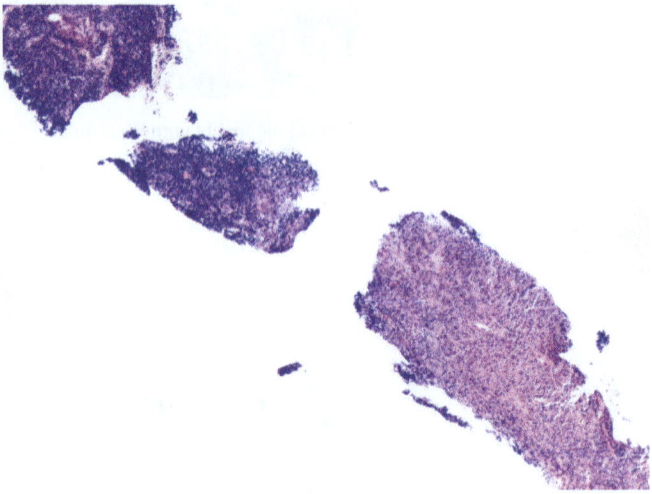

Fig. 9.36. DLBCL, external iliac lymph node. The relatively eosinophilic appearance of the fragment at the lower right contrasts with the basophilic fragments to the upper left.

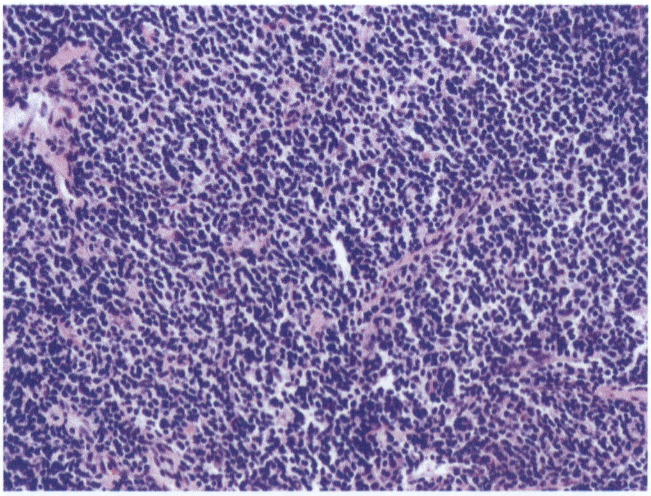

Fig. 9.37. The basophilic fragments show uninvolved lymphoid tissue with a marked predominance of small lymphocytes containing scant cytoplasm.

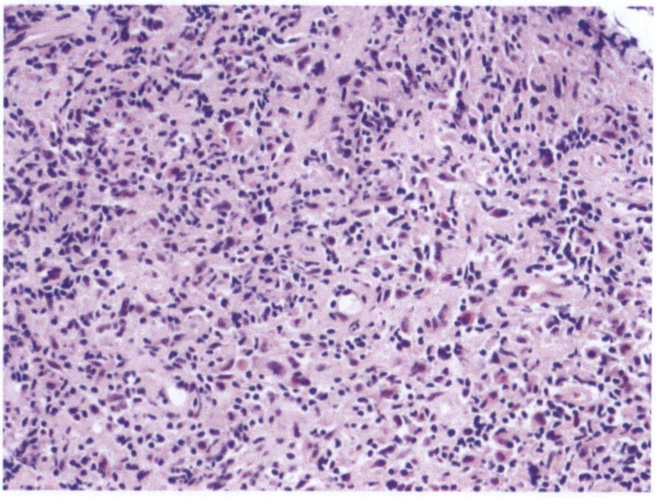

Fig. 9.38. The more eosinophilic fragments contain a diffuse neoplastic infiltrate composed of large abnormal lymphocytes with small, reactive lymphocytes admixed.

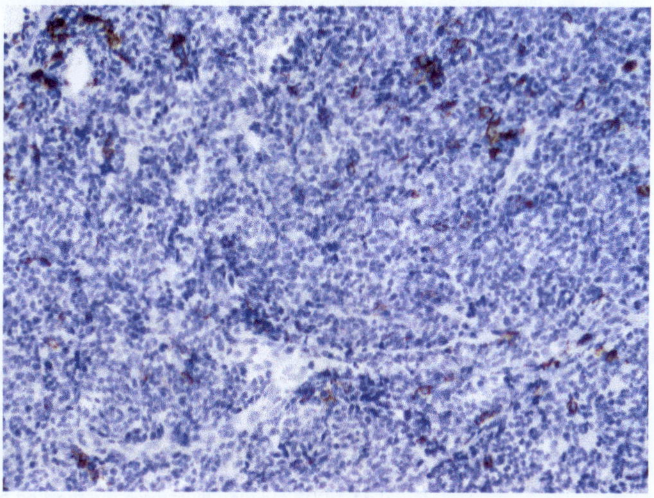

Fig. 9.39. DLBCL. CD20 highlights only rare small B cells in the uninvolved lymphoid tissue.

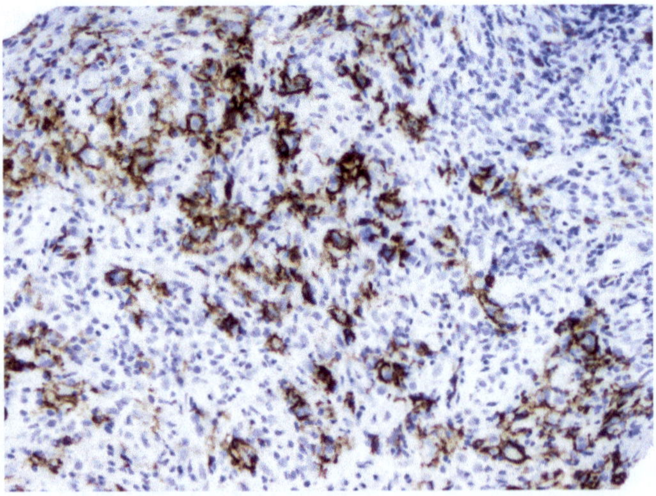

Fig. 9.40. In contrast, the neoplastic infiltrate shows positivity of the large abnormal cells for CD20, confirming their B cell lineage.

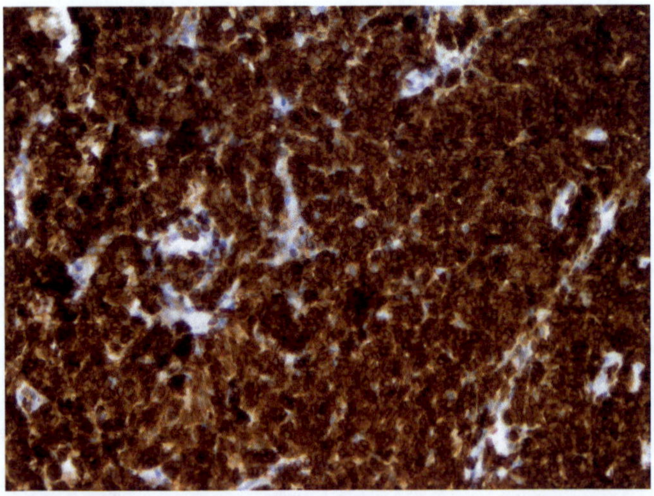

Fig. 9.41. CD3 staining illustrates the marked predominance of small T cells in what is most likely uninvolved paracortical lymph node tissue.

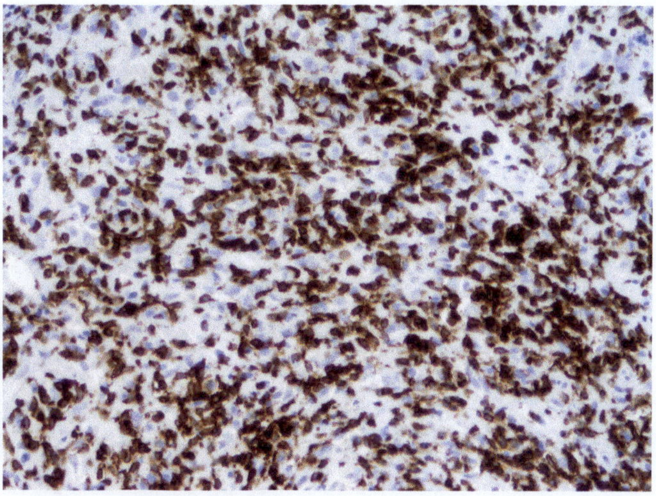

Fig. 9.42. DLBCL. Moderate numbers of small CD3 positive T cells comprise the reactive background for the neoplastic infiltrate.

CASE 8: 65-year-old man with left leg pain and foot drop. He had been diagnosed with diffuse large B cell lymphoma 11 months earlier and had had a good response to standard chemotherapy (CHOP + rituximab). PET scan showed increased FDG (2-deoxy-2-[18F]fluoro-D-glucose) uptake in left L5-S1 nerve roots, left piriformis, and sciatic nerve, as well as in left presacral and right inguinal lymph nodes. A needle biopsy of a right inguinal lymph node was performed to confirm recurrence of lymphoma.

Diagnosis: Diffuse large B cell lymphoma (DLBCL), recurrence (**Figs. 9.43**, **9.44**, and **9.45**).

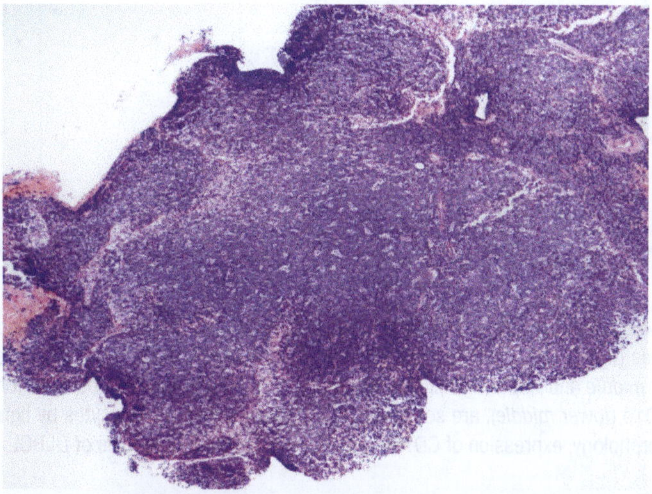

Fig. 9.43. DLBCL, inguinal lymph node. Tingible body macrophages lend a starry sky appearance to the diffuse homogenous infiltrate.

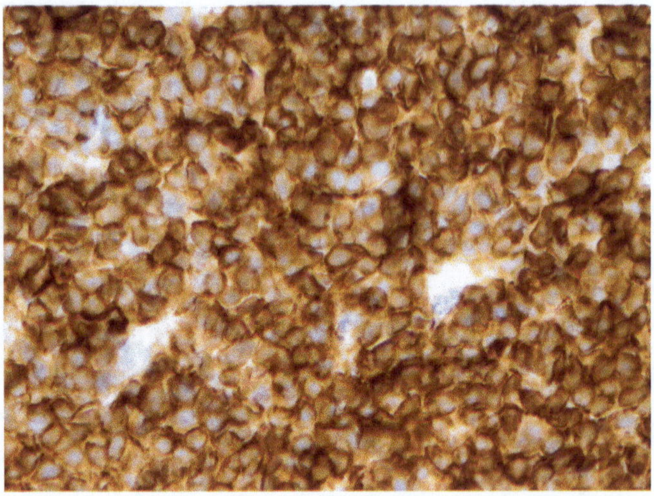

Fig. 9.44. CD79a staining demonstrates diffuse positivity of the large neoplastic B cells.

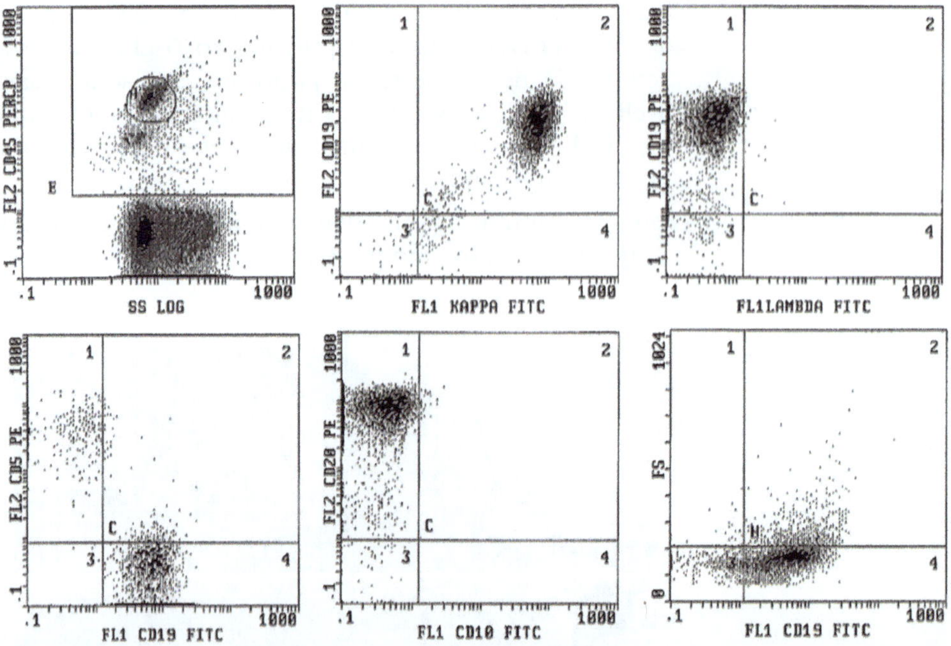

Fig. 9.45. Flow cytometric analysis shows a population of cells with CD45 and side-scatter properties typical of lymphocytes (*upper left*). The lymphocytes are predominantly CD19-positive B cells that express on their cell membranes (*upper middle* and *upper right*). The neoplastic cells, which are also positive for CD20 but negative for CD5 (*lower left*) and CD10 (*lower middle*), are somewhat larger than normal lymphocytes by light scatter criteria (*lower right*). Based on the morphology, expression of CD79a and monotypic Igκ, a diagnosis of DLBCL, recurrent, was rendered.

CASE 9: 57-year-old man with intermittent gross hematuria. Imaging studies showed a possible proximal left ureteral mass and lymphadenopathy. CT-guided needle biopsy of a left para-aortic lymph node was performed.

Diagnosis: Follicular lymphoma, grade 1 (**Figs. 9.46**, **9.47**, **9.48**, and **9.49**).

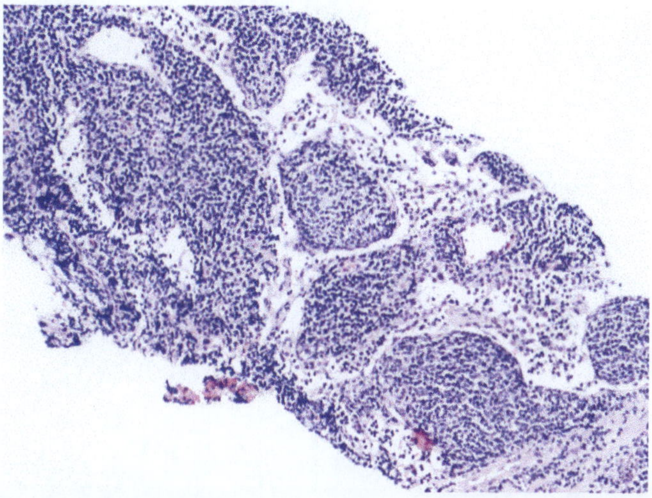

Fig. 9.46. Follicular lymphoma, grade 1, para-aortic lymph node. Nodularity of the neoplastic infiltrate is discernible at low power.

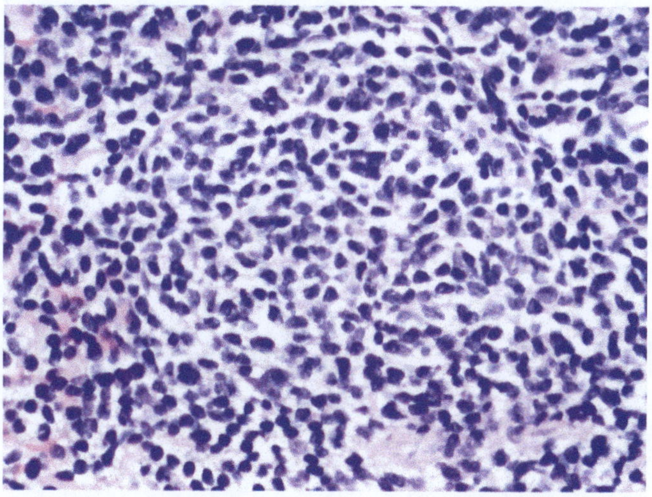

Fig. 9.47. Small centrocytes predominate within the neoplastic follicles.

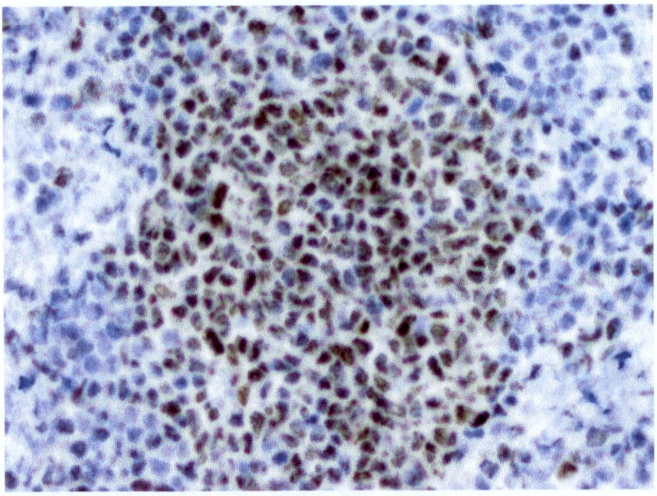

Fig. 9.48. Bcl6 expression confirms the germinal center differentiation of the small neoplastic lymphocytes.

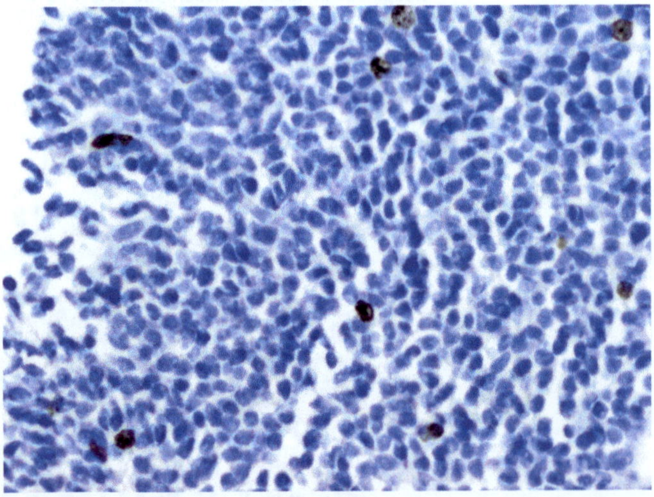

Fig. 9.49. Ki67 staining shows a very low proliferation rate and fits with the morphologic impression of a grade 1 follicular lymphoma.

CASE 10: 60-year-old man with supraventricular tachycardia. Right supraclavicular lymphadenopathy was noted, and given his history of a peripheral T cell lymphoma that had previously been treated with CHOP chemotherapy, suspicion of relapse was high. Ultrasound-guided needle biopsy of the right supraclavicular lymph node was performed.

Diagnosis: Peripheral T cell lymphoma, NOS, relapse (**Figs. 9.50**, **9.51**, **9.52**, and **9.53**).

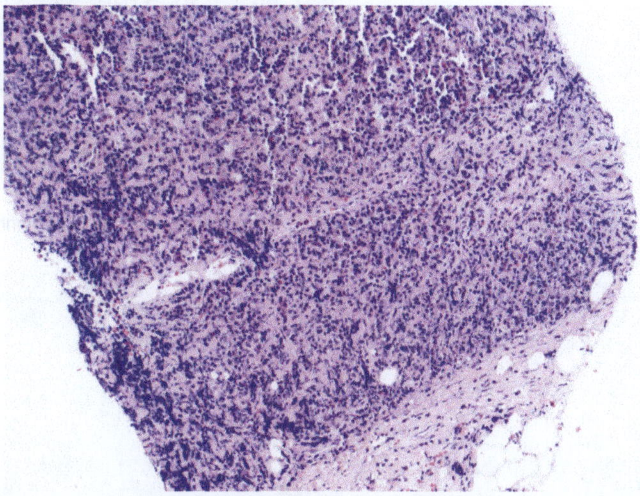

Fig. 9.50. Peripheral T cell lymphoma, supraclavicular lymph node. The neoplastic infiltrate is diffuse and heterogenous.

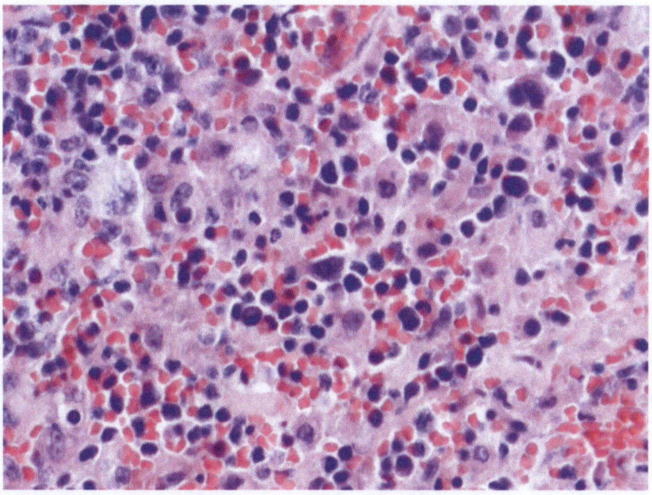

Fig. 9.51. Abnormal lymphocytes intermediate to large in size are present amidst a background of small lymphocytes, histiocytes, and plasma cells.

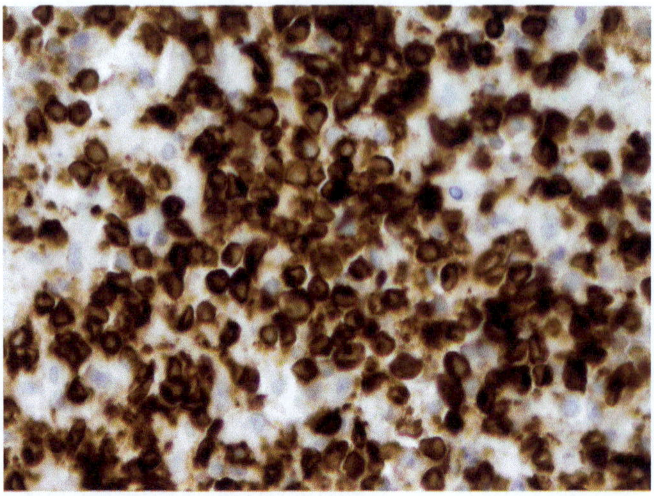

Fig. 9.52. CD3 stains the neoplastic (*larger*) and reactive (*smaller*) T cells.

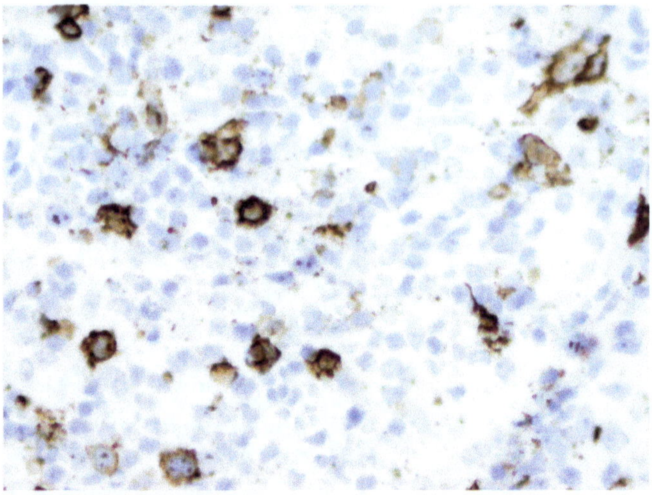

Fig. 9.53. CD20 staining highlights only scattered large B cells in the reactive infiltrate. In view of the previous diagnosis, these findings were sufficient to confirm recurrence of peripheral T cell lymphoma, NOS.

CASE 11: 47-year-old man with abdominal pain, dyspnea, and cold sweats. CT scan revealed bulky retroperitoneal lymphadenopathy, and a CT-guided biopsy was performed.

Diagnosis: Malignant germ cell neoplasm (**Figs. 9.54, 9.55, 9.56, 9.57**, and **9.58**).

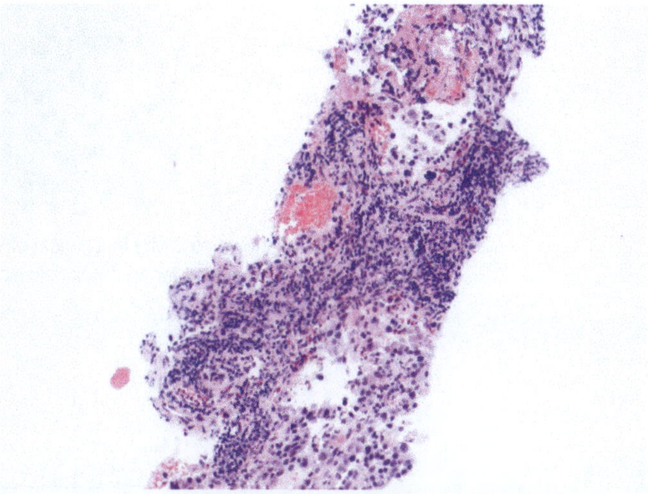

Fig. 9.54. Germ cell neoplasm, retroperitoneal lymph node. Larger cells are present in a sinusoidal distribution, with small lymphocytes predominating between the large cell foci.

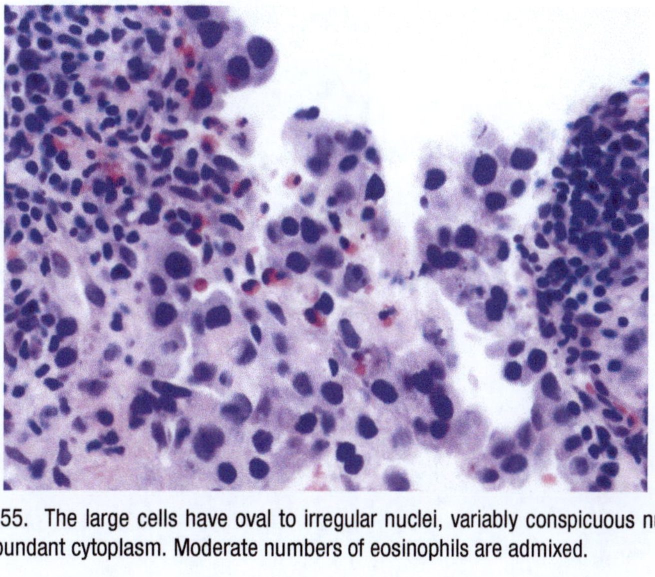

Fig. 9.55. The large cells have oval to irregular nuclei, variably conspicuous nucleoli, and abundant cytoplasm. Moderate numbers of eosinophils are admixed.

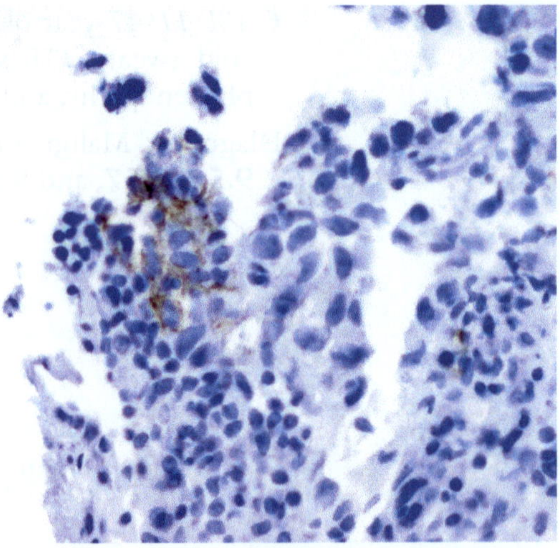

Fig. 9.56. CD30 shows positivity in a subset of the large cells, though its weak, variable nature would not be typical for an anaplastic large cell lymphoma.

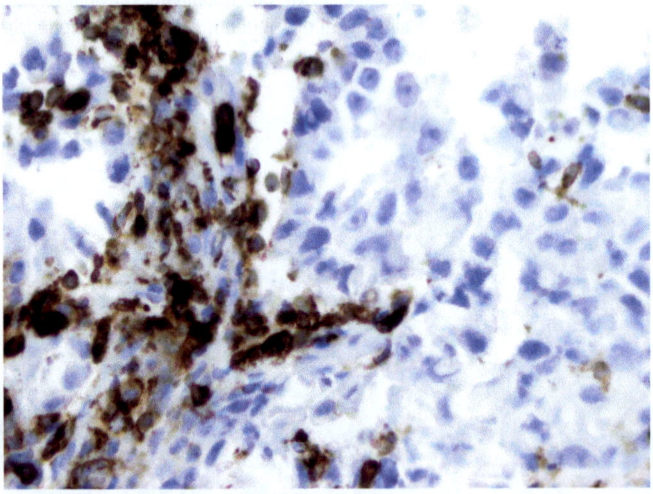

Fig. 9.57. CD45 highlights the small lymphocytes in the background, but the large neoplastic cells do not stain.

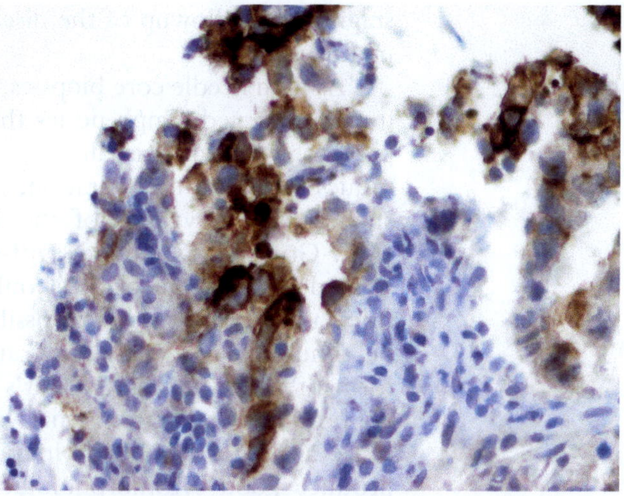

Fig. 9.58. The neoplastic cells are clearly positive for placental alkaline phosphatase making the diagnosis of a germ cell neoplasm.

Fine-Needle Aspiration Samples

With the increasing use of needle core biopsies, it is not unexpected that there is likewise an increasing use of fine-needle aspiration to obtain cellular material from lymph nodes and lymphoid infiltrates for diagnosis. The advantages of fine-needle aspiration biopsy are similar to those discussed for needle core biopsies, but unlike needle core biopsies, where the medium of examination is still a tissue section, fine-needle aspirates produce a cytological sample. Rendering accurate diagnoses on cytological preparations is more challenging and is highly specialized field that requires specialized training and skills.

It is not the intention to provide detailed discussion and instruction on how to diagnose needle aspirates, and the reader is referred to specialized texts on the subject. Suffice it to say that the range of specific entities that can be recognized in needle aspirates is significantly smaller and the diagnostic yield is less in comparison to needle core biopsies or excisional biopsies. Caution in the rendering of a new diagnosis of lymphoma based solely on a fine-needle aspirate cannot be overemphasized, and it is recommended that a lymph node excision should always be performed if the material obtained by aspiration is inadequate, if the findings are ambiguous, or if the clinical and radiological findings are not consistent with the cytological interpretation. Importantly, a strong reliance is placed on ancillary techniques such as immunohistochemistry, flow cytometry, and, in some cases, molecular analysis. However, the procedure is excellent and well suited for staging and followup of the disease and for monitoring of treatment response.

As with needle core biopsies, aspiration biopsy should be limited to enlarged lymph nodes that are either superficial and palpable or deep and visualized with imaging or ultrasound techniques. For routine aspiration, air-dried, methanol-fixed smears stained with a variant of the Romanovsky hematologic stain (May-Grünwald-Giemsa or Diff-Quick) and alcohol-fixed smears stained with Papanicolaou should be made. Make as many air-dried unstained smears as possible from the sample. These can be simultaneously rehydrated and fixed by immersion in 0.1% formal saline (van der Griendt's fixative) for 4–6 h. This protocol produces preparations that will tolerate heat-induced antigen retrieval procedures before immunohistochemical staining. They produce good cytomorphologic preservation and, importantly, eliminate the strong background staining encountered following other methods of fixation. Material remaining in the syringe after preparation of the smears can be washed out with phosphate buffered saline and prepared into cell blocks for immunohistochemistry. Additional passes to obtain material for flow cytometry and other investigations (e.g., bacterial and/or fungal culture) are often useful.

The aspiration biopsy is assessed for cellularity, composition, and cellular features. The first step in the diagnostic algorithm is assessment of whether the material is polymorphous, containing a mixture of cell types, or monomorphous, containing one predominant cell type.

Polymorphous Infiltrates

The majority of needle aspirates of lymph nodes are polymorphous, causing non-neoplastic conditions to figure heavily in the differential diagnoses.

The presence of a prominent population of neutrophils in a polymorphous cell population is indicative of an acute infective process, especially if the node is draining an inflamed site such as dental abscess, inflamed appendix, or tubo-ovarian abscess. At a later stage, purulent material composed of neutrophils and cell debris develops, and as the acute inflammatory process subsides, macrophages with phagocytosed material become prominent, and plasma cells mixed with lymphoid cells appear. While organisms may be revealed in a Gram stain, the debris present makes interpretation difficult, and bacterial culture is the best method of identifying the infecting organism.

Reactive hyperplasias pose a significant diagnostic problem, as a large number of specific entities need to be considered and the inability to assess architecture limits diagnostic accuracy. In general, aspirates of hyperplastic lymph nodes are cellular and comprise a mixture of cell types, the most prominent of which is the small lymphocyte. The lymphoid cells occur as dispersed, isolated, and single cells of variable size and appearance. Aggregates of small and large cells with FDC can be present, representing germinal centers, and plasma cells and tingible body macrophages are usually identifiable.

Follicular lymphoma requires distinction from reactive hyperplasia. This distinction can be difficult, and when in doubt, the results of flow cytometry can be of considerable assistance. Even if the presence of a clonal population of CD10-positive B cells is confirmed, grading of follicular lymphomas in cytologic specimens can be problematic.

Hodgkin lymphoma presents with a polymorphous infiltrate of epithelioid histiocytes, plasma cells, eosinophils, and atypical mononuclear cells. The diagnosis is made when typical RSC are present. The latter are CD45−/+, CD15+, CD30+, CD20−/+. **Table 9.1** provides the cellular features of some diagnostic entities with a polymorphous cellular infiltrate (**Table 9.2**).

Table 9.1
Needle core biopsies – advantages, disadvantages and handling

Advantages

- Easy and quick to perform under image guidance
- Can be done on an outpatient basis
- Targeted at pathological tissue rather than most accessible node/tissue
- Well tolerated, low morbidity
- Additional cores can be taken for flow cytometry and other investigations
- Able to obtain deep-seated material
- Allows immediate commencement of chemotherapy if required without waiting for recovery from surgery/invasive procedure
- Useful for staging, monitoring, and followup for recurrence

Disadvantages

- Lesser amount of diagnostic tissue
- Greater dependency on other investigative techniques including flow cytometry
- Potential loss of topographical and architectural features for assessment
- Danger of needle cores being used as replacement for complete excision of lymph nodes

Handling of specimen

- The small specimen should not be allowed to dry out; immediate immersion in 10% buffered formalin is required
- Fixation time of at least 4–6 h
- Cut sufficient sections onto silanized slides in the first instance in anticipation of immunohistochemistry requirements
- Separate core obtained for flow cytometry
- Should additional investigations be anticipated, request that radiologist obtain multiple cores

Table 9.2
Fine-needle aspirates – polymorphous smears

SLE – Hematoxylin/LE bodies in a background of small lymphocytes, plasma cells, tingible body macrophages, and necrosis
Kikuchi disease – Small and large transformed lymphocytes with crescentic histiocytes, necrotic/apoptotic debris, plasmacytoid monocytes, and apoptotic cells
Rheumatoid lymphadenopathy – Changes of florid hyperplasia with numerous plasma cells and Russell bodies
Dermatopathic lymphadenopathy – Melanin pigment in macrophages and prominent DRC
Infectious mononucleosis – Florid hyperplasia, stimulated lymphoid cells, immunoblasts, Reed–Sternberg-like cells, tingible body macrophages, plasma cells, mast cells, eosinophils; distinguish from FL
HIV lymphadenitis – Variable according to stage: florid hyperplasia to hypocellular in depletion stage with immunoblasts and plasma cells and tingible body macrophages
Granulomatous lymphadenitis – Granulomas in the form of epithelioid histiocytes, giant cells. Stain for AFB, fungi, pneumocystis, chlamydia, bacilli
Rosai-Dorfman disease – Abundant histiocytes with emperipolesis
Langerhans cell histiocytosis – Histiocytes with grooved nuclei, CD1a+/langerin+/S100+. Eosinophils present
Foreign body lymphadenitis – Histiocytes and presence of identifiable foreign material, e.g., silicone, detritic debris, lymphangiogram material
Follicular lymphoma – Difficult to distinguish from follicular hyperplasia, great reliance on flow cytometry results
Hodgkin lymphoma – Polymorphous population of epithelioid histiocytes, plasma cells, eosinophils, atypical mononuclear cells, and diagnostic RSC that are CD45−/+, CD15+, CD30+, CD20−/+.

Monomorphous Infiltrates

A predominantly monomorphous infiltrate in lymph node aspirates suggests a more limited differential diagnosis that includes the malignant lymphomas which produce a diffuse pattern of infiltration. Diffuse lymphomas can be diagnosed with a greater degree of confidence. The population of cells in the aspirate must be monotonous, i.e., cells of approximately equal size. When small (about the size of resting lymphocytes), CLL/SLL should be considered. The cells are CD23+/CD20+/CD43+/CD5+/cyclinD1−/Bcl6−.

A monomorphous population of intermediate-sized cells with irregular nuclei suggests mantle cell lymphoma. The lymphoma cells are cyclinD1+/CD45+/CD20+/CD5+/Bcl2+/CD23−.

A monomorphous population of large cells suggests large cell lymphoma, and metastatic carcinoma and melanoma should be excluded. In well-prepared smears, lymphoma cells do not form clusters, but the cells may overlap in poorly prepared preparations and cause confusion with metastatic tumor. The presence of basophilic spherules of cytoplasm called lymphoglandular bodies is helpful to identify the infiltrate as being lymphoid in nature.

DLBCL is CD45+/CD20+/CD79a+/Bcl6+/CD10+ with light-chain restriction. Cytokeratin and HMB45 are negative.

Burkitt lymphoma comprises a monotonous population of intermediate-sized cells with round nuclei, fine to coarse chromatin, and displays two to five distinct nucleoli. The scanty to moderate amount of cytoplasm is deeply basophilic and contains prominent lipid vacuoles. Tingible body macrophages may be present, and necrotic debris, mitotic figures, and apoptotic bodies are often seen. The tumor cells are CD20+/CD79a+/Bcl6+/Bcl2−/CD23−/CD5− and may stain for LMP-1 and EBER (especially in endemic cases). They show a very high Ki67 count that approaches 100%.

The presence of large atypical cells in a mixed cell infiltrate that may be mononuclear or multinucleated raises the possibility of Hodgkin lymphoma and anaplastic large cell lymphoma. They can be distinguished by the background cells present in Hodgkin lymphoma and the RSC immunophenotype. In ALCL, small lymphocytes and some epithelioid histiocytes form the background, and atypical cells are CD45−/+, EMA+/−, ALK+, CD30+, CD20−.

Other monomorphous infiltrates that may be diagnosed include plasmacytoma/plasma cell myeloma and lymphoblastic lymphoma. The T cell lymphomas are very difficult to diagnose on the basis of needle aspirates even with the aid of flow cytometry unless the smear shows convoluted cells as in mycosis fungoides and Sezary syndrome (**Table 9.3**).

Table 9.3
Fine-needle aspirates – monomorphous smears

CLL/SLL – Small lymphocytes, CD23+, CD20+, CD43+, CD5+, cyclinD1−, Bcl6−
MCL – Intermediate sized with slightly irregular nuclei, cyclinD1+, CD43+, CD20+, CD5+, Bcl2+, CD23−, Bcl6−
DLBCL – Large lymphoid cells, lymphoglandular bodies, CD45+, CD20+, variably CD10 and Bcl6 positive, light-chain restriction, CK−, HMB45−
Burkitt lymphoma – Intermediate-sized cells with two to five nucleoli, CD20+, Bcl6+, CD10+, Ki67 approaching 100%, variably EBER+ and LMP1+, CD23−, cyclinD1−
ALCL – Large atypical cells, hallmark cells, small lymphocytes with occasional epithelioid histiocytes, CD45−/+, EMA+, ALK+, CD30+, CD4+/−
Plasmacytoid plasmacytic lymphoma – Plasmacytoid cells mixed with small lymphocytes, CD38+, CD138+, CD45+, CD20−/+, CD79a+, Ig restriction
Lymphoblastic lymphoma, precursor T cell type – Lymphoblasts with folded nuclei and one to two nucleoli, TdT+, CD3+, CD4+, CD8+, CD20−, CD79a−

Subject Index

Note: The letters 'f' and 't' following the locators refer to figures and tables respectively.

A.S-Y. Leong, *A Pattern Approach to Lymph Node Diagnosis*,
DOI 10.1007/978-1-4419-7176-0,

C

D

E

F

G

H

I

K

L

N

R

S

T

MIX
Papier aus verantwortungsvollen Quellen
Paper from responsible sources
FSC® C105338

If you have any concerns about our products,
you can contact us on
ProductSafety@springernature.com

In case Publisher is established outside the EU,
the EU authorized representative is:
Springer Nature Customer Service Center GmbH
Europaplatz 3, 69115 Heidelberg, Germany

Printed by Libri Plureos GmbH
in Hamburg, Germany